Medical and Psychological Effects of Concentration Camps on HOLOCAUST SURVIVORS

Series Editor
ISRAEL W. CHARNY

Bibliographic Researcher
IZA LAPONCE

Volume 4
Genocide: A Critical Bibliographic Review

Medical and Psychological Effects of Concentration Camps on HOLOCAUST SURVIVORS

Edited by

Robert Krell & Marc I. Sherman

With a Foreword by Elie Wiesel

Routledge
Taylor & Francis Group
LONDON AND NEW YORK

Medical and Psychological Effects of Concentration Camps on Holocaust Survivors
Volume 4 in the Series
Genocide: A Critical Bibliographic Review

First published 1997 by Transaction Publishers

Published 2017 by Routledge
2 Park Square, Milton Park, Abingdon, Oxon OX14 4RN
711 Third Avenue, New York, NY 10017, USA

First issued in paperback 2018

Routledge is an imprint of the Taylor & Francis Group, an informa business

Library of Congress Catalog Number: 97-3110

Library of Congress Cataloging-in-Publication Data

Medical and psychological effects of concentration camps on Holocaust survivors / edited by Robert Krell and Marc I. Sherman ; with a foreword by Elie Wiesel.
p. cm. — (Genocide ; v. 4)
"Institute on the Holocaust and Genocide"—T.p. verso.
ISBN 1-56000-290-5 (alk. paper)
1. Holocaust survivors—Mental health—Bibliography. 2. Holocaust survivors—Health and hygiene—Bibliography. 3. Holocaust suriviors—Psychology—Bibliography. 4. World War, 1939–1945—Concentration camps—Psychological aspects—Bibliography. 5. Holocaust, Jewish (1939–1945)—Psychological aspects. I. Krell, Robert. II. Sherman, Marc I. III. Wiesel, Elie, 1928– . IV. Institute on the Holocaust and Genocide (Jerusalem) V. Series.
Z7164.G45M43 1997
016.61685'21—dc21 97-3110
CIP

ISBN 13: 978-1-138-51201-6 (pbk)
ISBN 13: 978-1-56000-290-1 (hbk)

Contents

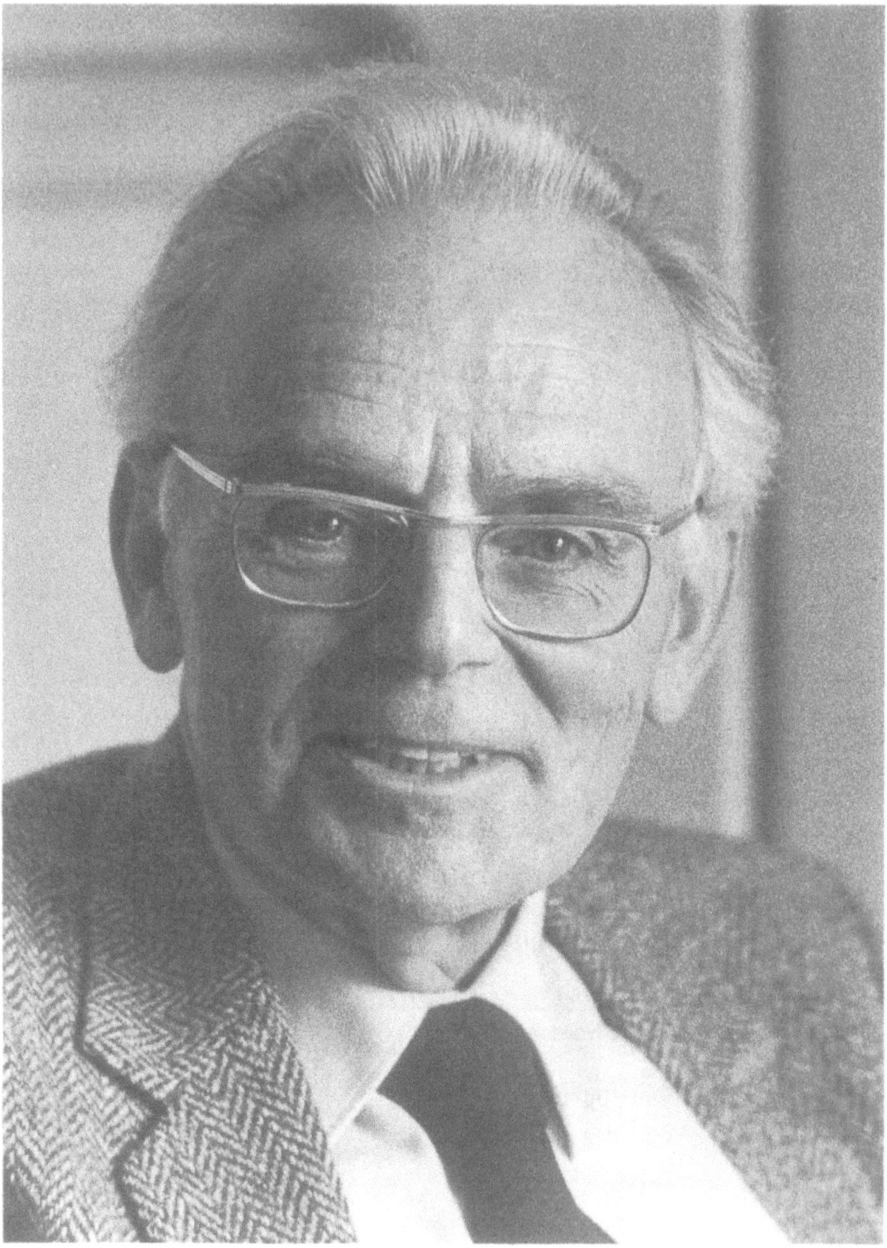

Leo Eitinger, M.D.
December 12, 1912–October 15, 1996

"The Eitinger Bibliography" Dedication to Leo Eitinger

This research bibliography is offered in honor of Professor Leo Eitinger of Oslo, Norway.

Regrettably, even as this book goes to press, we have received word of the passing of dear Leo Eitinger. He was, of course, aware of this volume, and wrote his response to this dedication as it appears on pp. xi–xii. This work was very important to Leo Eitinger; he helped in the last months with some citations; and he asked to send us his farewell just prior to his death knowing that publication of the book would follow shortly.

Professor Eitinger was born in Czechoslovakia in 1912. Already a medical doctor, with the start of the war he fled to Norway in 1939. It proved not far enough.

He was caught and deported to Auschwitz and bore the number 105268 on his left forearm.

Elie Wiesel writes in *Night*[1]: "Toward the middle of January, my right foot began to swell because of the cold. I was unable to put it on the ground. I went to have it examined. The doctor, a great Jewish doctor, a prisoner like ourselves, was quite definite: I must have an operation! If we waited, the toes—and perhaps the whole leg—would have to be amputated" (p. 74).

Dr. Eitinger did not perform the operation but assisted and held Elie Wiesel's hands, the only "anaesthetic" available in Auschwitz.

Professor Eitinger did not remember his patient, there were so many, and they looked so alike. Years later, he was invited to the Wiesel's home. Elie Wiesel had recognized him in Oslo where he went to lecture. Patients seldom forget their doctors!

Professor Eitinger studied the consequences of the war on its victims, but did not investigate survivors from the camps until years years after liberation. He subsequently wrote the book, *Concentration Camp Survivors in Israel and Norway*, published in 1964.

He was a pioneer in researching a subject from which many shied away. Dr. Eitinger has contributed insights into the experience of massive psychologic trauma for his entire life and inspired others to do similar work. His many books and papers are, of course, listed in this volume.

Let me share with you his comments from a lecture[2] to mental health professionals who try to help elderly survivors:

> Survivors of Nazi Concentration camps have their share of problems which are difficult to bear and difficult to solve. With the passage of time health deteriorates, strength is reduced, capacities dwindle. The traumatic experiences return therefore in reinforced strength. Survivors are of course in need of help for all their somatic ailments, but still more for their psychological isolation, their feeling of having lost their anchorage in the world and in humanity, their feeling that nobody cares if they are alive or not. If we manage to reverse this tragic evolution by establishing at least traces of real interhuman relationship and reduce the deep existential isolation, then we have made an important step—perhaps not bigger than the first step on the moon, but surely more important for a fellow human being, more important because it reduces the total sum of suffering in this world—and this is—so I believe—the most important task and activity for all of us. (p. 5)

It is with great respect that I, a child survivor of the Holocaust dedicate to him, an adult survivor, this work.

Robert Krell, M.D.
Professor Emeritus,
University of British Columbia

Notes

1. Wiesel, Elie (1960). *Night*. New York: Bantam Books.
2. Eitinger, Leo (1992). "Identification, Treatment and Care of the Aging Survivor. In Kenigsberg, Rositta E., and Lieblich, Cathy M. (eds.), *The First National Conference on Identification, Treatment and Care of the Aging Holocaust Survivor, March 29-31, 1992: Selected Proceedings*. Miami, FL: Holocaust Documentation and Education Center and Southeast Florida Center on Aging, Florida International University, pp. 5-15.

Response to Dedication

I am deeply moved and grateful to Professor Krell for his dedication and for joining my name with that of this important research bibliography.

May I add a few words about my background: By an incredible piece of luck I got for a few months the then life-saving work in the office of the main prisoners' "hospital" in Auschwitz. I learned nearly everything about the camp's death machinery, the hundreds of prisoners killed every day and about the arriving transports with thousands of Jews never registered and sent directly to the gas chambers. I saw all the lies, the deceit, and the perfidy of the SS doctors and the sufferings and maltreatment of the patients before they were murdered. I learned everything about the so-called "health care" in Auschwitz, but I saw also the dedication of the prisoner doctors, always under the most incredibly difficult situations.

All these impressions I could not forget, and felt that I had to share them with my colleagues immediately after my liberation. Thus health care in the concentration camp Auschwitz became the topic of my first publication on concentration camp prisoners. It was a factual report which in spite of its very "dry" and nearly emotionless description had become so incredible already when I myself read the proofs of it that I found it necessary to add a postscript stressing that there were no exaggerations in it. I felt, however, not strong enough to describe more of the sufferings or to study the still too near and too painful problems of the survivors.

I tried to understand the influence of difficult life situations on the individual's mental health through different pathways, first the living conditions of school children in a small Norwegian town completely ravaged by firebombing, then the influence of military service in peacetime on young Norwegian men.

Slowly approaching my personal experiences, I studied all the refugees who had been in contact with psychiatric institutions during the first ten years after the war. All of them had been in German camps during World War II. While working with the refugee-survivors, I learned that listening and trying to understand and to help survivors was good personal therapy for a psychiatrist-survivor. And then in 1957 it was my good fortune to become a member of an all-around medical-psychiatric-psychological team of university teachers, whose task it was to investigate thoroughly ex-prisoners.

Since then I have not been able to abandon the question of concentration camp survivors. I have interviewed and investigated survivors from nearly all European countries living in Norway and Israel. I have been in all the mental hospitals of Israel and found the survivors living there. I have examined the morbidity and mortality of all the Norwegians who had been in concentration camps outside Norway during the war. I have followed the few Norwegian Jewish survivors, practically from the day of their arrest until thirty years after the liberation.

The number of books and papers on the psychological effects of concentration camps published in the international literature had reached several hundred, and a bibliography was needed for further scientific work. During my sabbatical year (in 1979) which I had the privilege and pleasure to spend with Professor Breznitz at the Ray D. Wolfe Centre for Study of Psychological Stress at Haifa University, I tried to collect—as far as possible under the given circumstances—the literature on "my topic," to read it, and classify it. Psychologist, Miriam Rieck, continued the work in 1980 and the first—and necessarily incomplete—bibliography was published by the University of Haifa in 1980. After having worked with Professor Krell on the second edition of the bibliography in 1985, he has taken upon himself the difficult task to revise, enlarge, and bring up to a high scientific standard the present edition. I am happy and grateful that he now has accepted this responsibility and do hope that this volume will be of help to old and new students, particularly scholars whose work attempts to describe and to understand the psychological effects of the Holocaust—if this ever will be possible.

Leo Eitinger, M.D.
Professor Emeritus, University of Oslo

Foreword

Note by Series Editor:

Elie Wiesel was sixteen years old in Buna when he required treatment for his badly injured leg which had been infected and swollen. A Jewish doctor, himself a prisoner in the camp, who helped treat young Wiesel in the raw surroundings of the camp's "infirmary" was none other than Dr. Leo Eitinger. Young Elie Wiesel's leg was saved...and since the Holocaust he has devoted his life heroically not only to being a Voice of the Survivors of the Holocaust, but a Voice from the Holocaust to All Humanity.

Elie Wiesel's appreciation of Dr. Eitinger is in its origins the time-honored thanks of a patient to his doctor, but in this it becomes even more the thanks of all of us to a very special Doctor of Holocaust Survivors, and of our Humanity.

The Holocaust can never be atoned, but perhaps it is lighting a way to a new conception of an imperative of Human Decency. —Israel W. Charny

This volume is an offering and Leo Eitinger—his friends call him Shua—is worthy of it. Indeed, I would say that no one is worthier of such a tribute. For it deals with an area in which he, as a forerunner, has done wonders in exploring the wounded soul and the burning memory of survivors before bringing them relief and consolation.

I know, some may say that, as far as Eitinger is concerned, I am not objective. That is true. Nor do I wish to be.

What are we for one another? More than a comrade, more than a companion, I am his ally just as he is mine in our constant struggle against forgetfulness, hatred, and indifference. We both are faithful to our friendship which makes me proud.

Dare I recall our common past? We were together in Auschwitz and in Buchenwald where the despair of the living was equaled by the solitude of the dying. A quarter of a century later, we met again in Oslo. Since then, the contact between us has never been interrupted.

What do you admire in him with more affection and deeper gratitude? Is it his sense of integrity mixed with compassion? Or is it his admirable passion for that which makes the human being human, in other words: at the same time vulnerable and obstinate in the face of suffering? Or is it perhaps his capacity to pierce the wall of silence that surrounds and envelops the voices of so many Jewish Holocaust survivors. Professor Leo Eitinger is an example for his medical colleagues and an inspiration for his students and readers. But he is far more: he represents a conscience that remains eternally awake, attempting to know and understand all about the life and the survival of men and women who saw death and evil at work, enduring their cruelty without succumbing to it. Was it an accident that he was among the very first to involve himself with the psychology, with the psychotherapy of survivors? And to defend and treat all victims of torture anywhere? In all matters related to human suffering, he remains a discoverer and a guide.

Other psychiatrists have invented theories, for the most part poorly founded and even absurd, about the "guilt-feelings" of Auschwitz survivors who they tend to treat as mentally ill. For Eitinger, they are more than mental patients. He sees in them singular men and women who could have lost their sanity and their faith but did not lose them. Never does he allow anyone to hurt or harm them. Never does he talk down to them nor to speak about them condescendingly. He is and always will be their defender against those who, void of humility, listen to their tales of horror and humiliation, only to judge them.

More than they, and better than they, he understands and loves them. And that is only natural. Isn't he their brother, I mean our brother.

Elie Wiesel

Introductory Notes to the Bibliography

In order to acquaint the user of this bibliography with the topic, two introductory articles are offered. The first is titled "Psychiatry and the Holocaust" and examines the general impact of the Holocaust on psychiatry. The second, "Survivors and Their Families: Psychiatric Consequences of the Holocaust" deals with the impact of the Shoah on individuals.

The references in the body of the bibliography are listed in many languages. In order to simplify matters, we have provided translations in English to assist the reader.

The citations are drawn from the medical, psychiatric, psychological, and social work literature. A few citations may appear marginally related, but they were included if they were thought to contribute to the knowledge of "psychologic consequences." We have chosen in some cases to be over-inclusive rather than offer an editorial comment through exclusion. It remains for the researcher who uses these materials to examine their worth critically. The references are listed alphabetically and chronologically by date of publication.

This research bibliography had its origins in a first edition compiled by Professor Eitinger and Miriam Rieck in 1979-1980. Since I had previously collated hundreds of references by 1980, we agreed to combine the two collections with one edition subsequently published in 1985. This is the third edition.

I owe a debt of gratitude to many who helped research the existing literature and provided relevant references. I received advice and help from Margo Lane, the University of British Columbia Department of Psychiatry librarian; Peter Suedfeld, University of British Columbia Professor of Psychology; and Lisa Michelle Freeman, researcher. A special thanks to my secretary and research assistant, Francesca Wilson, for patiently entering the data which forms the content of this book.

This publication was assisted by a grant from the Vancouver Holocaust Centre for Education and Remembrance, Vancouver, B.C. The guidance of Professor Israel W. Charny of the Institute on the Holocaust and Genocide, Jerusalem, Series Editor, is gratefully acknowledged.

I am indebted to my wife, Marilyn, and our children for their patience with my preoccupations. They know it was important for me to complete this task.

Robert Krell

User's Guide to the Bibliography

This multilingual bibliography of the literature on Holocaust survivors in the fifty years from 1990 to 1995 contains 2461 citations from journal articles, books, chapters of books, conference proceedings as well as master's theses and doctoral dissertations.* The languages included are English, German, Polish, French, Norwegian, Spanish, Italian, Swedish, Hebrew, Czech, and Serbo-Croatian. English translations in brackets immediately follow virtually all foreign language citations.** Hebrew language citations are transliterated into Latin characters.

The bibliographic style used in this volume follows the style used in the previous volumes in the series, *Genocide: A Critical Bibliographic Review*, for which the *Publication Manual of th Psychological Association* was consulted for many structural rules including the alphabetized arrangement of the bibliography.

An annotated bibliography of selected books in the field is presented in the final section of this bibliography to offer researchers an additional analysis of major literature on the subject.

The format of each citation is designed for clarity, consistency, and thoroughness. Journal citations contain the full journal name while chapter citations contain the editors of the books in which they appear. Citations from proceedings include extensive information on dates and places of symposia, colloquia, and conferences. This will enable researchers to understand the extent of scholarship in the field. Doctoral dissertations cited include extensive bibliographic information including the university, total pages and location of the abstract in *Dissertations Abstract International.*

An author index at the end of the bibliography includes authors, editors, and institutional names. The numbers cited in the index refer to citation numbers, whole page numbers (i.e., p. 10) are given for the references that appear in the two introductory essays.

---

* A few citations dated 1996 have also been included, but formally this bibliography covers the period 1945–1995.

** We are deeply appreciative of the translations from Polish, French, and German by Judith Wertheimer, M.Ph., Holon, Israel.

Researchers interested in locating additional information about other aspects of the Holocaust and genocide are referred to Sherman, Marc I., and Charny, Israel W. (Eds.), *Holocaust and Genocide Bibliographic Database, Version 2.2* available from the Institute on the Holocaust and Genocide, Jerusalem (see address, telephone, fax and E-mail below). This is a PC database utilizing the Pro-Cite bibliographic database manager. It is available at major libraries including the United States Holocaust Memorial Museum in Washington, the Simon Wiesenthal Center in Los Angeles, the Wannsee-Conference Museum in Berlin and Yad Vashem in Jerusalem. It can also be purchased directly from the Institute on the Holocaust and Genocide, Jerusalem at a much reduced price for Holocaust researchers.

Many aspects of the Holocaust and genocide are reviewed in depth in the previous volumes in this series. Each chapter provides an encyclopedic summary of knowledge in the field and an annotated bibliography. The three volumes in the series are:

Charny, Israel W. (Ed.) *(1988). Genocide: A Critical Bibliographic Review. Vol. 1.* New York: Facts on File and London: Mansell. 273 pp.

Charny, Israel W. (Ed.) (1991). *Genocide: A Critical Bibliographic Review. Vol 2.* New York: Facts on File and London: Mansell. 432 pp.

Charny, Israel W. (Ed.). (1994). *The Widening Circle of Genocide. Genocide: A Critical Bibliographic Review. Vol. 3.* New Brunswick, NJ: Transaction. 375 pp.

The following bibliographic databases which are available on CD-ROM through major university research libraries will be of use to readers who seek additional information on medical and psychological aspects of the Holocaust:

Medline. Bethesda, MD: United States National Library of Medicine, 1966–Present (available on SilverPlatter).

Medline is the medical database of the U.S. National Library of Medicine. It is an international database covering literature from over 3,400 journals published worldwide. The database also includes selected chapters and articles from books.

PsycLit. Washington, DC: American Psychological Association, 1974-present (available on SilverPlatter).

PsycLit is the database of the American Psychological Association. It contains bibliographical citations to all the major fields of psychology in more than 30 languages taken from journals, books, and chapters of books published in over 45 countries.

Sociofile. Sociological Abstracts, Inc. 1974-Present (available on SilverPlatter).

> *Sociofile* is the bibliographic database to international literature in all areas of sociology.

Dissertation Abstracts. Ann Arbor, MI: University Microfilms Inc., 1861-Present (available on ProQuest).

> *Dissertation Abstracts* offers access to completed doctoral dissertations submitted to North American universities and colleges as well as selected European institutions.

Researchers interested in accessing references to books can use the following Library of Congress subject headings when searching on-line library catalogues:

Holocaust survivors—Psychology
Holocaust survivors—Mental Health
Human experimentation in Medicine—Germany—1933–1945
Children of Holocaust survivors—Psychology
Concentration camps—Germany—Psychological aspects

Researchers using this bibliography are invited to submit additional citations as well as those inadvertently omitted. Please send them to the following addresses:

Robert Krell, M.D., F.R.C.P.(C)
Professor Emeritus (Psychiatry)
University of British Columbia
Child & Family Psychiatric Clinic
4480 Oak Street, C4
B.C. Children's Hospital
Vancouver, B.C. V6H 3V4, Canada
Fax: 1-604-875-2907

Marc I. Sherman, M.L.S.
Director, Holocaust & Genocide Bibliographic Database
Institute on the Holocaust and Genocide
P.O.B. 10311
91102 Jerusalem, Israel
Fax: 972-2-672-0424
E-mail: TRA@TAULIB.TAU.AC.IL

We hope that this volume will enable readers to gain new insights into the medical and psychological problems experienced by survivors of the Holocaust and their families.

Marc I. Sherman

Notes on the Editors

Robert Krell, M.D., F.R.C.P.(C), Senior Editor of this book, was born in The Hague, Holland on August 5, 1940. He was hidden from 1942 to 1945 with the Munnik family, Albert, Violette, and Nora who have been recognized as Righteous Gentiles.

His parents survived individually in hiding but their families had all been murdered. In 1951, the Krells moved to Vancouver, British Columbia.

Robert graduated from the University of British Columbia with an M.D. in 1965, interned in Philadelphia and trained in psychiatry at Temple University Hospital and Stanford University Hospital.

Upon his return to U.B.C., he became a Professor of Psychiatry. As part of his practice he treated Holocaust survivors and their families as well as Dutch survivors of Japanese concentration camps.

He served for 20 years in the Canadian Jewish Congress, becoming National Vice-President from 1989-1992. He co-founded a Holocaust Education Symposium for high school students in 1975, an audio-visual testimony project which has taped 120 Vancouver survivors, and founded in 1985 the Vancouver Holocaust Centre Society for Remembrance and Education which opened its Holocaust Education Centre in 1994.

Being himself a child survivor of the Holocaust, he has assisted in the formation of child survivor groups, first in Los Angeles in 1983, then in Vancouver in 1989. He served on the International Advisory Council of the Hidden Child Conference which organized the 1991 Gathering in New York attended by 1,500 child survivors.

He and his wife have 3 daughters, 4 nephews, and 3 nieces.

Marc I. Sherman, M.L.S., Co-Editor of this book is Director of the Academic Research Information System (ARIS) at the Research Authority of Tel Aviv University, and Director of the Holocaust and Genocide Bibliographic Database at the Institute on the Holocaust and Genocide in Jerusalem.

Born in 1956 in Brooklyn, New York, he has a B.A. in history from George Washington University and a Master's degree in Library Science from Syracuse University. He is Associate Editor of the series *Genocide: A Critical Bibliographic Review*, and has co-edited *Human Rights: An International and Comparative Law Bibliography*, 1985, Westport, CT: Greenwood Press. He lives in Israel with his pretty and clever wife, Polly, who sometimes does not understand his devoted insanity to projects like this, and with their firstborn, a son, Arieh Levi, who came into this world as this volume was brought to its conclusion.

Israel W. Charny, Ph. D., Series Editor for this volume, is the originator of the series *Genocide: A Critical Bibliographic Review*, of which this is Volume 4, and himself edited the first three volumes: Volume 1, 1988, London: Mansell Publishing & New York: Facts on File; Volume 2, 1991, London: Mansell Publishing & New York: Facts on File; Volume 3, 1994, also entitled *The Widening Circle of Genocide*, New Brunswick, NJ: Transaction Publishers.

He is the author of *How Can We Commit the Unthinkable? Genocide: The Human Cancer*, published by Westview Press in 1982, followed by a paperback edition by Hearst Books (distributed by William Morrow Co.) in 1983, and forthcoming in a Portuguese edition by Editora Rosa Dos Tempos in Rio de Janeiro in 1997.

He also edited *Toward the Understanding and Prevention of Genocide* published by Westview Press in 1984. In 1985 he created the international newsletter, *Internet on the Holocaust and Genocide*, which he edited from 1985 to 1995, at which time the publication was transferred from the Institute on the Holocaust and Genocide in Jerusalem to the Centre for Comparative Genocide Studies at Macquarie University in Sydney, Australia.

He is Executive Director of the Institute on the Holocaust and Genocide in Jerusalem; and Professor of Psychology & Family Therapy and Director, Program for Advanced Studies in Integrative Psychotherapy, Dept. of Psychology & Martin Buber Center, Hebrew University of Jerusalem.

Two Introductory Essays

by

Robert Krell

1

Psychiatry and the Holocaust

Robert Krell

The genocidal destruction of European Jewry, known as the Holocaust, represents the single most disturbing catastrophe in this catastrophe-filled 20th century. Knowledge of the Holocaust has forced a serious re-evaluation of contemporary theology and philosophy, spawned a vast literature in many fields and has placed on the human agenda the central issue of survival into the 21st century, namely the reconciliation of civilization (civilized behavior) with technology.

Upon the fertile field of European antisemitism, Hitler combined centuries of Jew-hatred with Nazi racist theories to establish the political will to create the machinery of mass murder.

For psychiatry, the Holocaust encompasses a complex of significant events, including the exodus of European psychiatrists and psychoanalysts from Germany and Austria[1,2]; the role of German psychiatry in the experimentation with wholesale slaughter[3] and subsequent genocide; and the resistance of post-war psychiatry to deal appropriately with survivors in matters of compensation and of treatment. *It is the story of tremendous moral failures in medicine generally and psychiatry particularly, failures which have been too little examined.* The Holocaust, above all, was a massive assault on principles normally held to be decent and fair, and that included an inherent faith in a civilized nation's legal and medical system. These systems were dismantled in only a very few years. And precious few jurists or physicians complained when it was still possible to do so.

Brieger[4] described the gradual corrosion of medicine in Germany, surely amongst the finest in the world at that time. He relates that on March 31, 1933, Jewish physicians holding University, hospital, or faculty positions at the Charité Hospital in Berlin, were told they need not appear for work the following day. All together, 96 Jews were dismissed of a total staff of 277. There were no protests from the non-Jewish physicians.

The Nazi persecutions caused the immigration and/or escape of persons with considerable influence in psychiatry. Frieda Fromm-Reichman, born in Karlsruhe, Germany left in 1933 for the United States. Heinz Hartmann emigrated to Switzerland in 1938 and settled in the United States in 1941. Margaret Schoenberger Mahler, born in Sopron, Hungary, settled in New York in 1937. Rudolph Lowenstein, born in Lodz, Poland and who studied in Berlin and Paris, first served in the French army and finally settled in the USA in 1943. Sigmund Freud fled Vienna for the safety of London in 1938 as did Anna Freud following her arrest and release by the Gestapo. Ernst and Marianne Kris followed Freud to England. Hilde Bruch and Franz Kallman fled Germany for the United States in 1934 and 1936 respectively, and Silvano Arieti left Pisa in 1939 escaping via Switzerland to the United States. George Tarjan, the first foreign medical graduate to be American Psychiatric Association President (1984) fled Hungary in 1939, and Joel Elkes was studying in England when war broke out. Dr. Elchanan Elkes, his father, was elected head of the Jewish Council in the Kovno Ghetto of Kovno, Lithuania. He was killed at Dachau on July 25, 1944.[5]

All who fled lost members of their immediate families, with profound impact on their personal lives and perhaps on their subsequent psychiatric careers. "We have now had the first reports about the aunts, and it is the worst possible" (p. 279), wrote Anna Freud to Kata Levy in March 1946.[6] Freud's four elderly sisters had all been murdered in 1942, Marie in Theresienstadt, Rosa in Auschwitz, and Dolfi and Pauline in Treblinka.

Margaret Mahler's mother was killed in Auschwitz.[7] George Tarjan's sister and brother-in-law managed to escape Hungary in 1940, but his parents were left behind and murdered, and his younger brother died on the death march from Auschwitz, a loss which preoccupied Tarjan all his life.[8]

Anna Freud's biographer, Elizabeth Young-Bruehl[6] noted that, "In the hiatus between the International Congress in 1938 and the one in 1949, the membership of the International dropped by 64, and most of those people were Nazi victims. On the anniversary of Karl Landauer's death, she recalled his years as the President of the German Psychoanalytic Society and wrote to his daughter, who later trained with her in London" (p. 281). Karl Landauer died in Bergen Belsen.[9] Eva Landauer and her mother survived.

Anna Freud's observations on six children, orphans from the concentration camp Theresienstadt, led to a classic paper on group support.[10] She observed that the parentless Theresienstadt children had bonded to each other with great warmth and caring.

Out of the inferno that was Nazi Europe emerged a few survivors who were to have a considerable influence in psychiatry, including Leo Eitinger[11] of Oslo, Norway and Viktor Frankl[12] of Vienna, Austria.

In the United States, Holocaust survivors who are psychiatrists include Anna Ornstein, Paul Ornstein, Henry Krystal, Dori Laub and Emanuel Tanay. Several survivors have recently published memoirs including Yehuda Nir[13] and Rita Rogers.[14] In Canadian psychiatry, Erwin Koranyi and Voijtech A. Kral had survived the Holocaust, whereas in Israel there were Hillel Klein, Judith Rappaport and Franz Brull, amongst others. Psychologists with a survivor background include Daniel Kahneman, Bruno Bettelheim, Hans Strupp, Peter Suedfeld, Ervin Staub, Fritz Redl, and Reuven Feuerstein.

Psychiatrists who survived, and survivors who became psychiatrists, were not necessarily the first to contribute to the psychiatric literature on the Holocaust. The initial observations came from others. Presumably the wounds were too fresh, the grief too great. Over time, survivor/psychiatrists have written and/or spoken publicly, perhaps aware of Arieti's[15] words, "The destiny of mankind may to a large extent depend on the understanding that future generations have of the Holocaust and on the way they respond to this new awareness of the full potential of evil" (p. 163).

THE WAR YEARS AND AFTERMATH (1945-1965)

An account of the conditions in the Belsen camp on April 17, 1945 was provided by Collis.[16] "When the corpses were more accurately counted, the figure was nearer 8,000-10,000 than 3,000. In many cases, the dead lay in naked walls of bodies around the huts, many of which were filled, literally filled, with the dead and dying. Next to nothing had been done for these people for months. For a week they had almost no water" (p. 814). Bondy[17], an inmate of Buchenwald prior to the war (1938), used his personal experience of the prewar camps to suggest what might be found at liberation and considered methods of dealing with the camp inmates after the defeat of Nazi Germany. He states, "In writing this paper I felt a great uncertainty about the after-effects of internment. As far as I know, not much is known about this subject. We do not know how deeply the stay in a concentration camp or in other camps influences the whole character structure, how long it takes to overcome the difficulties, and what methods of treatment could be used" (p. 475).

Of particular interest is the fact that Bondy's "obscure" article is in the same journal as Bettelheim's[18] "famous" article. Bettelheim, on the basis of a similar pre-war incarceration, reached conclusions which have influenced the psychologic literature and maligned survivors for two generations.

Bettelheim's opinions were that inmates regressed to infancy, that the worst lived and the best died, and that social supports were absent. He then suggested how the Jewish victims should have acted as if his personal survival was secured by his actions. A long list of credible critics challenged his incredible writings. He continued undaunted for decades despite ample evidence that his initial psychologic observations of inmates in the concentration camps Dachau in 1938 and Buchenwald in 1939 were in any case not relevant to inmates who survived the death camps of 1942-1945.

In a particularly compelling article, Ernest Rappaport[19], a Block 13-neighbor of Bettelheim's Block 12 in Buchenwald, expressed his astonishment at his fellow inmate's interpretations of the situation. Rappaport generously attributes Bettelheim's controversial statements to not having acquired a sufficient distance from the experience and having "to obtain inner relief from his residual anxiety" (p. 722). Des Pres[20] and Eitinger[21] are not so generous in their criticism.

While Bondy, Rappaport and Bettelheim were imprisoned, the Nazi sterilization and "euthanasia" program was in full gear. Alexander[22] described the prewar murder programs of "the mentally defective, psychotics (particularly schizophrenics), epileptics and patients suffering from infirmities of old age and from various organic neurologic disorders such as infantile paralysis, Parkinsonism, multiple sclerosis and brain tumors" (p. 40). All arrangements, including the killing was under the direction of a committee of physicians headed by Dr. Karl Brandt. Dr. Hallervorden, a neuropathologist, and the recipient of five hundred brains from the killing centers indicated to Dr. Alexander[22] that, "The cause of psychiatry was permanently injured by these activities, and that psychiatrists have lost the respect of the German people forever" (p. 41). Dr. Hallervorden concluded, "Still, there are interesting cases in this material" (p. 41).

Psychiatric expertise continued to play a role in the selection of human subjects, and by 1942, "medical" experiments were not only carried out in concentration camps but openly presented at medical meetings. The search for a death attributable to natural causes, such as acute miliary tuberculosis, led to the intravenous injections of suspensions of live tubercule bacilli exclusively into Jewish children imprisoned at the Neuengamme concentration camp.

Alexander[22] reported that, "By February 1942, it was assumed in German scientific circles that the Jewish race was about to be completely exterminated"; and "It was therefore proposed that a collection of 150 body casts and skeletons of Jews be preserved for perusal by future students of anthropology" (p. 43). This was done for Dr. August Hirt, Professor of Anatomy at the University of Strasbourg, and the entire collection of bodies fell into the hands of the United States Army.

As to whether physicians could have resisted, Alexander cites the resistance of Dutch physicians to the orders of Seiss-Inquart, Reich Commissar For The Occupied Netherlands Territories. *The medical profession refused to co-operate and he deported 100 Dutch physicians to concentration camps. Yet no Dutch physician participated in the Nazi programs of euthanasia or non-therapeutic sterilization.*

Fredric Wertham[3] summarized the psychiatric profession's participation in mass murder, starting with Dr. Max de Crinis, Professor of Psychiatry at the University of Berlin and the Director of the Psychiatric Department of the aforementioned Charité Hospital. Along with de Crinis, at the heart of the killing operation was Werner Villinger, Head of the Department of Child Psychiatry at Tübingen, then Psychiatric Director at Bethel, an institution for epileptics and mentally disabled persons and Professor of Psychiatry at the University of Breslau at the time of the killings. According to Wertham, he was invited to a White House conference on children and youth in 1950.

Dr. Carl Schneider was Professor of Psychiatry at the University of Heidelberg, Kraepelin's position a generation earlier. He assumed a leadership role as expert for the processing of death questionnaires and selection of candidates for extermination.

De Crinis, Villinger and Schneider all committed suicide upon revelation of their involvement. Dr. Pfannmueller of the state hospital, Eglfing-Haar, simply starved children to death. In 1948 he was sentenced to six years in jail of which he served two. Details of medical experiments are recorded in Mitscherlich and Mielke's[23] account of twenty physicians on trial in 1946 before a war crimes tribunal at Nuremberg. Physician involvement is further documented by Olbrycht[24], and Sehn.[25] Lifton[26a,26b] interviewed 28 Nazi doctors and explored the medicalization of killing. He postulated the crossing of a boundary "between violent imagery and periodic killing of victims (as of Jews in pogroms) on the one hand, and the systematic genocide in Auschwitz on the other" (p. 285).

There were psychiatrists in the camps. Most died. Tas[9] was in the 'privileged' section of Bergen Belsen, privileged meaning that 70% of 3,000 died in one year, rather than 100% in a few weeks. Tas describes efforts at psychotherapy with children as well as psychosocial intervention in the family camp section. Kral[27] was in Theresienstadt and subsequently described his observations.

In the immediate post-war period, interviews with a psychological orientation were rare. Interviews were conducted primarily for the purpose of relocation, physical assistance, evidence for war crimes, and also for the historical record. Boder[28] conducted psychological interviews of 70 persons directly onto wire tape in the survivor's original language; these were then translated and transcribed. He states in his introduction to a book of eight interviews: "The verbatim records presented in this book make uneasy reading. And yet, they are not the grimmest stories that could be told - I did not interview the dead" (p. 126).

His own unease is revealed in a striking exchange between himself and a young survivor, Abe Mohnblum, 18 years old at the time of the interview. Mohnblum questions the knowledge of psychologists in understanding human nature. He states, "After all that I have seen, I know that we know nothing yet." Boder defends psychology. "Oh no. Never say that we know nothing. Some things are known and some things are not yet explored. There is very much more left to be studied in the realm of human relations. But if you say we know nothing - that is a falsehood" (p. 126). The exchange continues and Mohnblum does not back down. He ends the interview, "Well, we may still have an opportunity to discuss this when I talk about the time I was in Buchenwald" (p. 126). It is apparent that Mohnblum has discovered something of the human condition beyond the imagination of Dr. Boder. A lesser individual might have been cowed into silence as were so many survivors.

Early writers include Friedman[29] who addressed the therapy of survivors: "Perhaps future generations will be amazed and will judge harshly, not only the phenomena of the apocalyptic destruction that took place in our time, but also our apathetic attitude, our attempts to rationalize and explain away these tragic events" (p. 167). While exhorting the caretaker to address the problems of survivors, Friedman[30] falls prey to theoretical speculation which not only illustrates the weakness of existing theory and terminology, but is ultimately silly and insulting. While acknowledging "that in a desperate struggle for survival all the forces of the libido are concentrated on the instinct of self-preservation," Friedman nevertheless speculates on "the possibility that the continuous death threats reawakened old castration fears, prohibiting the indulgence in sex, as if the inmates felt that by refraining from sexual activity they would avoid punishment here too, the punishment of the gas chamber and the crematorium" (p. 604).

In marked contrast, Rappaport[19] states unequivocally, "My assumption now is that these psychic traumata go beyond any human concept. I am referring, of course, to the trauma suffered by Jewish survivors of the German concentration camps and I want to point out that statements made by psychoanalysts that 'external events,' no matter how overwhelming, precipitate a neurosis only when they touch on specific unconscious conflicts need revision so far as the survivors of the camps are concerned" (p. 720).

Between 1947 and 1951, approximately 120,000 Jews settled in the United States, the majority being survivors from Europe. An estimated 40,000 Jews came to Canada between 1945 and 1960, mostly survivors. And Israel took in nearly 100,000 prior to 1948 and perhaps 300,000-400,000 after. The Jewish survivors of Nazi occupied Europe were not all concentration camp inmates. The actual numbers found by the liberating armies in Germany's concentration camps probably totalled only 50,000. Others survived in hiding, with partisan units, or posing as gentiles. All survivors were displaced and uprooted for ever from home and family.[31]

The survival of anyone over 35 or under 15 was unlikely and concentration camp survivors were mainly youths and young adults, with a predominance of late arrivals to the camps. Very few survived 3-4 years in any concentration camp if they were known to be Jews. Whereas in war the vast majority of casualties are men, a genocidal war includes women, children and the elderly. Therefore, studies on Danish and Norwegian prisoners of war are primarily on men.[32,33] The subsequent Eitinger studies on Jewish survivors include men and women.[21]

The consequences of the camps, as well as the effects on those in hiding and in similar conditions of constant terror have been divided into early and late consequences. Late consequences usually meant that the observations were made 10-15 years after the war, hence it is of interest to note Rümke's[34] article written in 1951 but already titled, "The Late Consequences of Psychic Trauma." In it he describes a 44 year old former inmate of Vught and Sachsenhausen, who presented with (I translate): "A feeling as if a band were bound around the head, inability to concentrate, difficulty remembering, a feeling of restlessness, disturbed sleep, an inability to forget terrible experiences" (p. 2929) - all this in spite of returning to a loving family consisting of a wife and four children and his work. This early observation on a formerly healthy, non-Jewish Dutch survivor, lends credibility to the notion that it was primarily the impact of the trauma which caused the disturbances, not prewar personality flaws.

Bluhm[35] posed the question, "Which were the mental effects produced in a great number of people by an emergency which lasted for years? Did the mass of prisoners develop typical reactions which were essential for their survival?" (p. 6). She noted the use of "emotional frigidity," a state akin to depersonalization; self-observation and self-expression (in mind only); as well as attempts to maintain a sense of cleanliness in a world of filth. Her article consists of an examination of the written works of survivors. In an effort to explain some of the horrors, she discussed weak egos, regression to childhood, and identification with the aggressor. Unfortunately, no attempt is made to examine the possibility that the unimaginable horrors caused reactions not explainable through existing theories.

Sigmund Freud's doubt "that a terrifying experience can of itself produce a neurosis in adult life" (p. 720) is answered by Rappaport[19] who stated that, "He (Freud) could not have foreseen or imagined the terror practices of the S.S. which were designed to exhaust anybody's personality resources regardless of the presence or absence of specific conflicts in the unconscious. An insistence of investigators on finding some latent predisposition for the personality breakdown betrays their unwillingness to imagine the full impact of the terror" (p. 720).

A compensation law was passed in 1956 by the Federal Republic of Germany to provide to all individuals who were persecuted because of their race, religion or "weltanschauung" appropriate restitution. In order to receive compensation, the survivor had to prove that existing problems were a consequence of persecution.

Jewish survivors seldom could demonstrate neurologic damage and psychoanalysis failed to acknowledge the psychologic impact of trauma. The psychologic defects remained attributed to personality problems from before the war and this concept was heartily embraced by most German compensation psychiatrists appointed to examine survivors.

Niederland[36] cites numerous examples of rejected compensation claims. One example describes the opinion of the German university psychiatric clinic in M. overruling the affirmative testimony of two New York specialists with the statement, "There is a great deal of evidence that there exists a psychic maldevelopment in Mr. H.... We, see, however, no possibility of assuming a causal connection or possibility of such a connection between this maldevelopment and the persecution undergone by him until 1945" (p. 235). Niederland describes Mr. H. as 14 years of age in 1939 when the Nazis arrived in Poland. Subsequently his parents and two sisters were shipped to concentration camps and murdered. He was severely beaten daily for two months, was sent from camp to camp including Auschwitz and Mauthausen, and weighed seventy pounds at liberation.

In view of the "negative attitudes" on the part of so-called experts (not always German physicians), Niederland urged familiarization with the more common psychiatric disorders to be found in surviving victims. This post-persecution pathology had already been named the post-concentration camp syndrome. Niederland deliberately omitted mental symptoms due to organic brain damage or cerebral concussion caused by beatings. He focused on the responses of the psychic apparatus, the symptom-free interval (the existence of a relatively symptom-free period after liberation and before the emergence of new symptoms), and pointed out the overwhelming impact on personality of terror.

Eissler[37] expressed his anguish in a paper titled, "The murder of how many of one's children must a person be able to withstand symptom-free in order to have a normal constitution?"

Some psychiatric specialists simply deemed psychological sequelae less relevant than physical and neurological findings related to head injuries and other medical conditions which were considered a more legitimate claim to compensation.

Eitinger[21] was a prominent exponent of the organic etiology. It took several decades before he corrected his overemphasis on the organic and introduced a balanced perspective including the psychologic impact of severe trauma.

Part of the problem was that Eitinger's earliest research was on non-Jewish Norwegian resistance fighters who returned to intact homes and families. The Israeli group investigated later were Jews from many European countries, incarcerated for being Jewish, and also most of whom after liberation had neither home or family. About seventy percent were the sole survivors of their entire families. The Norwegian group were men. The Jewish group comprised men and women. In attempting to strike a balance between organic and psychic etiology, confusion arose. While emphasizing the organicity of head injuries, encephalitis, or spotted fever, Eitinger acknowledged that Jewish concentration camp inmates were not likely to have survived with these conditions. Only non-Jews survived to be examined for organic damage. With respect to sixty-two schizophrenics in his sample, while not wishing to suggest that a patient could develop such an "illness" because of his captivity, he summarized, "I have shown that more than half of the schizophrenic former concentration camp prisoners, who at the moment are in asylums in Israel, and about whom I was able to obtain fairly reliable information are suffering from a disorder which we can assume without doubt was brought about by the stay in concentration camps" (p. 143).

In his examination of twenty "neurotic" Israeli patients, he assumed that war conditions have not played a decisive role in the illness and that the "neuroses of these patients [are] independent of their war experience inasmuch as it is difficult to pose a direct causal connection" (p. 154). Yet, in the three typical neurotic cases Eitinger describes, one person lost her parents and five siblings by age 19, another lost his wife and two sons, and a third lost her husband but managed to hide her two sons.

Eitinger's conclusion was that, "The so-called concentration camp syndrome, with the symptomatology already described, seems to be correlated mainly to considerable mechanical and/or toxic traumatizing of the brain. This investigation thus supports the theory that this syndrome is of organogenic origin" (p. 189). But he allows, "The absence of this syndrome does not exclude the possibility that prolonged and deep mental traumata have been known to cause changes of personality of an irreversible nature (p. 189).

Whereas Niederland's survivor syndrome was based on psychologic observations, Eitinger's survivor syndrome focussed on the organic. Eitinger's initial observations gave way to valuable psychologic insights as described by Anton Gill[38] through interviews with Eitinger, himself a survivor of Auschwitz and Buchenwald. Hoppe[39] studied the life histories of 190 survivors and noted that all had been referred to him by legal advisors and their claims for restitution had frequently been rejected before by official examiners for German indemnification offices. In addition, the examining psychiatrist was often German, the examination brief and severely traumatic. A series of articles followed with generalizations sure to deter any other survivor from seeking compensation or therapeutic assistance from professionals. Engel[40] described a possible pattern equating work with torture, and Koenig[41] reported on chronic or persisting identity diffusion according to an Eriksonian model in a group of younger concentration camp inmates. He stated that, "A satisfactory theoretical framework for the understanding of the characterological changes in former adolescent camp survivors was developed" (p. 1083). Such theories do not reflect the postwar reality that the majority of survivors thrived on hard work and that the adolescent survivors were largely indistinguishable from their non-persecuted contemporaries.

Lederer[42] described the persecution syndrome after his examination of 50 patients claiming compensation, and held the opinion that the syndrome is of psychological origin. Trautman[43], on the basis of a series of interviews with two hundred survivors, reached the conclusion that the concentration camp syndrome cannot be regarded as either a traumatic neurosis or an anxiety neurosis. The experience for the survivor was that of prolonged panic, a real anxiety in response to the real danger of imminent death.

Chodoff[44] also minimized the notion of organic brain disease as an etiologic factor stating that, "Complaints of difficulty in remembering and concentrating (considered by Dr. Eitinger to be suggestive of brain disease) were present although they appear to play a more major role among Eitinger's patients than among those I examined" (p. 328). Chodoff suggests that, "Possibly, psychodynamic psychiatry has gone too far in its at least implied insistence that every state of emotional illness must result from the impact of a trauma on a personality somehow predisposed to react adversely to the trauma; cases of the kind described here must be taken into account before such explanations can be regarded as universal" (p. 327). Grobin[45] wrote that in his series of seventy examinations, there was a relative scarcity of serious organic disability among the victims. The seriously ill had died. Tuberculosis was an infrequent finding because tuberculous people were not admitted into Canada. Such problem people were left to the State of Israel. Klein et al[46] in Israel compared fifty inpatients who had suffered extreme conditions (concentration camps, ghettos, hiding) with forty inpatients who had spent World War II in Europe but under less extreme conditions. The backgrounds of all ninety patients were essentially similar. The researchers refrained from drawing conclusions, but indicated that the study was prompted in part when, "During the period of the Eichmann trial, severe psychological reactions, both in psychiatric patients and in otherwise 'healthy' camp survivors who had not, until then, shown major difficulties in adaptation, could be observed" (p. 334). There had been a reluctance to study concentration camp inmates in Israel, in part because of the attempt to assist survivors to adjust to the new homeland "rather than to delve into the immediate traumatic past which contained so much horror and destruction, not only for the direct victims, but for the Jewish population of Israel, too" (p. 334).

LATER OBSERVATIONS (1965–1985)

By 1965 it had become evident that the catastrophic trauma visited upon the persecuted did not require pre-morbid personalities or psychosocial antecedents to leave its permanent and indelible impact on the survivor. Observations on the children of survivors (the second generation)[47] had begun, drawing attention to the possible effects on the offspring of massively traumatized parents. Some of the available knowledge to that time was consolidated at the Wayne State University Conference on Massive Psychic Trauma[48] which was subsequently published. The articles, although uneven in quality, and perpetuating some earlier problems in understanding survivors, nevertheless provided a focus on the burdens of survivors.

Solkoff[49], in a critical review of 90 articles about children of survivors, noted the paucity of controls and the focus on survivors who were known to clinicians rather than those leading more or less healthy and productive lives.

Psychiatry failed to revise theory and devise terminology relevant to the survivor's experience (Krell[50]). Although the range of human responses to extreme stress is finite, the usual limits were surpassed, and the responses not understood. Frankl[51] and Lifton[52] sought to describe the excesses of human sadism and sufferings by coining phrases to describe the phenomenology of a new world of experience, so aptly titled "The Kingdom of Night" by Wiesel.[53]

The language of atrocity as described by Langer[54] required re-examination in light of the Holocaust. For example, in order to examine guilt, one must first know about the environment created by the perpetrator. Langer pointed out the situations in which people were forced to make a "choiceless choice" (p. 72): a woman forced to choose one child to live of two she carried in her arms on the arrival platform in Auschwitz; a head of the Jewish Council in the Ghetto ordered to deliver one thousand Jews daily for deportation or the Germans would take two thousand; a 16 year old who can stay with his mother and die, or flee, perhaps to live; - *these are not choices*.

Leon Kahn[55] describes parting from his mother: "Our parting will remain forever on my mind and conscience" (p. 72). Forced at age 15 to choose between an attempt to survive with his father and brother or face certain death with his mother and grandmother, he opted to join the partisans. Wiesel's father died in his arms in the concentration camp. Kahn's father died in his arms in the forest. Holocaust survivors who express guilt often witnessed the death of a loved one and thought they could or should have done more, even when it was absolutely impossible to do so.

According to Carmelly[56], at the very least, survivor's guilt should be divided into passive guilt (those who happened to be alive at liberation), and active guilt (those who committed immoral acts or chose not to help when it was possible).

For much of the 70's, therapists labored with little information[57] in the face of considerable countertransference.[58]

In three editions of the *Comprehensive Textbook of Psychiatry*[59] throughout the 60's and 70's there is no information about Holocaust survivors. The *American Handbook of Psychiatry*[60] has one article in its second edition. A four-volume encyclopedic work, the *Basic Handbook of Child Psychiatry*[61] contains no information either on children who survived the Holocaust, or about the children of Holocaust survivors.

The textbooks read by a generation of trainees in psychiatry have no information on these victims. It is possible that editors were subject to personal resistance similar to that described in 61 psychotherapists surveyed by Danieli.[62]

The therapists who treated Holocaust survivors experienced guilt feelings for having led a comfortable life, experienced anger on learning what happened, and horror to the point of changing the subject in order to hear no more.

Resistance to working with victims of trauma remained a problem for therapists not only with Holocaust survivors, but also with survivors of sexual abuse, rape and torture. It was not until 1980 when PTSD was included in the DSM III that trauma research flourished as a subject of psychiatric and psychologic investigation. The literature on Holocaust survivors was relevant to this resurgence of interest and it was re-examined by contemporary researchers.

The 80's have also witnessed the emergence of observations on a comparatively ignored group of Holocaust survivors, the child survivors. Moskovitz[63] described twenty four such children interviewed by her as adults. The fate of children has been documented, and movingly described by child and adolescent survivors such as Kosinski[64] and Wiesel.[53] In a review of Holocaust literature, Ezrahi[65] noted that Kosinski's novel in which the subject is a child "taps the most primary sources of fear and terror that are sublimated even in much of Holocaust literature. Somehow, until Kosinski, childhood had retained its innocence in tragedy" (p. 118).

Child survivors have escaped attention because most were hidden and remained 'in hiding' in order to blend in as citizens of their adoptive lands, and because they were discouraged by adults to speak of their past.[66] Now, well into their 50's and 60's, they too are confronting the realities of a tragic past. Michel Goldberg[67], Saul Friedlander[68], and Andre Stein[69] are among the children who in adult life have shattered decades of silence.

Learning about child survivors reveals information relevant to the total survivor population. Firstly, it demonstrates the damage wrought among those not in concentration camps but in hiding. Secondly, it points out the importance of Keilson's[70] descriptions delineating the phase of persecution, the actual phase of incarceration or hiding, and the post-war period. Keilson's theories demonstrate that the quality of post-war experience was crucial to the functioning of the survivor, particularly the youngest ones. The area of adaptation and coping requires careful continuing investigation. The adaptive maneuvers of traumatized children examined longitudinally into adulthood, may provide strategies for the management of severe trauma.[71,72,73,74]

CONCLUSIONS

The Holocaust had a massive and lasting impact on psychiatry. German psychiatrists were involved in the murder of "defective children" and adults, mass murder which eventually led to genocide. Nazi ideology forced the expulsion of Jewish psychiatrists and psychoanalysts who enriched North American psychiatry but who also suffered grievous personal losses, a fact which may have influenced their post-war careers. Thousands of physicians were murdered, including numerous psychiatrists.

The psychiatric literature[75] of the Holocaust reflects missed opportunities. A closer examination of the earliest psychiatric investigations into the sequelae of concentration camp incarceration might have alerted the investigator to the existence of post-traumatic stress disorder several decades before its eventual inclusion into the DSM III in 1980. Earlier recognition may have provided improved treatment opportunities.[76] Terry[77] and Ornstein[78] regret the usage of the entity "survivor syndrome" which to them seems to have precluded a more careful, individual consideration of the survivor. Krystal and Eitinger, who have struggled for two generations to better understand survivors and the impact of their experiences have made considerable progress. Krystal's[79] contributions emphasize the survivor's need to integrate through effective mourning while Eitinger's[80] lucid clarification of his later thinking and findings correct some of his earlier confusing observations.

Chodoff[81] had summarized the essential ingredients for potentially successful insight- oriented psychotherapy by illustrating the special difficulties for the survivor and for his therapist. A variety of modifications have evolved over time in the treatment of survivors, from Bastiaans'[82] pioneering efforts in Holland with intensive abreactive treatment to less intrusive therapies more suited perhaps to the aging survivor and present-day functioning.[83,84,85] Some therapists, more involved with the second generation, began to include parents in modified or actual family therapy with varying degrees of success.[86,87,88] Davidson's[89] lucid observations could serve as a handbook to the treatment of trauma survivors.

One area of potential therapeutic importance is the in-depth examination of the meaning and relevance of memory and its recapture.[90,91] The survivor experiences daily the return of fragments of memory through dreams and nightmares and relevant triggers (sirens, barking). Each occurrence sets in motion a disturbing and disorienting series of events which may lead to preoccupation and depression. The obtaining of a chronologic account, an orderly exercise to place the fragments in context, seems to have a positive and lasting therapeutic effect.[92]

Such an account captured on video tape is permanent, can be played for interested family, and has historical value in Holocaust education programs.

The impact of the Holocaust will not disappear with the passing of the last survivor, nor for that matter, the last killer. *The Holocaust remains with us, a permanent stain on the human experience and on the individual psyche. Psychiatrists can ill afford to ignore its impact on psychiatry. This particular trauma deserves continued scrutiny. From it we may still draw knowledge to assist not only aging survivors of the Holocaust but victims of contemporary genocides, persecution and torture.*

It is helpful to remember Elie Wiesel's caution[93] that at an earlier time, "The literature of testimony still commanded respect. As yet nobody was explaining to the dead how they should have gone to their deaths, or to the survivors how they should be living their lives. One did not pass judgment.

Not yet..." (p. 238). However, Wiesel is not opposed to study, in fact, "On the contrary, I say that it (the Holocaust) must be studied more and more in all its forms and all its expressions. There is no more urgent theme for this analytical and self-analytical generation. But it must be approached with fear and trembling. And above all, with humility" (p. 239).

REFERENCES

1. Fermi, Laura (1968). *The Illustrious Immigrants*. Chicago, IL: The University of Chicago Press.

2. Coser, Louis (1984). *Refugee Scholars in America*. New Haven, CT: Yale University Press.

3. Wertham, Frederic (1966). *A Sign for Cain - An Exploration of Human Violence*. London: Robert Hale.

4. Brieger, Gert H. (1980). The medical profession. In: Friedlander, Henry, and Milton, Sybil (Eds.), *Bureaucracy and Genocide*. Millwood, NJ: Kraus International.

5. Tory, Avram (1990). *Surviving the Holocaust - The Kovno Ghetto Diary*. Cambridge, MA: Cambridge University Press.

6. Young-Bruehl, Elizabeth (1988). *Anna Freud - A Biography*. New York: Summit Books.

7. Stepansky, Paul E. (1988). *The Memoirs of Margaret S. Mahler*. New York: The Free Press.

8. Pasnau, Robert O., and Work, Henry H. (1993). George Tarjan, MD 1912-1991. *American Journal of Psychiatry*, 150, 691-694.

9. Tas, J. (1951). Psychological disorders among inmates of concentration camps and repatriates. *Psychiatric Quarterly*, 5, 679-690.

10. Freud, Anna, and Dann, Sophie (1951). An experiment in group upbringing. In: Eissler, Ruth S.; Freud, Anna; Hartmann, Heinz; and Kris, Ernst (Eds.), *Psychoanalytic Study of the Child. Vol. 6.* New York: International Universities Press, pp. 127-168.

11. Eitinger, Leo (1962). Concentration camp survivors in the post-war world. *American Journal of Orthopsychiatry*, 32(3), 367-375.

12. Frankl, Viktor E. (1959). *From Death Camp to Existentialism: A Psychiatrist's Path to a New Therapy*. Boston, MA: Beacon Press.

13. Nir, Yehuda (1989). *The Lost Childhood*. New York: Brace Jovanovich.

14. Mack, John, and Roger, Rita (1988). *The Alchemy of Survival - One Woman's Journey*. Boston, MA: Addison Wesley.

15. Arieti, Silvano (1979). *The Parnas*. New York: Basic Books.

16. Collis, W.R.F. (1945). Belsen camp: A preliminary report. *British Medical Journal*, 814-816.

17. Bondy, Curt (1943). Problems of internment camps. *Journal of Abnormal and Social Psychology*, 38(4), 453-475.

18. Bettelheim, Bruno (1943). Individual and mass behavior in extreme situations. *Journal of Abnormal and Social Psychology*, 38(4), 417-452.

19. Rappaport, Ernest A. (1968). Beyond traumatic neurosis: A psychoanalytic study of late reactions to the concentration camp trauma. *International Journal of Psychoanalysis*, 49, 719-731.

20. Des Pres, Terrence (1979). The Bettelheim problem. *Social Research*, 46(4), 619-647.

21. Eitinger, Leo (1972). *Concentration Camp Survivors in Norway and Israel*. The Hague: Martinus Nijhoff.

22. Alexander, Leo (1949). Medical science under dictatorship. *The New England Journal of Medicine*, 241(2), 39-47.

23. Mitscherlich, Alexander; and Mielke, Fred (1949). *Doctors of Infamy: The Story of Nazi Medical War Crimes*. New York: Henry Schuman.

24. Olbrycht, Jan (1987). The Nazi health office actively participated with the SS administration in Auschwitz. In: *Auschwitz Anthology. Vol. 1: Inhuman Medicine. Part 1*. Warsaw: International Auschwitz Committee, pp. 147-205.

25. Sehn, Jan (1970). The case of the Auschwitz physician J.P. Kremer. In: *Auschwitz Anthology. Vol. 1: Inhuman Medicine. Part 1*. Warsaw: International Auschwitz Committee, pp. 206-258.

26a. Lifton, Robert Jay (1982). Medicalized killing in Auschwitz. *Psychiatry*, 45(4), 283-297.

26b. Lifton, Robert Jay (1986). *The Nazi Doctors: Medical Killing and the Psychology of Genocide*. New York: Basic Books.

27. Kral, Vojtech A. (1951). Psychiatric observations under severe chronic stress. *American Journal of Psychiatry*, 108, 185-192.

28. Boder, David P. (1949). *I Did Not Interview the Dead*. Urbana, IL: University of Illinois Press.

29. Friedman, Paul (1948). The effects of imprisonment. *Acta Medica Orientalia*, 7, 163-167.

30. Friedman, Paul (1949). Some aspects of concentration camp psychology. *American Journal of Psychiatry*, 105, 601-605.

31. Krell, Robert (1979). Holocaust families: The survivors and their children. *Comprehensive Psychiatry*, 20, 560-568.

32. Thygesen, Paul, and Kieler, Jørgen (1952). Famine disease: Mental deterioration. In: Helweg-Larsen, Per; Hoffmeyer, Henrik; Kieler, Jørgen; Hess Thaysen, Eigil; Hess Thaysen, Jørn; Thygesen, Paul; and Hertel Wulff, Munke, *Famine Disease in German Concentration Camps, Complications and Sequelae: With Special Reference to Tuberculosis, Mental Disorders and Social Consequences*. Copenhagen: Ejnar Munksgaard, pp. 235-250. [Also published as *Acta Psychiatrica et Neurologica Scandinavica*, Supplementum 83.]

33. Eitinger, Leo (1963). Preliminary notes on a study of concentration camp survivors in Norway. *Israel Annals of Psychiatry* and Related Disciplines, 1(1), 59-67.

34. Rümke, H.C. (1951). Late werkingen van psychotraumata [Late consequences of psychic trauma]. *Nederlands Tijdschrift Voor Geneeskunde*, 95, 2928-2937.

35. Bluhm, Hilda O. (1948). How did they survive? Mechanisms of defense in Nazi concentration camps. *American Journal of Psychotherapy*, 2, 3-32.

36. Niederland, William G. (1961). The problem of the survivor: Some remarks on the psychiatric evaluation of emotional disorders in survivors of Nazi persecution. *Journal of the Hillside Hospital*, 10, 233-247.

37. Eissler, Kurt R. (1963). Die Ermordüng von wievielen seiner Kinder muss ein mensch symptomfrei ertragen Können, um eine normale Konstitution zu haben? [The murder of how many of his children must a person be able to endure symptom-free in order to have a normal constitution?] *Psyche: Zeitschrift für Psychoanalyse und ihre Anwendungen*, 17, 241-291.

38. Gill, Anton (1988). *The Journey Back from Hell: Conversations with Concentration Camp Survivors*. London: Grafton Books.

39. Hoppe, Klaus (1971). Chronic reactive aggression in survivors of extreme persecution. *Comprehensive Psychiatry*, 12(3), 230-237.

40. Engel, Werner H. (1962). Reflections on the psychiatric consequences of persecution: An evaluation of restitution claimants. *American Journal of Psychotherapy*, 16, 191-203.

41. Koenig, Werner (1964). Chronic or persisting identity diffusion. *American Journal of Psychiatry*, 120(11), 1081-1084.

42. Lederer, Wolfgang (1965). Persecution and compensation: Theoretical and practical implications of the "persecution syndrome." *Archives of General Psychiatry*, 12, 464-474.

43. Trautman, Ernest (1964). Fear and panic in Nazi concentration camps: A biosocial evaluation of the chronic anxiety syndrome. *International Journal of Social Psychiatry*, 10(2), 131-141.

44. Chodoff, Paul (1963). Late effects of the concentration camp syndrome. *Archives of General Psychiatry*, 8, 323-333.

45. Grobin, W. (1965). Medical assessment of late effects of National Socialist persecution. *Canadian Medical Association Journal*, 92, 911-917.

46. Klein, Hillel; Zellermayer, Julius; and Shanan, Joel (1963). Former concentration camp inmates on a psychiatric ward. *Archives of General Psychiatry*, 8, 334-342.

47. Rakoff, Vivian; Sigal, John J.; and Epstein, Nathan (1966). Children and families of concentration camp survivors. *Canada's Mental Health*, 14, 24-26.

48. Krystal, Henry (1968). *Massive Psychic Trauma*. New York: International Universities Press.

49. Solkoff, Norman (Ed.) (1981). Children of survivors of the Nazi Holocaust: A critical review of the literature. *American Journal of Orthopsychiatry*, 51, 29-42.

50. Krell, Robert (1984). Holocaust survivors and their children: Comments on psychiatric consequences and psychiatric terminology. *Comprehensive Psychiatry*, 25(5), 521-528.

51. Frankl, Viktor E. (1962). *Man's Search for Meaning: An Introduction to Logotherapy*. Boston, MA: Beacon Press.

52. Lifton, Robert Jay (1979). Survivor experience and traumatic syndrome. In: *The Broken Connection: On Death and the Continuity of Life*. New York: Simon and Schuster, pp. 163-178.

53. Wiesel, Elie (1986). *Night*. New York: Bantam Books.

54. Langer, Lawrence L. (1982). *Versions of Survival: The Holocaust and the Human Spirit*. Albany: State University of New York Press.

55. Kahn, Leon (1978). *No Time to Mourn*. Vancouver, BC: Laurelton Press.

56. Carmelly, Felicia (1975). Guilt feelings in concentration camp survivors: Comments of a "survivor." *Jewish Community Service*, 52(2), 139-144.

57. Krell, Robert (1990). Holocaust survivors: A clinical perspective. *Psychiatric Journal of the University of Ottawa*, 15(1), 18-21.

58. Rabkin, Leslie (1975). Countertransference in the extreme situation: The family therapy of survivor families. In: Wolberg, Lewis R., and Aronson, Marvin L. (Eds.), *Group Therapy, 1975: An Overview*. New York: Stratton Intercontinental.

59. Freedman, Alfred; and Kaplan, Harold (Eds.) (1967). *Comprehensive Textbook of Psychiatry*. Baltimore, MD: William and Wilkins.

60. Arieti, Silvano (Ed.) (1975). *American Handbook of Psychiatry*. New York: Basic Books.

61. Noshpitz, Joseph (Ed.) (1979). *Basic Handbook of Child Psychiatry*. New York: Basic Books.

62. Danieli, Yael (1981). *Therapists' Difficulties in Treating Survivors of the Nazi Holocaust and Their Children*. Unpublished doctoral dissertation, New York University, 216 pp. *Dissertation Abstracts International*, 42(12-B), p. 4927. (University Microfilms no. AAC 8210968).

63. Moskovitz, Sarah (1983). *Love Despite Hate: Child Survivors of the Holocaust and Their Adult Lives*. New York: Schocken.

64. Kosinski, Jerzy (1965). *The Painted Bird*. New York: Bantam Books.

65. Ezrahi, Sidra (1973). Holocaust literature in European languages. In: *Encyclopedia Judaica Year Book 1972-1973*. Jerusalem: Keter, pp. 106-119.

66. Krell, Robert (1985). Introduction to "Child survivors of the Holocaust: 40 years later." *Journal of the American Academy of Child Psychiatry*, 24(4), 378-380.

67. Goldberg, Michel (1982). *Namesake*. New Haven, CT: Yale University Press.

68. Friedlander, Saul (1980). *When Memory Comes*. New York: Avon Books.

69. Stein, André (1984). *Broken Silence: Dialogues From the Edge*. Toronto, ONT: Lester and Orpen Dennys.

70. Keilson, Hans (1992). *Sequential Traumatization in Children*: A Clinical and Statistical Follow-up Study on the Fate of the Jewish War Orphans in the Netherlands. Jerusalem: The Hebrew University: Magnes Press.

71. Rutter, Michael (1987). Psychosocial resilience and protective mechanisms. *American Journal of Orthopsychiatry*, 57, 316-331.

72. Garmezy, Norman (1991). Resilience in children's adaptation to negative life events and stressed environments. *Pediatric Annals*, 20, 459-466.

73. Krell, Robert (1993). Child survivors of the Holocaust: Strategies of adaptation. *Canadian Journal of Psychiatry*, 38(6), 384-389.

74. Terr, Lenore (1991). Childhood traumas: An outline and overview. *American Journal of Psychiatry*, 148, 10-20.

75. Eitinger, Leo; Krell, Robert; and Rieck, Miriam (1985). *The Psychological and Medical Effects of Concentration Camps and Related Persecutions on Survivors of the Holocaust: A Research Bibliography*. Vancouver, BC: University of British Columbia Press.

76. Krell, Robert (1989). Alternative therapeutic approaches to Holocaust survivors. In: Marcus, Paul, and Rosenberg, Alan (Eds.), *Healing Their Wounds: Psychotherapy with Holocaust Survivors and Their Families*. New York: Praeger, pp. 215-226.

77. Terry, Jack (1984). The damaging effects of the "survivor syndrome." In: Luel, Steven A., and Marcus, Paul (Eds.), *Psychoanalytic Reflections on the Holocaust: Selected Essays*. New York: Ktav, pp. 135-148.

78. Ornstein, Anna (1985). Survival and recovery. *Psychoanalytic Inquiry*, 5(1), 99-130.

79. Krystal, Henry (1981). Integration and self-healing in post-traumatic states. *Journal of Geriatric Psychiatry*, 142(2), 165-189.

80. Eitinger, Leo (1981). Denial in concentration camps. *Nordisk Psykiatrisk Tidsskrift*, 5, 148-156.

81. Chodoff, Paul (1980). Psychotherapy of the survivor. In: Dimsdale, Joel E. (Ed.), *Survivors, Victims and Perpetrators: Essays on the Nazi Holocaust*. Washington, DC: Hemisphere, pp. 205-216.

82. Bastiaans, Jan (1979). De behandeling van oorlogsslachtoffers [The treatment of war victims]. *TGO Tijdschrift voor Therapie, Geneesmiddel en Onderzoek*, 1, 352-358.

83. Marcus, Paul, and Rosenberg, Alan (1989). *Healing Their Wounds: Psychotherapy with Holocaust Survivors and Their Families*. New York: Praeger.

84. Krell, Robert (1994). The psychiatric treatment of Holocaust survivors. In: Charny, Israel W. (Ed.), *The Widening Circle of Genocide, Vol. 3 of Genocide: A Critical Bibliographic Review*. New Brunswick, NJ: Transaction, pp. 245-271.

85. Eitinger, Leo (1993). Identification, treatment and care of the aging Holocaust survivor: A keynote address. In: Kenigsberg, Rositta E., and Lieblich, Cathy M. (Eds.), *The First*

National Conference on Identification, Treatment and Care of the Aging Holocaust Survivor, March 29-31, 1992: Selected Proceedings. Miami, FL: Holocaust Documentation and Education Center and Southeast Florida Center on Aging, Florida International University, pp. 5-15.

86. Russel, Axel (1974). Late psychosocial consequences in concentration camp survivors families. *American Journal of Orthopsychiatry*, 44(4), 611-619.

87. Davidson, Shamai (1980). Transgenerational transmission in the families of Holocaust survivors. *International Journal of Family Psychiatry*, 1(1), 95-112.

88. Krell, Robert (1982). Family therapy with children of concentration camp survivors. *American Journal of Psychotherapy*, 36(5), 513-522.

89. Davidson, Shamai (1992). *Holding on to Humanity - The Message of the Holocaust Survivors: The Shamai Davidson Papers*. (Ed.: Charny, Israel W.) New York: New York University Press.

90. Hogman, Flora (1985). Role of memories in lives of World War II orphans. *Journal of American Academy of Child Psychiatry*, 24(4), 390-396.

91. Fresco, Nadine (1984). Remembering the unknown. *International Review of Psycho-Analysis*, 11(4), 417-427.

92. Krell, Robert (1985). Therapeutic value of documenting child survivors. *Journal of American Academy of Child Psychiatry*, 24(4), 397-400.

93. Wiesel, Elie (1979). *A Jew Today*. New York: Vintage Books.

2

Survivors and Their Families: Psychiatric Consequences of the Holocaust

Robert Krell

The end of World War II revealed a problem of staggering proportions. Until the liberation of the death camps, no one had anticipated such horror. Frenzied activity ensued to salvage the physical existence of the pitiful remnants of survivors. The psychological consequences manifested themselves shortly after and on a scale hitherto unknown. A series of clinical observations provided a first glance at the psychogenic origins of a wide variety of symptoms in survivors.[1,2] No psychiatric terminology existed to describe the emotional consequences of concentration camp incarceration, nor were there treatment strategies.

While North American psychiatrists were exploring the psychodynamic issues, their European colleagues were more preoccupied with the obvious organic damage of malnutrition and beatings.[3,4] For a time, the psychologic trauma was overshadowed by the emphasis on organic studies. It became evident that physical damage could not account for all sufferings of the survivor. Restitution payments required psychiatric examination. Despite overwhelming evidence to the contrary, the emotional issues remained secondary in importance because of strongly held beliefs that adult emotional trauma is pre-determined in childhood.[5,6] At best, psychiatrists simply denied the psychological impact of the massive trauma and did not recognize its importance. At worst, psychiatrists who adhered only to the theory of constitutional etiology, acted on behalf of the German Government in examination for compensation. Their foregone conclusion was that persecution *per se* was unlikely to be the determinant to emotional problems deserving compensation.

Eissler[7] exposed this "perversion of psychiatry" and stated, "When a physician refers to concentration camp experiences as 'disagreeable,' he has given away his secret contempt. When he commits an error to the detriment of a victim by misrepresenting the meaning of a medical term, or when he fails to concern himself with the true duration of the persecution to which the survivor has been exposed, then one can be quite certain that he has become the victim of a dangerous regression" (p. 1358).

The survivors examined for restitution and/or referred for therapy were described and a constellation of commonly encountered symptoms became known as "the concentration camp syndrome." Although at first the syndrome was considered a variant of traumatic neurosis, psychiatrists soon recognized the enormity of the massive psychologic stress as the precipitant. Chodoff[8] stated, "When one considers the intensity of the stress undergone by these patients, there seems little necessity to postulate any pre-existing personality weakness or predisposition" (p. 327).

Over time, researchers such as Eitinger[9] who had previously espoused the organic position, recognized the importance of psychogenic factors. Simultaneously, there was a profusion of psychodynamic explanations.[10,11] Chodoff[12] pointed out, "There have been a number of psychoanalytic attempts to explicate the psychodynamics responsible for the persisting symptoms. These attempts are interesting, but the fact that most derive from relatively superficial reparation examinations rather than from intensive psychoanalytic scrutiny vitiate their value" (p. 943).

THE PSYCHIATRIC TERMINOLOGY

The concentration camp syndrome became a generally accepted construct commonly observed in survivors. Equally accepted were the notions that most survivors have problems with aggression and survivor guilt, the two problems identified by Krystal and Niederland as pathogenic forces in 92% of survivors examined by them.[13] It is possible that some of these concepts have been uncritically incorporated into the literature. The suspiciousness, nightmares, occasional or chronic depressions, anxiety attacks and psychosomatic problems found in most survivors are actually logical responses to a bizarre and extreme trauma. The symptoms reflect a unique and devastating life experience which, in turn, raises fundamental questions as to the understanding of psychopathology. In fact, one might suggest that a survivor free of nightmares, paranoia and anxiety, exhibits a degree of abnormality. Examining problems of aggression and survivor guilt[14] more closely raises concerns about the usage of common psychodynamic interpretations of aggression and guilt when applied to Holocaust survivors.

Identification with the aggressor, a psychoanalytic concept formulated by Anna Freud[15] in 1936, refers to a child's mastery of anxiety by imitating the anger of a parent or teacher. The terminology she had formulated to describe impersonating an aggressor in childhood did not anticipate the sadistic aggression of Nazi perpetrators. Some Jewish survivors examined by psychiatrists[16] were nevertheless described as having "identified with the aggressors" in some behaviors. Given the nature of death camps, to label victims as "Nazi-like" is inappropriate. After all, any such identification was not to master anxiety but to ensure survival. Possibly clinicians have such difficulty understanding the sadism of the perpetrators that they attempt to understand them through the victims. Rather than examining the aggressors (which is difficult), one examines the victims who have "identified with the aggressor" (which is easier).

Survivor guilt has been assumed present in nearly all survivors of the Holocaust. *It is more likely that guilt is present in nearly all therapists of survivors*. Several studies[17,18] suggest that survival guilt is not uniformly present, and when it is, frequently it is an accompaniment to depression. A majority of survivors indicate that they thought survival was due to luck, change, the help of God or fate. The awareness of the limitations of personal initiative cannot be readily reconciled with guilt which requires at least the perception that one could have acted differently.

THE PROBLEMS WITH THERAPY

Therapy with survivors is extraordinarily complicated. Berger[19] points to three major difficulties: "The need to fail or be punished often leads to failure in therapy; massive denial of the events of the persecution, sometimes supported by the therapist's own need to deny, often presents an impenetrable barrier; there is often an amnesia for the period preceding the persecution (that is for the crucial early experiences). These reports suggest that therapy with survivors cannot follow conventional psychoanalytic lines" (pp. 242-243).

The reference to therapist denial must be taken seriously in the context of therapy with survivors and their children. It has become evident that therapist denial runs rampant in the treatment of survivors' children. Kestenberg[20] reports that a questionnaire distributed to analysts for comments on treatment of the offspring of Holocaust survivors revealed that, "Some were startled by the question because it never occurred to them to link their patient's dynamics to the history of their parent's persecution" (p. 313). Hochman[21], in treating a child of survivors, mentions candidly that it was in the third year of analysis, "before I realized this was an important issue in the case," referring to the fact that both parents were German/Jewish refugees and both sets of grandparents were in concentration camps. These are but two examples of many which illustrate that the treatment of Holocaust survivors is compromised by therapists who, were they treating other patients, *would* take a detailed history of family background and influences.

What makes it possible for otherwise skilled therapists to bypass Holocaust information? Perhaps fear lies at the heart of the matter; not anxiety over the unknown, but fear of what is known. Few therapists were prepared to treat survivors because of the knowledge of what they might hear if they dared ask. A probing therapist may not only provoke the survivor's rage but his own unresolved feelings of guilt and utter helplessness, a helplessness reinforced by the fact that there is no terminology and no framework of therapy to guide him. There are extraordinary pressures to which a therapist may be subject.[22,23]

Given the failures of psychoanalytic treatment of survivors, one wonders why it took so long to devise different approaches. The creative application of psychodynamic principles might have provided new insights. Lifton[24] attempted to provide a theoretical framework from which to view the survivor. In the process of refining psychiatric terminology, he has remarked on the hostility which exists towards survivors. Lifton suggests that as an accompaniment to the Holocaust experience which is so far beyond our grasp and comprehension, "There is a subjective sense of death taint which both the survivor and others feel in relationship to the survivor" (p. 186).

In the process of attempting therapy, psychiatrists have often reported failures of treatment with the onus on the survivors' failure to make use of therapists.

For survivor-parents, the birth of a child signalled a confusion, a mixture of despair and hope. A child was the living reminder of those who were lost, born into a world of proven evil, yet representing a triumph over Nazism. In order not to burden the child, survivor/parents frequently withheld information about the tragedy with mixed success.[25]

Observations on the family interaction of survivor/families, revealed a definite impact on the children, the second generation.[26] The evidence of transmission of Holocaust effects spawned group and family therapy techniques which had better clinical results than individual therapy.[27,28a,28b,29]

Participation in Holocaust education in which survivors provide eyewitness accounts to students appears to be healing and therapeutic as does the documentation of personal accounts. Participants report that teaching youngsters what actually happened is one of the few opportunities to make meaningful an event that had no discernible meaning previously. Bearing witness in order to prevent a future tragedy has provided some survivors with a forum in which the telling of their stories is richly rewarded by attentive students who write them to visit their schools and who shower them with gratitude for their participation in the form of letters and poems.[30]

THE ASSUMPTION OF PSYCHOPATHOLOGY

The psychiatric literature has reflected badly on the survivor and suffers from over-generalizations. One can perhaps understand the reluctance of some survivors to come for therapy. Krystal[31] wrote, "Many of the male survivors tend to be permanently inhibited in their ability for sexual initiative and potency, in a manner reminding us of the ethological concept of the 'defeated male' (p. 3). In this characterological change, there is an acceptance of the castrated slave role." Hoppe[32] diagnosed a woman patient, "Besides a chronic reactive depression the patient suffers from chronic reactive aggression and hate addiction" (p. 214). The descriptions of individual patients were unfortunately generalized widely to the survivor population. It has not escaped the attention of survivors that there are many preconceived notions held by mental health professionals, mostly negative.

For many years, the exploration of the victim's psychopathology obscured the remarkable adaptations made by some survivors. Various findings have been challenged in critical reviews[33,34] and in later research.[35] There exists the likelihood that the transmission of effects from generation to generation may include positive attributes, not only the oft-described negative consequences.

When psychopathology is present in second generation children, it may indeed be serious and difficult to treat.[36] However, there is no discernible universal effect which determines that all children of survivors will be the carriers of parental suffering. Those children aware of the parental experience often assume the burden of the past with dignity. As to whether that legacy is more likely to bring positive contributions to human welfare or swell the rosters of mental health clinics, the final word is not in. It is important to consider carefully non-clinical samples of these children, now adult, in order to re-examine the sometimes biased perspective.

CONCLUSION

Fifty years of observations on survivors of the concentration camps and other survivors of the Holocaust (in hiding, partisans, slave labor camps) has provided a new body of medical and psychiatric literature. Survivors of various kinds have always been of interest and concern to the psychiatrist. Many psychiatric disorders are rooted in the loss of a loved one, leaving behind someone to survive that loss. Mourning and depression are among the commonly researched phenomena in psychiatric writings. Generally speaking, no previous observations, research, or clinical expertise had prepared the psychiatrist and psychologist for the experiences of multiple loss and the severity of trauma suffered by Holocaust survivors. The scope and scale surpassed the imagination.

The imprint of the trauma is permanent. Nevertheless, many survivors have not only adapted to their past but carved out a meaningful future. The burden of their memories has been passed on, sometimes purposefully, sometimes unknowingly, to their children. It is the children who are presently engaged in some of the more meaningful research on survivors; perhaps as one method of coming to grips with their parent's experience.[37]

The rapidly expanding literature signals an attempt to understand the psychological complexity of survivor pathology and, at this late date, of survivor health. Few reliable tools exist to tease out that which is unique about this colossal event in terms of its impact and consequences. The effort must continue.

Clinicians today face the challenge of treating the aging survivor[38] whose illness or hospitalization, may re-trigger Holocaust-related memories. The second generation children, now in their 30's and 40's are raising families of their own. Some of their personal problems remain raw and unresolved, and may influence the third generation. Not to be ignored is the direct impact of the grandparents' experiences as related to their grandchildren.

For those who work with patients and clients as mental health professionals, familiarity with survivor literature is required in the event that they are called to assist such a person or family.

Elie Wiesel[39], in an address to physicians and nurses, summarized what we might do to help. I paraphrase his words: "Listen to them. Listen to them carefully. Become the repository of their stories. The survivors need to be heard and in the process you will discover, they have more to teach you, than you them."

REFERENCES

1. Friedman, Paul (1949). Some aspects of concentration camp psychology. *American Journal of Psychiatry*, 105, 601-605.

2. Niederland, William G. (1968). The problem of the survivor: The psychiatric evaluation of emotional disorders in survivors of the Nazi persecution. In: Krystal, Henry (Ed.), *Massive Psychic Trauma*. New York: International Universities Press, pp. 8-22.

3. Eitinger, Leo (1961): Pathology of the concentration camp syndrome. *Archives of General Psychiatry*, 5, 371-379.

4. Strøm, Axel (1968). *Norwegian Concentration Camp Survivors*. Oslo: Universitetsforlaget, and New York: Humanities Press.

5. Niederland, William G. (1968). The psychiatric evaluation of emotional disorders in survivors of Nazi persecution. In: Krystal, Henry (Ed.), *Massive Psychic Trauma*. New York: International Universities Press, pp. 8-22.

6. Meerloo, Joost A. (1963). Neurologism and denial of psychic trauma in extermination camp survivors. *American Journal of Psychiatry*, 120, 65-66.

7. Eissler, Kurt R. (1967). Perverted psychiatry? *American Journal of Psychiatry*, 123, 1352-1358.

8. Chodoff, Paul (1963). Late effects of the concentration camp syndrome. *Archives of General Psychiatry*, 8, 323-333.

9. Eitinger, Leo (1966). Concentration camp survivors in Norway and Israel. In: David, Henry P. (Ed.), *Migration, Mental Health and Community Services: Proceedings of a Conference Convened by the American Joint Distribution Committee, Co-sponsored by the World Federation for Mental Health, and Held in Geneva, Switzerland, November 28-30, 1966*. Geneva: American Joint Distribution Committee, pp. 14-22.

10. Grauer, H. (1969). Psychodynamics of the survivor syndrome. *Canadian Psychiatric Association Journal*, 14(6), 617-622.

11. Hoppe, Klaus (1966). The psychodynamics of concentration camp victims. *Psychoanalytic Forum* 1(1), 76-85.

12. Chodoff, Paul (1975). Psychiatric aspects of the Nazi persecution. In: Arieti, Silvano (Ed.), *American Handbook of Psychiatry*. New York: Basic, pp. 932-946.

13. Krystal, Henry, and Niederland, William G. (1968). Clinical observations on the survivor syndrome. In: Krystal, Henry (Ed.), *Massive Psychic Trauma*. New York: International Universities Press, pp. 327-348.

14. Krell, Robert (1984). Holocaust survivors and their children: Comments on psychiatric consequences and psychiatric terminology. *Comprehensive Psychiatry*, 25(5), 521-528.

15. Freud, Anna (1979). *The Ego and the Mechanisms of Defence*. London: Hogarth Press.

16. Sachs, Lisbeth J., and Titievsky, Jaime (1967). On identification with the aggressor: A clinical note. *Israel Annals of Psychiatry and Related Disciplines*, 5, 181-184.

17. Tuteur, Werner (1966). One hundred concentration camp survivors: Twenty years later. *Israel Annals of Psychiatry and Related Disciplines*, 4(1), 78-90.

18. Leon, Gloria Rakita; Butcher, James; Kleinman, Max; Goldberg, Alan; and Almagor, Moshe (1981). Survivors of the Holocaust and their children: Current status and adjustment. *Journal of Personality and Social Psychology*, 41(3), 503-516.

19. Berger, David M. (1977). The survivor syndrome: A problem of nosology and treatment. *American Journal of Psychotherapy*, 31(2), 238-251.

20. Kestenberg, Judith S. (1972). Psychoanalytic contributions to the problem of children of survivors from Nazi persecution. *Israel Annals of Psychiatry and Related Disciplines*, 10, 311-325.

21. Hochman, John (1978). On the analysis of a child of Holocaust survivors with some notes on countertransference problems. *Bulletin of the Southern California Psychoanalytical Institute and Society*, 33.

22. Rabkin, Leslie (1975). Countertransference in the extreme situation: The family therapy of survivor families. In: Wolberg, Lewis R., and Aronson, Marvin L. (Eds.), *Group Therapy: An Overview*. New York: Stratton Intercontinental.

23. Danieli, Yael (1982). Countertransference in the treatment and study of Nazi Holocaust survivors and their children. *Victimology*, 5(2-4), 355-367.

24. Lifton, Robert Jay (1968). The survivors of the Hiroshima disaster and the survivors of Nazi persecution. In: Krystal, Henry (Ed.), *Massive Psychic Trauma*. New York: International Universities Press, pp. 168-203.

25. Krell, Robert (1979). Holocaust families: The survivors and their children. *Comprehensive Psychiatry*, 20, 560-568.

26. Rakoff, Vivian; Sigal, John J.; and Epstein, Nathan (1966). Children and families of concentration camp survivors. *Canadian Mental Health*, 14, 24-26.

27. Russell, Axel (1982). Family/marital therapy with second generation Holocaust survivor families, questions and answers. In: Gurman, E. (Ed.), *The Practice of Family Therapy. Vol. 2*. New York: Brunner/Mazel, pp. 233-237.

28a. Davidson, Shamai (1980). The clinical effects of massive psychic trauma in families of Holocaust survivors. *Journal of Marital and Family Therapy*, 6(1) 11-21.

28b. Davidson, Shamai (1992). *Holding on to Humanity - The Message of the Holocaust Survivors: The Shamai Davidson Papers*. (Ed.: Charny, Israel W.) New York: New York University Press.

29. Krell, Robert (1982). Family therapy with children of concentration camp camp survivors. *American Journal of Psychotherapy*, 36, 513-522.

30. Krell, Robert (1989). Alternative therapeutic approaches to Holocaust survivors. In: Marcus, Paul, and Rosenberg, Alan (Eds.), *Healing Their Wounds: Psychotherapy with Holocaust Survivors and Their Families*. New York: Praeger, p. 215.

31. Krystal, Henry (1968). Patterns of psychological damage. In: Krystal, Henry (Ed.), *Massive Psychic Trauma*. New York: International Universities Press, pp. 1-7.

32. Hoppe, Klaus (1968). Psychotherapy with survivors of Nazi persecution. In: Krystal, Henry (Ed.), *Massive Psychic Trauma*. New York: International Universities Press, pp. 204-219.

33. Solkoff, Norman (1981). Children of survivors of the Nazi Holocaust: A critical review of literature. *American Journal of Orthopsychiatry*, 51, 29-43.

34. Solkoff, Norman (1992). Children of survivors of the Nazi Holocaust: A critical review of literature. *American Journal of Orthopsychiatry*, 62(3), 342-358.

35. Russel, Axel; Plotkin, Donna; and Heapy, Nelson (1985). Adaptive abilities in nonclinical second-generation Holocaust survivors and controls: A comparison. *American Journal of Psychotherapy*, 29(4), 564-579.

36. Axelrod, Sylvia; Schnipper, Ofelia L.; and Rau, John H. (1980). Hospitalized offspring of Holocaust survivors: Problems and dynamics. *Bulletin of the Menninger Clinic*, 44(1), 1-14.

37. Rose, Susan, and Garske, John (1987). Family environment, adjustment and aging among children of Holocaust survivors. *American Journal of Orthopsychiatry*, 57(3), 332-344.

38. Kenigsberg, Rositta E., and Lieblich, Cathy M. (Eds.) (1992). *The First National Conference on Identification, Treatment and Care of the Aging Holocaust Survivor, March 29-31, 1992: Selected Proceedings*. Miami, FL: Holocaust Documentation and Education Center and Southeast Florida Center on Aging, Florida International University.

39. Wiesel, Elie (1982). *The Holocaust patient*. A Lecture at Cedars-Sinai Hospital preserved on audiovisual tape. Cedars-Sinai Hospital, Los Angeles, California.

Bibliography of Medical

and

Psychological

Effects of Concentration Camps

on

Holocaust Survivors

Bibliography of Medical and Psychological Effects of Concentration Camps on Holocaust Survivors

1 Aarts, Petra (1988). *Literatuur studie naar intergenerationele transmissie van vervolvings trauma by joodse oorlogsslachtoffers: Een geschiedenis van vandaag* [Literature study of intergenerational transmission of persecution trauma in Jewish war victims: A history of today]. Unpublished doctoral dissertation, Free University, Amsterdam.

2 Aarts, Petra (1994). Oorlog als erfenis: De overdracht van oorlogstrauma's op naoorlogse generaties [The legacy of war: Intergenerational transmission of trauma]. *Amsterdams Sociologisch Tijdschrift*, 21(1), 176-196.

3 Abalan, F.; Martinez-Gallardo, R.; and Bourgeois, M. (1989). Secuelas neuropsiquiatricas e la deportation en los campos de concentracion nazis durant la segunda guerra mundial [Neuropsychic sequelae of deportation to Nazi concentration camps during the second world war]. *Actas Luso-Espanolas de Neurologia, Psiquiatria y Ciencias Afines*, 17(1), 36-43.

4 Abel, Theodore (1951). The sociology of concentration camps. *Social Forces*, 30(2), 150-155.

5 Aberbach, David (1989). Creativity and the survivor: The struggle for mastery. *International Journal of Psycho-Analysis*, 16(3), 273-286.

6 Abramovitch, Henry (1986). There are no words: Two Greek Jewish survivors of Auschwitz. *Psychoanalytic Psychology*, 3(3), 201-216.

7 Abramowitz, Moshe Z.; Lichtenberg, Pesach; Marcus, Esther-Lee; and Shapira, Baruch (1994). Treating a Holocaust survivor without addressing the Holocaust: A case report. In: Brink, Terry L. (Ed.), *Holocaust Survivors' Mental Health.* New York: Haworth, pp. 75-80. [Published as a special issue of *Clinical Gerontologist*, 14(3).]

8 Adamczyk, Anatol (1980). Ostatnie dni w szpitalu obozu w Litomierzycach [The last days in the hospital of the Leitmeritz camp]. *Przegląd Lekarski*, 37(1), 184-186.

9 Adams, Kathryn Betts; Mann, Ellen Steinberg; Prigal, Rebecca Weintraub; Fein, Adel; Souders, Trisha L.; and Gerber, Barbara Sookman (1994). Holocaust survivors in a Jewish nursing home: Building trust and enhancing personal control. In: Brink, Terry L. (Ed.), *Holocaust Survivors' Mental Health.* New York: Haworth, pp. 99-117. [Published as a special issue of *Clinical Gerontologist*, 14(3).]

10 Adelman, Anne (1995). Traumatic memory and intergenerational transmission of Holocaust narratives. In: Solnit, Albert J.; Neubauer, Peter B.; Abrams, Samuel; and Dowling, A. Scott (Eds.), *Psychoanalytic Study of the Child. Vol. 50.* New Haven, CT: Yale University Press, pp. 343-367.

11 Adelsberger, Lucie (1956). *Auschwitz, ein Tatsachenbericht* [Auschwitz, A Factual Account]. Berlin: Lettner. 176 p.

12 Adelsberger, Lucie (1974). Psychologische Beobachtungen im Konzentrationslager Auschwitz [Psychological observations in the Auschwitz concentration camp]. *Schweitzerische Zeitschrift für Psychologie*, 6, 124-131.

13 Adelson, Daniel (1962). Some aspects of value conflict under extreme conditions. *Psychiatry*, 25(3), 273-279.

14 Adler, H.G.; Langbein, Herman; and Lingens, Ella (Eds.) (1962). *Auschwitz: Zeugnisse, und Berichte* [Auschwitz: Testimonies and Reports]. Frankfurt: Europäische Verlagsanstalt. 423 pp.

15 Ahlheim, Rose (1985). Bis ins dritte und vierte Glied: Das Verfolgungstrauma in der Enkelgeneration [Into the third and fourth generations: The trauma of persecution in the generation of grandchildren]. *Zeitschrift für Psychologie mit Zeitschrift für Angewandte Psychologie*, 39(4), 330-354.

16 Albeck, Joseph (1994). Intergenerational consequences of trauma: Reframing traps in treatment theory - a second generation perspective.

In: Williams, Mary Beth, and Sommer, John F., Jr. (Eds.), *Handbook of Post-Traumatic Therapy*. Westport, CT and London: Greenwood, pp. 106-125.

17 Aleksandrowicz, Dov (1973). Children of concentration camp survivors. In: Anthony, E. James, and Koupernik, Cyrille (Eds.), *The Child in His Family. Vol. 2: The Impact of Disease and Death*. New York: John Wiley & Sons, pp. 385-392.

18 Alexander, Leo (1948). Sociopsychologic structure of the S.S.: Psychiatric report of the Nuremberg trials for war crimes. *Archives of Neurology*, 59, 622-634.

19 Alexander, Leo (1948). War crimes: Their social-psychological aspects. *American Journal of Psychiatry*, 105, 170-177.

20 Alexander, Leo (1949). Medical science under dictatorship. *New England Journal of Medicine*, 241(2), 39-47.

21 Allodi, Federico A. (1991). Assessment and treatment of torture victims: A critical review. *Journal of Nervous and Mental Disease*, 179(1), 4-11.

22 Allodi, Federico A. (1994). Post-traumatic stress disorder in hostages and victims of torture. *Psychiatric Clinics of North America*, 17(2), 279-288.

23 Almagor, Moshe, and Leon, Gloria Rakita (1989). Transgenerational effects of the concentration camp experience. In: Marcus, Paul, and Rosenberg, Alan (Eds.), *Healing Their Wounds: Psychotherapy with Holocaust Survivors and Their Families*. New York: Praeger, pp. 183-195.

24 Althoff, Becky (1948). Observations on the psychology of children in a DP camp. *Journal of Social Casework*, 29, 17-22.

25 Amati-Sas, Silvia (1989). Avatars de l'angoisse de separation dans des conditions extrêmes [Avatars of separation anxiety under extreme conditions]. *Révue Française de Psychanalyse*, 53(1), 69-73.

26 Amati-Sas, Silvia (1990). Die Ruckgewinnung des Schamgefuhls [The reclamation of shame feelings]. *Psyche: Zeitschrift für Psychoanalyse und ihre Anwendungen*, 44(8), 724-740.

27 Ambash, Lois C. (1995). *Holocaust shards, Holocaust shreds: American meanings of the Holocaust*. Unpublished doctoral dissertation,

The Union Institute, Cincinnati, Ohio, 301 pp. *Dissertation Abstracts International*, 56(6-A), p. 2297. (University Microfilms no. AAC 9528742).

28 Amelunxen, U. (1971). Herabsetzung der Altersgrenzen in der Sozialversicherung für Verfolgte des National Sozialismus [Lowering the age limit in social insurance for people persecuted by the National Socialists]. In: Herberg, Hans-Joachim (Ed.), *Spätschäden nach Extrembelastungen* [Late Damage After Extreme Stress]. Herford: Nicolai, pp. 99-103. [II Internationalen Medizinisch-Juristischen Konferenz. Dusseldorf, 1969].

29 Améry, Jean (1986). *At the Mind's Limits: Contemplations by a Survivor on Auschwitz and its Realities*. New York: Shocken. 111 pp.

30 Amit, Yoram (1995). AMCHA's documentation services. In: Lemberger, John (Ed.), *A Global Perspective on Working with Holocaust Survivors and the Second Generation*. Jerusalem: JDC-Brookdale Institute of Gerontology and Human Development, AMCHA, and JDC-Israel, pp. 111-120.

31 Ammon, Gunter (1984). The dynamics of Holocaust. *Dynamische Psychiatrie*, 17(5-6), 404-415.

32 Anderson, Vicky L. (1993). Gender differences in altruism among Holocaust rescuers. *Journal of Social Behavior and Personality*, 8(1), 43-58.

33 Angell, Marc (1990). The Nazi hypothermia experiments and unethical research today. *New England Journal of Medicine*, 322(20), 1462-1464.

34 Annas, George J. (1994). The changing landscape of human experimentation: Nuremberg, Helsinki, and beyond. In: Michalczyk, John J. (Ed.), *Medicine, Ethics, and the Third Reich: Historical and Contemporary Issues*. Kansas City, MO: Sheed & Ward, pp. 106-128.

35 Annas, George J., and Grodin, Michael A. (Eds.) (1992). *The Nazi Doctors and the Nuremberg Code: Human Rights in Human Experimentation*. New York: Oxford University Press. 371 pp.

36 Ansell, Charles (1986). "Ilsa." *Psychotherapy Patient*, 2(4), 45-52.

37 Anthony, E. James (1973). Symposium: Children of the Holocaust. Editorial comment. In: Anthony, E. James, and Koepernik, Cyrille

(Eds.), *The Child in His Family. Vol. 2: The Impact of Disease and Death*. New York: John Wiley & Sons, pp. 352-356.

38 Antman, Steven R. (1983). *Offspring of Holocaust survivors and the process of self-actualization and related variables*. Unpublished doctoral dissertation, California School of Professional Psychology, Fresno, 144 pp. *Dissertation Abstracts International*, 46(8-B), p. 2794. (University Microfilms no. AAC 8523266).

39 Antonovsky, Aron; Maoz, Benjamin; Dowty, N.; and Wijsenbeek, H. (1971). Twenty five years later: A limited study of sequelae of the concentration camp experience. *Social Psychiatry*, 6(4), 186-193.

40 Apfelbaum, Emil (Ed.) (1946). *Maladie de Famine: Rècherches Cliniques sur la Famine Executées dans la Ghetto de Varsovie en 1942* [Hunger Disease: Clinical Research on Famine Performed in the Warsaw Ghetto in 1942]. Warsaw: American Joint Distribution Committee. 264 pp.

41 Apfelbaum, Emil (1979). Pathophysiology of the circulatory system in hunger disease. In: Winick, Myron (Ed.), *Hunger Disease: Studies by the Jewish Physicians in the Warsaw Ghetto*. New York: John Wiley & Sons, pp. 125-160.

42 Apostoł-Staniszewska, Jadwiga (1977). Refleksje z obozu kobiecego w Brzezince [Reminiscences from the Brzezinka concentration camp for women]. *Przegląd Lekarski*, 34(1), 200-207.

43 Apostoł-Staniszewska, Jadwiga (1981). Wobec śmierci w Brzezince i w Ravensbrück [Facing death at the Birkenau and Ravensbruck concentration camps]. *Przegląd Lekarski*, 38(1), 163-168.

44 Apostoł-Staniszewska, Jadwiga (1987). Reflexionen aus dem Frauenlager in Birkenau [Reflections from the concentration camp for women in Birkenau]. In: Hamburger Institut für Sozialforschung (Eds.), *Die Auschwitz-Hefte. Texte der polnischen Zeitschrift "Przegląd Lekarski" über historische, psychische und medizinische Aspekte des Lebens und Sterbens in Auschwitz. Band 1* [The Auschwitz Journal. Text of the Polish Journal "Medical Review" on Historical, Psychic and Medical Aspects of Life and Death in Auschwitz. Volume 1]. Weinheim and Basel: Beltz, pp. 219-225.

45 Appelberg, Esther (1972). Holocaust survivors and their children. In: Linzer, Norman (Ed.), *The Jewish Family: Authority and Tradition in Modern Perspective*. New York: Commission on Synagogue Relations, Federation of Jewish Philanthropies, pp. 109-122.

46 Appy, Johann-Gottfried (1993). The meaning of "Auschwitz" today: Clinical reflections about the depletion of a destructive symbol. In: Moses, Rafael (Ed.), *Persistent Shadows of the Holocaust: The Meaning to Those Not Directly Affected*. Madison, CT: International Universities Press, pp. 3-28.

47 Arieti, Silvano (1981). The prerequisites of Nazi barbarism. *Israel Journal of Psychiatry and Related Sciences*, 18(4), 283-297.

48 Arns, W., and Wahle, H. (1965). Über die Dauerschäden des Nervensystems nach einer Fleckfieberenzephalitis [On permanent damages of the nervous system after a typhus-encephalitis]. *Fortschritte der Neurologie, Psychiatrie*, 33, 113-144.

49 Aronzon, Rami (1994). Psychotherapy of a child survivor of Theresienstadt. *Echoes of the Holocaust*, 3, 52-60. [Bulletin of the Jerusalem Center for Research into the Late Effects of the Holocaust, Talbieh Mental Health Center, Jerusalem, Israel].

50 Arthur, Ranson J. (1982). Psychiatric syndromes in prisoners of war and concentration camp survivors. In: Friedman, Claude T.H., and Faguet, Robert A. (Eds.), *Extraordinary Disorders of Human Behavior*. New York: Plenum.

51 Askevold, Finn (1983). Gibt es ein generelles Kriegsschadensyndrom? [Does a general war damage syndrome exist?]. *Cahiers d'Information Médicales, Sociales et Juridiques*, 19, 155-157.

52 Aslanov, A. (1964). Die Rolle der Störungen der Tätigkeit des Höheren Nervensystems in der Pathogenese der neuropsychischen Folgen der Deportation in den Nazikonzentrationslagern (Störungen festgestellt bei Deportierten und Kriegsgefangenen) [The role of disturbances of higher nervous system functions in the pathogenesis of neuro-psychic sequelae of deportation in the Nazi concentration camps (disturbances determined in deported persons and prisoners of war)]. In: *Ätio-Pathogenese und Therapie der Erschöpfung und vorzeitigen Vergreisung* [The Aetiology and Therapy due to Exhaustion and Premature Aging]. Wien: Verlag der FIR, pp. 584-591. [IV Internationaler Medizinischer Kongress. Bucharest, 22-27 Juni 1964].

53 Assael, Marcel, and Givon, Marianne (1982). Hezdaknut nitzoley hashoah b'aretz [Aging of Holocaust survivors in Israel]. *Gerontologia*, 21(2), 55-64.

54 Assael, Marcel, and Givon, Marianne (1984). The aging process in Holocaust survivors in Israel. *American Journal of Social Psychiatry*, 4(1), 32-36.

55 Auerhahn, Nanette C., and Laub, Dori (1984). Annihilation and restoration: Post-traumatic memory as pathway and obstacle to recovery. *International Review of Psychoanalysis*, 11(3), 327-344.

56 Auerhahn, Nanette C., and Laub, Dori (1987). Play and playfulness in Holocaust survivors. In: Neubauer, Peter B., and Solnit, Albert J. (Eds.), *Psychoanalytic Study of the Child. Vol. 42*. New Haven, CT: Yale University Press, pp. 45-58.

57 Auerhahn, Nanette C.; Laub, Dori; and Peskin, Harvey (1993). Psychotherapy with Holocaust survivors. *Psychotherapy*, 30(3), 434-442.

58 Auerhahn, Nanette C., and Prelinger, Ernst (1983). Repetition in the concentration camp survivor and her child. *International Review of Psychoanalysis*, 10(1), 31-46.

59 Aviram, Alexander; Silverberg, Donald S.; and Carel, Rafael S. (1987). Hypertension in European immigrants to Israel: A possible effect of the Holocaust. *Israel Journal of Medical Sciences*, 23(4), 257-263.

60 Axelrod, Sylvia; Schnipper, Ofelia L.; and Rau, John H. (1980). Hospitalized offspring of Holocaust survivors: Problems and dynamics. *Bulletin of the Menninger Clinic*, 44(1), 1-14.

61 Ayalon, Ofra; Eitinger, Leo; Lansen, Johan; Sunier, Armand; and others. (1983). *The Holocaust and its Perseverance: Stress, Coping and Disorder*. Assen, The Netherlands: Van Gorcum. 64 pp. [Proceedings of a symposium held May 13, 1982, in honor of the 70th birthday of Dr. Armand Sunier, leader of the post-World War II reconsruction of the Jewish mental health services in the Netherlands].

62 Aziz, Philippe (1976). *Doctors of Death*. 4 vols. Geneva: Ferni Publishers. [*Vol. 1: Karl Brandt, The Third Reich's Man in White; Vol. 2: Joseph Mengele, The Evil Doctor; Vol. 3: When Man Became a Guinea Pig for Death; Vol. 4: In the Beginning was the Master Race*].

63 Baader, Gerhard (1992). Psychiatrie und Vernichtungsstrategien in der NS-Ideologie [Psychiatry and extermination strategies in Nazi ideology]. In: Jockush, Ulrich, and Scholz, Lothar (Eds.), *Verwaltetes Morden im Nationalsozialismus: Verstrickung, Verdrängung, Verantwortung von Psychiatrie und Justiz* [Administered Killings at the Time of National Socialism: Involvement, Suppression, Responsibility of Psychiatry and Judicial System]. Regensburg: Roderer, pp. 18-25.

64 Baader, Gerhard (1992). Psychiatry and extermination strategies in Nazi ideology. In: Jockush, Ulrich, and Scholz, Lothar (Eds.), *Administered Killings at the Time of National Socialism: Involvement, Suppression, Responsibility of Psychiatry and Judicial System*. Regensburg: Roderer, pp. 18-25.

65 Bachar, Eytan; Cale, Michael; Eisenberg, Jacques; and Dasberg, Haim (1994). Aggression expression in grandchildren of Holocaust survivors: A comparative study. *Israel Journal of Psychiatry and Related Sciences*, 31(1), 41-47.

66 Bachar, Eytan; Dasberg, Haim; and Ben-Shakhar, Gershon (1995). Demandingness and belligerence in hospitalized depressed Holocaust concentration camp survivors as perceived by the staff. *Israel Journal of Psychiatry and Related Sciences*, 32(4), 262-267.

67 Baeyer, Walter R. von (1961). Erlebnisbedingte Verfolgungsschäden [Damaged caused by experienced persecution]. *Nervenarzt*, 32(12), 534-538.

68 Baeyer, Walter R. von (1971). Über die Auswirkungen der Verfolgung und Konzentrationslagerhaft vom Standpunkt des Psychiaters [On the effect of persecution and concentration camp internment from the point of view of the psychiatrist]. In: Herberg, Hans-Joachim (Ed.), *Spätschäden nach Extrembelastungen* [Late Damage After Extreme Stress]. Herford: Nicolai, pp. 176-181. [II Internationalen Medizinisch-Juristischen Konferenz. Dusseldorf, 1969].

69 Baeyer, Walter R. von (1977). Pathogenetische Bedeutung psychosozialer Extrembelastung für die Entstehung endogener Psychosen [On the pathogenetic significance of extreme psychosocial stress in the development of endogenous psychoses]. *Nervenarzt*, 48(9), 471-477.

70 Baeyer, Walter R. von, and Binder, Werner (1982). *Endomorphe Psychosen bei Verfolgten. Statistische-klinische Studien an Entschädigungsgutachten* [Endomorphic Psychoses in Persecuted Persons: Statistical-Clinical Studies of Compensation Judgments]. New York: Springer. 185 pp.

71 Baeyer, Walter R. von; Häfner, Heinz; and Kisker, Karl-Peter (1963). Zur Frage des "symptomfreien Intervalles" bei erlebnisreaktiven Störungen Verfolgter (Erfahrungen aus zwei Begutachtungen) [On the problem of the "symptomless interval" of disturbances caused by persecution (experiences from two examinations)]. In: Paul, Helmut, and Herberg, Hans-Joachim (Eds.), *Psychische Spätschäden nach politischer Verfolgung* [Psychological Late Damages Following Political Persecution]. Basel: Karger, pp. 125-153.

72 Baeyer, Walter R. von; Häfner, Heinz; and Kisker, Karl-Peter (1963). "Wissenschaftliche Erkenntnis" oder "Menschliche Wertung" der erlebnisreaktiven Schäden Verfolgter ["Scientific insight" or "human evaluation" of damage caused by experienced persecution]. *Nervenarzt*, 34(3), 120-123.

73 Baeyer, Walter R. von; Häfner, Heinz; and Kisker, Karl-Peter (1964). *Psychiatrie der Verfolgten: Psychopathologische und gutachtliche Erfahrungen an Opfern der nationalsozialistischen Verfolgung und vergleichbarer Extrem belastungen* [Psychiatry of the Persecuted: Psychopathological and Evaluative Experiences with Victims of Nazi Persecution and Comparable Stress Conditions]. Berlin: Springer. 397 pp.

74 Baeyer, Walter R. von, and Kisker, Karl-Peter (1960). Abbiegung der Persönlichkeitsentwicklung eines Jugendlichen durch nationalsocialistische Verfolgungen. Paranoide Fehlhaltung [Deviations in the development of the personality of a juvenile caused by National Socialistic persecution. Paranoid maladjustment]. In: March, Hans (Ed.), *Verfolgung und Angst in ihren leib-seelischen Auswirkungen. Dokumente* [Persecution and Anxiety in Their Psychosomatic Forms of Expression. Documentation]. Stuttgart: Klett, pp. 11-27.

75 Baider, Lea; Peretz, Tamar; and Kaplan De-Nour, Atara (1992). Effect of the Holocaust on coping with cancer. *Social Science and Medicine*, 34(1), 11-15.

76 Baider, Lea; Peretz, Tamar; and Kaplan De-Nour, Atara (1993). Holocaust cancer patients: A comparative study. *Psychiatry*, 56(4), 349-355.

77 Baider, Lea, and Sarell, Moshe (1984). Coping with cancer among Holocaust survivors in Israel: An exploratory study. *Journal of Human Stress*, 10(3), 121-127.

78 Balaz, V., and Balazova, E. (1978). Die klinisch physiologischen Mechanismen der gegenwärtigen aktiven Folgen des Krieges für die Gesundheit der Widerstandskämpfer und die damit verbundenen therapeutischen Probleme [The effect of clinical physiological mechanisms of contemporary active war sequelae on the health of resistance fighters and the therapeutic problems connected with them]. In: *Medizinische Untersuchungen der Spätfolgen des Krieges und des NS-Regimes bei Jugendlichen und Kindern von ehemaligen KZ-*

Häftlingen und Verfolgten [Medical Research of the Late Effects of the War and National Socialism Regime on Youth and Children of Former Concentration Camp Inmates and Persecuted Persons]. Wien: Internationale Föderation der Widerstandskämpfer. [VI Internationaler Medizinischer Kongress der FIR. Prague, 1976].

79 Balazs, M. (1994). Hypothermia Kiserletek a dachaui Koncentracioş taborban [Hypothermia experiments in the Dachau concentration camp]. *Orvosi Hetilap*, 135(40), 2208-2209.

80 Banach, Grażyna, and Dominik, Małgorzata (1985). Psychiatryczne następstwa obozów hitlerowskich w drugim pokoleniu byłych więźniów [Psychiatric sequelae of Hitler's concentration camps in the progeny of former prisoners]. *Przegląd Lekarski*, 42(1), 29-34.

81 Barab, G. (1956). Tguvot meuharot etsel meshuhrarei mahanot rikuz [Belated reactions in former concentration camp inmates]. *Harefuah*, 50, 228-229.

82 Bardige, Betty Lynn S. (1983). *Reflective thinking and prosocial awareness: Adolescents face the Holocaust and themselves*. Unpublished doctoral dissertation, Harvard University, Cambridge, Massachusetts, 219 pp. *Dissertation Abstracts International*, 44(5-B), p. 1614. (University microfilms no. 8320158).

83 Barnhoorn, J.A.J. (1954). *Verhongering als mogelijke oorzaak van nerveuse, psychische en psychosomatische stoornissen: Wet buitengewoon pensioen 1940-1945, voor deelnemers aan het verzet, alsmede voor hun nagelaten betrekkingen* [Starvation as a Possible Cause of Nervous, Psychic and Psychosomatic Disturbances: The Special Pension 1940-1945 for Participants in the Resistance and Their Dependants]. The Hague: Buitengewone Pensioenraad. 28 pp.

84 Barocas, Harvey A. (1971). A note on the children of concentration camp survivors. *Psychotherapy Patient*, 8, 189-190.

85 Barocas, Harvey A. (1975). Children of purgatory: Reflections on the concentration camp survival syndrome. *International Journal of Social Psychiatry*, 21(2), 87-92.

86 Barocas, Harvey A. (1984). Discussion of "Children of the Holocaust and their children's children: Working through current trauma in the psychotherapeutic process," by Terez Virag. *Dynamic Psychotherapy*, 2(1), 61-63.

87 Barocas, Harvey A., and Barocas, Carol B. (1973). Manifestations of concentration camp effects on the second generation. *American Journal of Psychiatry*, 130(7), 820-821.

88 Barocas, Harvey A., and Barocas, Carol B. (1979). Wounds of the fathers: The next generation of Holocaust victims. *International Journal of Psycho-Analysis*, 6(3), 331-340.

89 Barocas, Harvey A., and Barocas, Carol B. (1980). Separation-individuation conflicts in children of Holocaust survivors. In: Quaytman, Wilfred (Ed.), *Holocaust Survivors: Psychological and Social Sequelae*. New York: Human Sciences Press, pp. 6-14. [Published as a special issue of *Journal of Contemporary Psychotherapy*, 11(1)].

90 Bar-On, Dan (1990). Children of perpetrators of the Holocaust: Working through one's own moral self. *Psychiatry*, 53(3), 229-245.

91 Bar-On, Dan (1992). "Am I different from my Father?" An interview with two daughters of perpetrators of the Third Reich. In: Jockush, Ulrich, and Scholz, Lothar (Eds.), *Administered Killings at the Time of National Socialism: Involvement, Suppression, Responsibility of Psychiatry and Judicial System*. Regensburg: Roderer, pp. 82-101.

92 Bar-On, Dan (1992). "Bin ich anders als mein Vater?" - Ein Interview mit zwei Töchtern von Tätern im Dritten Reich ["Am I different from my Father?" An interview with two daughters of perpetrators of the Third Reich]. In: Jockush, Ulrich, and Scholz, Lothar (Eds.), *Verwaltetes Morden im Nationalsozialismus: Verstrickung, Verdrängung, Verantwortung von Psychiatrie und Justiz* [Administered Killings at the Time of National Socialism: Involvement, Suppression, Responsibility of Psychiatry and Judicial System]. Regensburg: Roderer, pp. 86-110.

93 Bar-On, Dan (1993). First encounter between childen of survivors and children of perpetrators. *Journal of Humanistic Psychology*, 33(4), 6-14.

94 Bar-On, Dan (1995). *Fear and Hope: Three Generations of the Holocaust*. Cambridge, MA: Harvard University Press. 372 pp.

95 Bar-On, Dan (1995). Four encounters between descendents of survivors and descendents of perpetrators of the Holocaust: Building social bonds out of silence. *Psychiatry*, 58(3), 225-245.

96 Bar-On, Dan, and Gaon, Amalia (1991). "We suffered too": Nazi children's inability to relate to the suffering of victims of the Holocaust. *Journal of Humanistic Psychology*, 31(4), 77-95.

97 Baron, Lawrence (1977). Surviving the Holocaust. *Journal of Psychology and Judaism*, 1(2), 25-37.

98 Baron, Lisa (1992). *Interpersonal adjustment, narcissism, and coping in children of Holocaust survivors*. Unpublished doctoral dissertation, Fordham University, Bronx, New York, 226 pp. *Dissertation Abstracts International*, 53(1-B), p. 556. (University Microfilms no. AAC 9215346).

99 Baron, Lisa; Reznikoff, Marvin; and Glenwick, David S. (1993). Narcissism, interpersonal adjustment, and coping in children of Holocaust survivors. *Journal of Psychology*, 127(3), 257-269.

100 Barral, P.; Carpentier, G.; and Dubor, P. (1961). Behandlung des Konzentrationslagersyndroms und der allgemeinen Mangelzustände durch die Fraktion "B" des serums [Treatment of the concentration camp syndrome and general states of deficiency with fraction "B" of the serum]. In: *Die Behandlung der Asthenie und der vorzeitigen Vergreisung bei ehemaligen Widerstandskämpfern und KZ-Häftlingen* [Treatment of Asthenics and Premature Aging in Former Resistance Fighters and Concentration Camp Inmates]. Wien: Verlag der FIR, pp. 165-185. [III Internationale Medizinische Konferenz. Liege, 17-19 März 1961].

101 Barral, P.; Carpentier, G.; and Dubor, P. (1961). Traitement du syndrôme post-concentrationnaire et des états de déficience générale par la fraction "B" du sérum [Treatment of the concentration camp syndrome and general states of deficiency with fraction "B" of the serum]. In: *La thérapeutique de l'asthénie et de la senescence prématurée chez les anciens déportés et résistants* [Treatment of Asthenics and Premature Aging in Former Resistance Fighters and Concentration Camp Inmates]. Wien: Editions de la Fédération Internationale des Résistants, pp. 173-194. [IIIème Conference Médicale Internationale. Liège, 17 - 19 Mars 1961]

102 Bartelski, Lesław M. (1985). Dzieci i wojna [Children and war]. *Przegląd Lekarski*, 42(1), 113-120.

103 Bar-Tur, Liora, and Levy-Shiff, Rachel (1994). Holocaust review and bearing witness as a coping mechanism of an elderly Holocaust survivor. In: Brink, Terry L. (Ed.), *Holocaust Survivors' Mental*

Health. New York: Haworth, pp. 5-16. [Published as a special issue of *Clinical Gerontologist*, 14(3).]

104 Bass-Wichelhaus, Helene (1995). The interviewer as witness: Countertransference, reactions, and techniques. In: Kestenberg, Judith S., and Fogelman, Eva (Eds.), *Children during the Nazi Reign: Psychological Perspective on the Interview Process*. Westport, CT: Praeger, pp. 175-188.

105 Bastiaans, Jan (1957). *Psychomatische Gevolgen van Onderdrukking en Verzet* [Psychosomatic Sequelae of Persecution and Resistance]. Amsterdam: Noord-Hollandsche Uitgevers Maatschappij. 485 pp.

106 Bastiaans, Jan (1969). The role of aggression in the genesis of psychosomatic disease. *Journal of Psychosomatic Research*, 13, 307-314.

107 Bastiaans, Jan (1970). Over de specificiteit en de behandeling van het KZ-syndroom [On the specifics and treatment of the concentration camp syndrome]. *Nederlands Tijdschrift voor Geneeskunde*, 23, 364-371.

108 Bastiaans, Jan (1972). General comments on the role of aggression in human psychopathology. *Psychotherapy and Psychosomatics*, 20 (5), 300-311.

109 Bastiaans, Jan (1974). Het KZ syndroom en de menselijke vrijheid [The KZ syndrome and human freedom]. *Nederlands Tijdschrift voor Geneeskunde*, 118, 1173-1178.

110 Bastiaans, Jan (1974). The KZ syndrome: A thirty year study of the effects on victims of Nazi concentration camps. *Revista Medico-Chirurgicala a Societatii de Medicini Si Naturalisti Din Iasi*, 78(3), 573-578.

111 Bastiaans, Jan (1974). Verlating en rouw [Desertion and mourning]. *Intermediair*, 20.

112 Bastiaans, Jan (1978). The optimal use of anxiety in the struggle for adaptation. In: Spielberger, Charles D., and Sarason, Irwin G. (Eds.), *Stress and Anxiety. Vol. 5*. Washington, D.C.: Hemisphere, pp. 219-231.

113 Bastiaans, Jan (1979). De behandeling van oorlogsslachtoffers [The treatment of war victims]. *TGO Tijdschrift voor Therapie, Geneesmiddel en Onderzoek*, 1, 352-358.

114 Bastiaans, Jan (1979). Control of aggression and psychotherapy. In: *Israel-Netherlands Symposium on the Impact of Persecution. Jerusalem, 16-24 October 1977.* Rijswijk, The Netherlands: Ministry of Cultural Affairs, Recreation and Social Welfare, pp. 25-37.

115 Bastiaans, Jan (1980). Vom Menschen im KZ und vom KZ im Menschen, ein Beitrag zur Behandlung des KZ-syndroms und dessen Spätfolgen [On people in the concentration camp and the concentration camp in people, a lecture on the management of concentration camp syndromes and their consequences]. In: Henseler, H., and Kuchenbuch, A. (Eds.), *Die Wiederkehr von Krieg und Verfolgung in Psychoanalysen* [The Recurrence of War and Persecution in Psychoanalysis]. Berlin.

116 Bastiaans, Jan (1984). De behandeling van oorlogsslachtoffers [The treatment of war victims]. *Arts & Wereld*, 17(1), 9-17.

117 Battegay, Raymond (1994). Überlebende des Holocaust: Eine Ausenseitengruppe [Survivors of the Holocaust: A group apart]. *Becheft zur Zeitschrift Gruppenpsychotherapie und Gruppendynamik*, 30, 86-99.

118 Baum, Rainer (1989). Die Bürde der Wahrheit. Juden und Nichtjuden in Osterreich und der Bundesrepublik Deutschland nach dem Krieg [The burden of truth: Jews and non-Jews in Austria and in the Federal Republic of Germany after the war]. *Kolner Zeitschrift für Soziologie und Sozialpsychologie*, 41(1), 123-148.

119 Baumel, Esther (1981). *The Jewish Refugee Children in Great Britain, 1938-1939*. Ramat Gan, Israel: Bar-Ilan University Press. 294 pp.

120 Baumel, Judith Tydor (1990). The Jewish refugee children from Europe in the eyes of the American press and public opinion 1934-1945. *Holocaust and Genocide Studies*, 5(3), 293-312.

121 Baumel, Judith Tydor (1995). Social interaction among Jewish women in crisis during the Holocaust: A case study. *Gender and History*, 7(1), 64-84.

122 Baumgarten-Wessel, M.E. (1977). *Wet uitkeringen vervolgingsslachtoffers 1940-1945* [The compensation-law for persecuted people 1940-1945]. Faculty of Law Thesis, Skriptie Rijksuniversiteit Leiden, Faculteit der Rechtsgeleerdheid, Leiden.

123 Beardwell-Wieleżyńska, Myrtle (1967). Obóz koncentracyjny w Bergen-Belsen bezpośrednio po wyzwoleniu [The concentration camp in Bergen-Belsen immediately after the liberation]. *Przegląd Lekąrski*, 23(1), 105-112.

124 Becker, M. (1963). Extermination camp syndrome. *New England Journal of Medicine*, 268, 1145.

125 Becker, Ernest (1969). The pawnbroker: A study in basic psychology. In: *Angel in Armor: A Post-Freudian Perspective on the Nature of Man*. New York: Braziller, pp. 73-99.

126 Beery, Merav (1995). *Hakesher beyn aspectim shel revacha naphshit sub'yectivit etzel nitzoley shoah lebeyn hagil sh'bo hayoo b'tkufat hashoah* [The relationship between aspects of subjective wellbeing of Holocaust survivors and the survivors' ages at the time of the Holocaust]. Unpublished master's thesis, Department of Psychology, Tel Aviv University, Tel Aviv, Israel. 113 pp.

127 Beider, J. (1984). Sequelles tardives et retardées de la catastrophe concentrationnaire [Late and delayed effects of the concentration camp catastrophe]. *Annales Medico Psychologiques*, 142(2), 277-283.

128 Bekkering, P.G. (1981). Kinderen als oorlogsslachtoffers [Children as war victims]. *Nederlands Tijdschrift voor Geneeskunde*, 125(18), 713-714.

129 Belaisch, J. (1961). Die Hormontherapie beim Deportierten im Jahre 1961 [The hormonal therapy in a deportee in 1961]. In: *Die Behandlung der Asthenie und der vorzeitigen Vergreisung bei ehemaligen Widerstandskämpfern und KZ-Häftlingen* [Treatment of Asthenics and Premature Aging in Former Resistance Fighters and Concentration Camp Inmates]. Wien: Verlag der FIR, pp. 101-106. [III Internationale Medizinische Konferenz. Liege, 17-19 März 1961].

130 Bellert, Józef (1971). The Polish Red Cross camp hospital after the liberation of the camp in Auschwitz. In: *Auschwitz Anthology. Vol. 2: In Hell They Preserved Human Dignity. Part 2*. Warsaw: International Auschwitz Committee, pp. 123-143.

131 Ben-Baruch, M. (1981). Re-evaluation of the right of Holocaust survivors to exist through a social work approach. In: *Israel-Netherlands Symposium on the Impact of Persecution. Dalfsen, Amsterdam, 14-18 April 1980*. Rijswijk, The Netherlands: Ministry of Cultural Affairs, Recreation and Social Welfare, pp. 117-119.

132 Bendiner, E. (1981). Korczak: Pediatrician on the road to hell. *Hospital Practice*, 16(7), 125-139.

133 Ben Gershom, Ezra (1990). From Haeckel to Hackethal: Lessons from Nazi medicine for students and practitioners of medicine. *Holocaust and Genocide Studies*, 5(1), 73-87.

134 Benner, Patricia; Roskies, Ethel; and Lazarus, Richard (1980). Stress and coping under extreme conditions. In: Dimsdale, Joel E. (Ed.), *Survivors, Victims and Perpetrators: Essays on the Nazi Holocaust*. Washington, D.C.: Hemisphere, pp. 219-258.

135 Bensheim, H. (1960). Die KZ-Neurose rassich Verfolgter. Ein Beitrag zur Psychopathologie der Neurosen [The concentration camp neurosis of racially persecuted persons. A contribution to the psychopathology of neuroses]. *Nervenarzt*, 31, 462-471.

136 Ben-Sira, Zeev (1983). Loss, stress and readjustment: The structure of coping with bereavement and disability. *Social Science and Medicine*, 17(21), 1619-1632.

137 Ben-Sira, Zeev (1984). Chronic illness, stress and coping. *Social Science and Medicine*, 18(9), 725-736.

138 Berenstein, Isidoro (1987). Die endliche und die undliche Analyse: 50 Jahre danach [Analysis terminable and interminable: 50 years later]. *Jahrbuch der Psychoanalyse*, 20, 31-61.

139 Berezin, Martin A. (1981). Introduction: The aging survivor of the Holocaust. *Journal of Geriatric Psychiatry*, 14(2), 131-133.

140 Berger, David M. (1977). The survivor syndrome: A problem of nosology and treatment. *American Journal of Psychotherapy*, 31(2), 238-251.

141 Berger, David M. (1985). Recovery and repression in concentration camp survivors: Psychodynamic re-evaluation. *Canadian Journal of Psychiatry*, 30(1), 54-59.

142 Berger, Deborah E. (1980). *Children of Nazi Holocaust survivors: A coming of age*. Unpublished master's thesis, Goddard College, Plainville, Vermont. [Available from the Simon Wiesenthal Center Library, Los Angeles, California].

143 Berger, Joseph (1984). Late onset psychosis in concentration camp survivors. *Emotional First Aid: A Journal of Crisis Intervention*, 1(3), 11-13.

144 Berger, Leslie (1988). The long-term psychological consequences of the Holocaust on the survivors and their offspring. In: Braham, Randolph L. (Ed.), *The Psychological Perspectives of the Holocaust and of its Aftermath*. Boulder, CO: Social Sciences Monographs; and New York: Csengeri Institute for Holocaust Studies of the Graduate School and University Center of the City University of New York, pp. 175-221.

145 Berger, Robert L. (1990). Nazi science: The Dachau hypothermia experiments. *New England Journal of Medicine*, 322(20), 1435-1440.

146 Berger, Robert L. (1994). Ethics in scientific communication: Study of a problem case. *Journal of Medical Ethics*, 20(4), 207-211.

147 Berger, Robert L. (1994). Nazi science: The Dachau hypothermia experiments. In: Michalczyk, John J. (Ed.), *Medicine, Ethics, and the Third Reich: Historical and Contemporary Issues*. Kansas City, MO: Sheed & Ward, pp. 101-105.

148 Berger, Ronald J. (1994). Remembering the Holocaust: Some observations on collective memories and survivor oral/life histories. *Sociological Imagination*, 31(2), 117-124.

149 Berger, Ronald J. (1995). Agency, structure, and Jewish survival of the Holocaust: A life history study. *Sociological Quarterly*, 36(1), 15-36.

150 Berghoff, E. (1964). Zum Begriff der sogenannten Lagerschäden und deren Auswirkungen [On the concept of the so-called camp damages and its effects]. In: *Ätio-Pathogenese und Therapie der Erschöpfung und vorzeitigen Vergreisung* [The Aetiology and Therapy Due to Exhaustion and Premature Aging]. Wien: Verlag der FIR, pp. 119-120. [IV Internationaler Medizinischer Kongress. Bucharest, 22-27 Juni 1964].

151 Bergmann, Maria V. (1982). Thoughts on superego pathology of survivors and their children. In: Bergmann, Martin S., and Jucovy, Milton E. (Eds.), *Generations of the Holocaust*. New York: Basic Books, pp. 287-309.

152 Bergmann, Martin S. (1982). Recurrent problems in the treatment of survivors and their children. In: Bergmann, Martin S., and Jucovy, Milton E. (Eds.), *Generations of the Holocaust*. New York: Basic Books, pp. 247-266.

153 Bergmann, Martin S. (1983). Therapeutic issues in the treatment of Holocaust survivors and their children. *American Journal of Social Psychiatry*, 3(1), 21-23.

154 Bergmann, Martin S. (1985). Reflections on the psychological and social function of remembering the Holocaust. *Psychoanalytic Inquiry*, 5(1), 9-20.

155 Bergmann, Martin S. (1995). The Jewish and German roots of psychoanalysis and the impact of the Holocaust. *American Imago*, 52(3), 243-259.

156 Bergmann, Martin S.; Furst, Sidney S.; Grossman, Frances G.; and Wangh, Martin (1984). Psychoanalysis and reflections on the Holocaust: A roundtable. In: Luel, Steven A., and Marcus, Paul (Eds.), *Psychoanalytic Reflections on the Holocaust: Selected Essays*. New York: Ktav, pp. 209-229.

157 Bergmann, Martin S., and Jucovy, Milton E. (Eds.) (1982). *Generations of the Holocaust*. New York: Basic Books. 338 pp.

158 Bergmann, Martin S., and Jucovy, Milton E. (1982). Prelude. In: Bergmann, Martin S., and Jucovy, Milton E. (Eds.), *Generations of the Holocaust*. New York: Basic Books, pp. 3-29.

159 Bergmann, Martin S., and Jucovy, Milton E. (Eds.) (1990). *Generations of the Holocaust*. New York: Columbia University Press. 356 pp.

160 Berl, F. (1948). The adjustment of displaced persons. *Jewish Association of Social Services Quarterly*, 24, 254.

161 Berman, Adolf (1976). The fate of children in the Warsaw ghetto. In: Gutman, Israel, and Rothkirchen, Livia (Eds.), *The Catastrophe of European Jewry: Antecedents, History, Reflections*. Jerusalem: Yad Vashem, pp. 400-421.

162 Berou, L.; Dimitriu, A.; and Iacobini, P. (1964). Über die Morbidität ehemaliger politischer Häftlinge, verschleppter Personen und antifaschistischer Kämpfer der Widerstandsbewegung in der rumänischen Volksrepublik und über therapeutische Massnahmen sozialen Charakters in unserem Lande [On the morbidity of formal political prisoners, deported persons and anti-fascist fighters in the resistance movement in the Rumanian republic and about therapeutic measures of social character in our country]. In: *Ätio-Pathogenese und Therapie der Erschöpfung und vorzeitigen Vergreisung* [The

Aetiology and Therapy Due to Exhaustion and Premature Aging]. Wien: Verlag der FIR, pp. 573-578. [IV Internationaler Medizinischer Kongress. Bucharest, 22-27 Juni 1964].

163 Bettelheim, Bruno (1943). Individual and mass behavior in extreme situations. *Journal of Abnormal and Social Psychology*, 38(4), 417-452.

164 Bettelheim, Bruno (1979). *Surviving and Other Essays*. New York: Knopf. 432 pp.

165 Betzendahl, W. (1949). Über die Frage der Spätfolgen von Fleckfieber und Wolhynienfieber [On the problem of late sequelae of typhus and of trench-fever]. *Allgemeine Zeitschrift für Psychiatrie und Psychisch-Gerichtliche Medizin*, 124, 130-161.

166 Beyrak, Nathan (1995). Helping witnesses tell their story. In: Lemberger, John (Ed.), *A Global Perspective on Working with Holocaust Survivors and the Second Generation*. Jerusalem: JDC-Brookdale Institute of Gerontology and Human Development, AMCHA, and JDC-Israel, pp. 121-134.

167 Bialonski, H. (1959). Das Rehabilitationswesen im In- und Ausland [The rehabilitation system in the country and abroad]. In: Schench, E.G., and Nathusius, W. von (Eds.), *Extrem Lebensverhaltnisse und ihre Folgen. Bericht über den 4. Ärtzekongress für Pathologie, Therapie und Begutachtung der Heimkehrenkrankheiten in Düsseldorf, 1959* [Extreme Life Conditions and Their Effects. Report on the 4th Physician's Conference on Pathology, Therapy and Survey of Returnee's Diseases in Dusseldorf, 1959]. Verband der Heimkehrer, pp. 70-96.

168 Białówna, Irena (1979). Z historii reviru w Brzezince [The Brzezinka concentration camp and its hospital for women]. *Przegląd Lekarski*, 36(1), 164-175.

169 Białówna, Irena (1987). Aus der Geschichte des Reviers im Frauenlager in Birkenau [The Brzezinka concentration camp and its hospital for women]. In: Hamburger Institut für Sozialforschung (Eds.), *Die Auschwitz-Hefte. Texte der polnischen Zeitschrift "Przegląd Lekarski" über historische, psychische und medizinische Aspekte des Lebens und Sterbens in Auschwitz. Band 1* [The Auschwitz Journal. Text of the Polish Journal "Medical Review" on Historical, Psychic and Medical Aspects of Life and Death in Auschwitz. Volume 1]. Weinheim and Basel: Beltz, pp. 173-184.

170 Biberstein, Aleksander (1977). Przyczynek do dziejów obozu w Krakowie-Płaszow [A contribution to the history of the Krakow-Plaszow Nazi concentration camp]. *Przegląd Lekarski*, 34(1), 195-198.

171 Biderman, Aya, and Krell, Robert (1992). The patient who is a Holocaust survivor. *Israel Journal of Medical Sciences*, 122(4), 258-261.

172 Bieder, J. (1984). Séquelles tardives et retardées de la catastrophe concentrationnaire [Late and belated aftereffects of disastrous experiences in concentration camps]. *Annales Medico-Psychologiques*, 142(2), 277-283.

173 Bienka, Stanisław (1985). Socjo-medyczne aspekty rodzin byłych więźniów hitlerowskich obozów koncentracyjnych [Socio-medical aspects of families of former prisoners of Hitler's concentration camps]. *Przegląd Lekarski*, 42(1), 20-24.

174 Bienstock, Bonita E. (1988). *Daughters and granddaughters of female concentration camp survivors: Mother-daughter relationships*. Unpublished doctoral dissertation, Florida Institute of Technology, Melbourne, 397 pp. *Dissertation Abstracts International*, 50(1-B), p. 340. (University Microfilms no. AAC 8907938).

175 Biermann, Gerd (1964). Identitätsprobleme jüdischer Kinder und Jugendlicher in Deutschland [Identity problems of Jewish children and youth in Germany]. *Praxis der Kinderpsychologie und Kinderpsychiatrie*, 13(6), 213-221.

176 Biermann, Gerd, and Biermann, Renate (1967). Kinder in Israel [Children in Israel]. *Praxis der Kinderpsychologie und Kinderpsychiatrie*, 16(3), 97-112.

177 Bilik, Dorothy S. (1977). *The immigrant survivor: Post-Holocaust consciousness in recent Jewish American fiction*. Unpublished doctorial dissertation, University of Maryland, College Park, 295 pp. *Dissertation Abstracts International*, 39(2-B), p. 880. (University Microfilms no. AAC 7812878).

178 Bilikiewicz, Tadeusz (1970). Reflections on the psychology of genocide. In: *Auschwitz Anthology. Vol. 1: Inhuman Medicine. Part 1*. Warsaw: International Auschwitz Committee, pp. 3-35.

179 Bistritz, Janice F. (1988). Transgenerational pathology in families of Holocaust survivors. In: Braham, Randolph L. (Ed.), *The*

Psychological Perspectives of the Holocaust and of its Aftermath. Boulder, CO: Social Sciences Monographs; and New York: Csengeri Institute for Holocaust Studies of the Graduate School and University Center of the City University of New York, pp. 129-144.

180 Blady Szwajger, Adina (1990). *I Remember Nothing More: The Warsaw Children's Hospital and the Jewish Resistance*. New York: Pantheon. 184 pp.

181 Blahá, František (1961). Arteriosklerose bei KZ-Häftlingen [Arteriosclerosis in concentration camp inmates]. In: *Die Behandlung der Asthenie und der vorzeitigen Vergreisung bei ehemaligen Widerstandskämpfern und KZ-Häftlingen* [Treatment of Asthenics and Premature Aging in Former Resistance Fighters and Concentration Camp Inmates]. Wien: Verlag der FIR, pp. 81-82. [III Internationale Medizinische Konferenz. Liege, 17-19 März 1961].

182 Blahá, František (1961). Kriegsfolgen an der menschlichen Gesundheit in der Tschechoslowakischen Sozialistischen Republik aus den Jahren 1938-1945 [Effects of war on persons' health in the Czechoslovakian republic of the years 1938-1945]. In: *Die Behandlung der Asthenie und der vorzeitigen Vergreisung bei ehemaligen Widerstandskämpfern und KZ-Häftlingen* [Treatment of Asthenics and Premature Aging in Former Resistance Fighters and Concentration Camp Inmates]. Wien: Verlag der FIR, pp. 239-240. [III Internationale Medizinische Konferenz. Liege, 17-19 März 1961].

183 Blahá, František (1964). Folgen des Krieges für die menschliche Gesundheit nach 20 Jahren [Effects of the war on human health 20 years later]. In: *Ätio-Pathogenese und Therapie der Erschöpfung und vorzeitigen Vergreisung* [The Aetiology and Therapy Due to Exhaustion and Premature Aging]. Wien: Verlag der FIR, pp. 241-244. [IV Internationaler Medizinischer Kongress. Bucharest, 22-27 Juni 1964].

184 Blahá, František (1971). Arteriosklerose, Hypertension und Herzinfarkt bei Kriegsbeschädigten [Arteriosclerosis, hypertension and myocardial infarction in war injured]. In: Herberg, Hans-Joachim (Ed.), *Spätschäden nach Extrembelastungen* [Late Damage After Extreme Stress]. Herford: Nicolai, pp. 109-114. [II Internationalen Medizinische-Juristischen Konferenz. Dusseldorf, 1969].

185 Blahá, František (1973). Ärztliche und soziale Beurteilung und Wiedergutmachung der Spätfolgen durch den 2. Weltkrieg auf den Gesundheitszustand nach 20 Jahren [Medical and social evaluation and restitution of sequelae of the 2nd World War on the state of health after 20 years]. In: *Ermüdung und vorzeitiges Altern: Folge von Extrembelastungen* [Exhaustion and Premature Aging: Result of Extreme Stress]. Leipzig: Barth, pp. 302-308. [V Internationaler Medizinischer Kongress der FIR. Paris, 21-24 September 1970].

186 Blahá, František (1973). Folgen des 2. Weltkrieges auf den Gesundheitszustand [Sequelae of the 2nd World War on the state of health]. In: *Ermüdung und vorzeitiges Altern: Folge von Extrembelastungen* [Exhaustion and Premature Aging: Result of Extreme Stress]. Leipzig: Barth, pp. 289-292. [V. Internationaler Medizinischer Kongress der FIR. Paris, 21-24 September 1970].

187 Blank, Lily W. (1996). *The relationship between the Holocaust and object relations in adult children of Holocaust survivors*. Unpublished doctoral dissertation, Adelphi University, The Institute of Advanced Psychological Studies, Garden City, New York, 115 p. *Dissertation Abstracts International*, 56(11-B), p. 6378. (University Microfilms no. AAC 9608300).

188 Blau, David, and Kahana, Ralph J. (Eds.) (1981). Special issue: "The aging survivor of the Holocaust." *Journal of Geriatric Psychiatry*, 14(2), 131-234.

189 Blau, David, and Kahana, Ralph J. (Eds.) (1983). Special issue: "Psychotherapy of the elderly." *Journal of Geriatric Psychiatry*, 16(1), 3-102.

190 Blazevic, D. (1964). Ätio-pathogenese und Therapie der Erschöpfung und vorzeitigen Vergreisung [The aetiology, pathogenesis and therapy of exhaustion and premature aging]. In: *Ätio-Pathogenese und Therapie der Erschopfung und vorzeitigen Vergreisung* [The Aetiology and Therapy Due to Exhaustion and Premature Aging]. Wien: Verlag der FIR, pp. 603-605. [IV Internationaler Medizinischer Kongress. Bucharest, 22-27 Juni 1964].

191 Bloch, Herbert A. (1947). The personality of inmates of concentration camps. *American Journal of Sociology*, 52, 335-341.

192 Bloch, M.B. (1971). Het post-concentratie kampsyndroom [The concentration camp syndrome]. *Nederlands Militair voor Geneeskunde Tijdschrift*, 24, 165.

193 Blokhin, V.N. (1955). Die Rückkehr der Invaliden des vaterländischen Krieges in das Berufsleben der USSR [The return of the invalids of the patriotic war into professional life in the USSR].

In: Michel, Max (Ed.), *Gesundheitsschäden durch Verfolgung und Gefangenschaft und ihre Spätfolgen: Zusammenstellung der Referate und Ergebnisse der Internationalen Sozialmedizinischen Konferenz über die Pathologie der Ehemaligen Deportierten und Internierten, 5-7 Juni 1954 in Kopenhagen* [Health Damages Caused by Persecution and Internment and the Late Effects: Compilation of the Papers and Results of the International Conference of Social Medicine on the Pathology of Former Deported and Interned Persons, 5-7 June 1954 in Copenhagen]. Frankfurt am Main: Röderberg, pp. 228-235.

194 Bloom, Sandra L. (1994). Hearing the survivor's voice: Sundering the wall of denial. *Journal of Psychohistory*, 21(4), 461-477.

195 Blos, Peter (1968). Children of social catastrophe: Sequelae in survivors and the children of survivors. In: *Minutes of Discussion Group 7. Meeting of the American Psychoanalytical Association*. New York: American Psychoanalytical Association.

196 Bluhm, Hilda O. (1948). How did they survive? Mechanism of defense in Nazi concentration camps. *American Journal of Psychotherapy*, 2, 3-32.

197 Blum, Harold P. (1995). The intergenerational taboo of Nazism: A response and elaboration of Volker Friedrich's paper, "Internalization of Nazism and its effects on German psychoanalysts and their patients." *American Imago*, 52(3), 281-289.

198 Blumenthal, Norman N. (1981). *Factors contributing to varying levels of adjustment among children of Holocaust survivors*. Unpublished doctoral dissertation, Adelphi University, The Institute of Advanced Psychological Studies, Garden City, New York, 187 pp. *Dissertation Abstracts International*, 42(4-B), p. 1596. (University Microfilms no. AAC 8120876).

199 Boder, David P. (1949). *I Did Not Interview the Dead*. Urbana, IL: University of Illinois Press. 220 pp.

200 Boder, David P. (1954). The impact of catastrophe: Assessment and evaluation. *Journal of Psychology*, 38(1), 3-50.

201 Boehme, H. von; Scharkoff, T.; and Scharkoff, H. (1969). Spätschäden nach abnormalen Lebensbedingungen [Late sequelae of abnormal life conditions]. *Zeitschrift für Alternsforschung*, 22, 55-68.

202 Boeken, N. (1979). Psychosocial care of victims of persecution in the Netherlands. In: *Israel-Netherlands Symposium on the Impact of*

Persecution. Jerusalem, 16-24 October 1977. Rijswijk, The Netherlands: Ministry of Cultural Affairs, Recreation and Social Welfare, pp. 45-61.

203 Bogaty, Nina L. (1986). *The post-Holocaust family: A psychohistorical investigation into the intergenerational transmission of trauma.* Unpublished doctoral dissertation, Rutgers, The State University of New Jersey, New Brunswick, 312 pp. *Dissertation Abstracts International*, 48(1-B), p. 256. (University Microfilms no. AAC 8709159).

204 Bogusz, Józef (1970). Experiments conducted by Nazi physicians with university degrees. In: *Auschwitz Anthology. Vol. 1: Inhuman Medicine. Part 1.* Warsaw: International Auschwitz Committee, pp. 36-42.

205 Bogusz, Józef (1974). Koncentracyjnych [Concentration camps]. *Przegląd Lekarski*, 31(1), 3-12.

206 Bogusz, Józef (1977). Słowo wstępne [Introduction: 17th issue dedicated to medical problems during the Nazi occupation]. *Przegląd Lekarski*, 34(1), 3-16.

207 Bogusz, Józef (1978). Historia niemieckich obozów koncentracyjnych podczas II Wojny światowej: Słowo wstępne [History of German concentration camps during World War II: Introduction]. *Przegląd Lekarski*, 35(1), 3-15.

208 Bogusz, Józef (1978). Polnische Errungenschaften in der Erforschung medizinischer Probleme der Nazi-Okkupationszeit [Polish achievements in the research of medical problems of the Nazi occupation]. In: *Medizinische Untersuchungen der Spätfolgen des Krieges und des NS-Regimes bei Jugendlichen und Kindern von ehemaligen KZ-Häftlingen und Verfolgten* [Medical Research of the Late Effects of the War and National Socialism Regime on Youth and Children of Former Concentration Camp Inmates and Persecuted Persons]. Wien: Internationale Föderation der Widerstandskämpfer. [VI Internationaler Medizinischer Kongress der FIR. Prague, 1976].

209 Bogusz, Józef (1982). Wpływ norymberskiego procesu lekarzy hitlerowskich na kształtowanie się pojęć o dokonywaniu badań na ludziach [Effects of the Nuremberg trials of SS physicians and the shaping of concepts on human experimentation]. *Przegląd Lekarski*, 38(1), 72-79.

210 Bogusz, Józef (1984). Uwagi lekarza o martyrologii Żydów polskich [Remarks of a physician about the martyrdom of the Polish Jews]. *Przegląd Lekarski*, 41(1), 54-62.

211 Bogusz, Józef (1985). Słowo wstępne [Introduction: 25th issue dedicated to medical problems during the occupation under Hitler]. *Przegląd Lekarski*, 42(1), 5-19.

212 Bogusz, Józef (1987). Der Einfluss des Nürnberger Ärzteprozesses auf die Begriffsbildung bei Experimenten an Menschen [Effects of the Nuremberg trials of SS physicians and the shaping of concepts on human experimentation]. In: Hamburger Institut für Sozialforschung (Eds.), *Die Auschwitz-Hefte. Texte der polnischen Zeitschrift "Przegląd Lekarski" über historische, psychische und medizinische Aspekte des Lebens und Sterbens in Auschwitz. Band 2* [The Auschwitz Journal. Text of the Polish Journal "Medical Review" on Historical, Psychic and Medical Aspects of Life and Death in Auschwitz. Volume 2]. Weinheim and Basel: Beltz, pp. 15-24.

213 Bogusz, Józef, and Ryn, Zdzisław (1985). Wojna i okupacja a medycyna. Miedzynarodowa sesja w Krakowie, 25-26 kwietnia 1985 r [War, the Nazi occupation and medicine. International meeting in Cracow, 25-26 April 1985]. *Przeglad Lekarski*, 43(1), 189-202.

214 Bohm, Tomas, and Kaplan, Suzanne (1985). Aktuellt om andragenerations fenomenet [The current topic of the second generation phenomenon]. *Psykisk Haelsa*, 26(3), 119-122.

215 Bolkosky, Sidney M. (1992). The victims who survived. In: Dobkowski, Michael, and Walliman, Isidor (Eds.), *Genocide in Our Times: An Annotated Bibliography with Analytical Introductions*. Ann Arbor, MI: Pierian, pp. 67-75.

216 Bondy, Curt (1943). Problems of internment camps. *Journal of Abnormal and Social Psychology*, 38(4), 453-475.

217 Bondy, Curt (1963). Versagungstoleranz und Versagungssituation [Psychological situations and threshold of breakdown]. In: Paul, Helmut; and Herberg, Hans-Joachim (Eds.), *Psychische Spätschäden nach politischer Verfolgung* [Psychological Late Damages Following Political Persecution]. Basel: Karger, pp. 7-19.

218 Bonnard, Augusta (1954). Some discrepancies between perception and affect as illustrated by children in wartime. In: Eissler, Ruth S.; Hartmann, Heinz; Freud, Anna; and Kris, Ernst (Eds.),

Psychoanalytic Study of the Child. Vol. 9. London: Imago, pp. 242-251.

219 Boozer, Jack S. (1980). Children of Hippocrates: Doctors in Nazi Germany. *Annals of the American Academy of Political and Social Science*, 450, 83-97.

220 Borgel, Maurice (1991). Traumatisme et activités de penser de l'analyste [Trauma and thinking activities of the analyst]. *Psychoanalystes*, 38, 11-24.

221 Borkowski, Włodzimierz (1984). Wspomnienia z "Krankenbaŭ" w Oświęcimiu [Reminiscences from the "sick ward" in Auschwitz]. *Przegląd Lekarski*, 41(1), 100-108.

222 Boucher, M. (1964). Chronische Asthenie und Flecktyphusrezidive bei den ehemaligen Deportierten (Brill'sche Krankheit) [Chronic asthenia and recurrent typhus in deportees (Brill's disease)]. In: *Ätio-Pathogenese und Therapie der Erschöpfung und vorzeitigen Vergreisung* [The Aetiology and Therapy Due to Exhaustion and Premature Aging]. Wien: Verlag der FIR, pp. 85-87. [IV Internationaler Medizinischer Kongress. Bucharest, 22-27 Juni 1964].

223 Bourgeon, Michael (1986). Beratungsarbeit mit Familien von Verfolgten aus der NS-Zeit [Experiences in counselling with families of victims of the Holocaust]. *Praxis der Kinderpsychologie und Kinderpsychiatrie*, 35(6), 222-228.

224 Bower, Herbert (1994). The concentration camp syndrome. *Australian and New Zealand Journal of Psychiatry*, 28(3), 391-397.

225 Boyd, Kenneth (1995). What can medical ethics learn from history? *Journal of Medical Ethics*, 21(4), 197-198.

226 Braham, Randolph L. (Ed.) (1988). *The Psychological Perspectives of the Holocaust and of its Aftermath*. Boulder, CO: Social Sciences Monographs; and New York: Csengeri Institute for Holocaust Studies of the Graduate School and University Center of the City University of New York. 225 pp.

227 Brainin, Elisabeth, and Kaminer, Hanna (1982). Psychoanalyse und Nationalsozialismus [Psychoanalysis and National Socialism]. *Psyche: Zeitschrift für Psychoanalyse und ihre Anwendungen*, 36(11), 989-1012.

228 Branik, E., and Rosenfeld-Prusak, K. (1992). Zur psychischen Situation von judischen Jugendlichen in Deutschland [The psychiatric status of Jewish adolescents in Germany]. *Zeitschrift für Kinder und Jugendpsychiatrie*, 20(4), 273-279.

229 Braude-Heller, Anna; Rotbalsam, Israel; and Elginger, Regina (1979). Clinical aspects of hunger disease in children. In: Winick, Myron (Ed.), *Hunger Disease: Studies by the Jewish Physicians in the Warsaw Ghetto*. New York: John Wiley & Sons, pp. 45-68.

230 Braun, Abraham (1974). Some remarks on persecution pathology. *Psychotherapy and Psychosomatics*, 24, 106-108.

231 Bravo, Anna; Davite, Lilia; and Jalla, Danielle (1990). Myth, impotence, and survival in the concentration camps. In: Samuel, Raphael, and Thompson, Paul (Eds.), *The Myths We Live By*. London: Routledge, pp. 95-110.

232 Breggin, Peter R. (1993). Psychiatry's role in the Holocaust. *International Journal on Risk and Safety in Medicine*, 4, 133-148.

233 Brenner, Ira (1988). Multisensory bridges in response to object loss during the Holocaust. *Psychoanalytic Review*, 75(4), 573-587.

234 Brenner, Ira, and Kestenberg, Judith S. (1996). *The Last Witness: The Child Survivor of the Holocaust*. New York: American Psychiatric Press. 272 pp.

235 Breznitz, Tamar (1979). Recent stress and bereavement in Israel. In: *Israel-Netherlands Symposium on the Impact of Persecution. Jerusalem, 16-24 October 1977*. Rijswijk, The Netherlands: Ministry of Cultural Affairs, Recreation and Social Welfare, pp. 76-80.

236 Brieger, Gert (1980). The medical profession. In: Friedlander, Henry, and Milton, Sybil (Eds.), *The Holocaust: Ideology, Bureaucracy and Genocide*. Millwood, NJ: Kraus International, pp. 141-150.

237 Brink, Terry L. (Ed.) (1994). *Holocaust Survivors' Mental Health*. New York: Haworth. 147 pp. [Published as a special issue of *Clinical Gerontologist*, 14(3).]

238 Brody, Sylvia (1973). The son of a refugee. In: Eissler, Ruth S.; Freud, Anna; Kris, Marianne; and Solnit, Albert J. (Eds.), *Psychoanalytic Study of the Child. Vol. 28*. New Haven, CT: Yale University Press, pp. 169-191.

239 Broesse-Strauss, Ingrid, and Steffen, Hartmut (1976). Zur Psychopathologie von Kindern NS-verfolgter Eltern. Zwei psychosomatische Fallstudien [On the psychopathology of children of parents persecuted by the NS regime: Two psychosomatic case studies]. *Zeitschrift für Kinder und Jugendpsychiatrie*, 4(1), 55-70.

240 Brost, U. (1967). Zur Praxis der Wiedergutmachung [On the practice of reparations]. In: *Die Beurteilung von Gesundheitsschäden nach Gefangenschaft und Verfolgung* [The Assessment of Health Damages Following Internment and Persecution]. Herford: Nicolai, pp. 73-76. [Internationalen Medizinisch-Juristischen Symposiums in Köln, 1967].

241 Brost, U. (1973). Beziehungen von Ernährung und Arbeit zur Häufigkeit des Diabetes; aufgezeigt an Todesursachenstatistiken [The relationship of nutrition and work to the frequency of diabetes demonstrated in statistics of death]. In: *Ermüdung und vorzeitiges Altern: Folge von Extrembelastungen* [Exhaustion and Premature Aging: Result of Extreme Stress]. Leipzig: Barth, pp. 33-36. [V. Internationaler Medizinischer Kongress der FIR. Paris, 21-24 September 1970].

242 Browning, Christopher R. (1988). Genocide and public health: German doctors and Polish Jews, 1939-1941. *Holocaust and Genocide Studies*, 3(1), 21-36.

243 Brozek, K. (1980). Dr. Jan Buzek. *Przegląd Lekarski*, 37(1), 187-189.

244 Bruggerman, John A. (1980). Tweede generatie oorlogsslachtoffers [The second generation war victims]. In: Frijling-Schreuder, Bets (Ed.), *Psychoanalytici aan het Woord* [Psychoanalysts and Their Word]. Deventer: Van Loghum Slaterus, pp. 248-257.

245 Bruggerman, John A. (1994). The significance of absent objects in the analysis of transgenerational conflicts. *Zeitschrift für Psychoanalytische Theorie und Praxis*, 9(3), 293-300.

246 Brüll, Franz (1969). The trauma: A theoretical consideration. *Israel Annals of Psychiatry and Related Disciplines*, 7(1), 96-108.

247 Bruwer, A. (1989). Thoughts after reading Robert Jay Lifton's *Nazi Doctors*. *Medicine and War*, 5(4), 184-196.

248 Brym, H.; Lønnum, Arve; and Oyen, O. (1971). Über die neuen Kriegspensionierungsgesetze in Norwegen [On the new war laws pension in Norway]. In: Herberg, Hans-Joachim (Ed.), *Spätschäden* *nach Extrembelastungen* [Late Damage After Extreme Stress]. Herford: Nicolai, pp. 311-316. [II Internationalen Medizinisch-Juristischen Konferenz. Dusseldorf, 1969].

249 Brzezicki, Eugeniusz; Gawalewicz, Adolf; Holuj, Tadeusz; Kępiński, Antoni; Kłodziński, Stanisław; and Wolter, Władysław (1968). Więźniowie funkcyjni w hitlerowskich obozach koncentracyjnych (diskusja) [Prisoners with a function in Nazi concentration camps: A discussion]. *Przegląd Lekarski*, 24(1), 253-261.

250 Brzezicki, Eugeniusz; Gawalewicz, Adolf; Holuj, Tadeusz; Kępiński, Antoni; Kłodziński, Stanisław; and Wolter, Władyslaw (1987). Die Funktionshäftlinge in den Nazi-Konzentrationslagern. Eine Diskussion [Prisoners with a function in Nazi concentration camps: A discussion]. In: Hamburger Institut für Sozialforschung (Eds.), *Die Auschwitz-Hefte. Texte der polnischen Zeitschrift "Przegląd Lekarski" über historische, psychische und medizinische Aspekte des Lebens und Sterbens in Auschwitz. Band 1* [The Auschwitz Journal. Text of the Polish Journal "Medical Review" on Historical, Psychic and Medical Aspects of Life and Death in Auschwitz. Volume 1]. Weinheim and Basel: Beltz, pp. 231-239.

251 Bucelli, Daniela, and Vallario, Luca (1989). Quando finisce la speranza: Il suicido di Primo Levi [When hope ends: The suicide of Primo Levi]. *Giornale Storico di Psicologia Dinamica*, 13(25), 91-105.

252 Budick, Cynthia (1985). *An investigation of the effect of Holocaust survivor parents on their children*. Unpublished doctoral dissertation, University of Rhode Island, Kingston, 282 pp. *Dissertation Abstracts International*, 46(11-B), p. 4005. University Microfilms no. AAC 8600679).

253 Budny, Jerzy (1968). Wpływ przebywania w obozie koncentracyjnym na uzębienie byłych więźniów [The influence of the stay in a concentration camp on the dental status of ex-prisoners]. *Przegląd Lekarski*, 25, 65-70.

254 Budny, Jerzy (1972). Dentition of former prisoners. In: *Auschwitz Anthology. Vol. 3: It Did Not End in Forty-Five. Part 2*. Warsaw: International Auschwitz Committee, pp. 42-80.

255 Bulka, Reuven (1981). Editor's perspective. *Journal of Psychology and Judaism*, 6(1), 5-6.

256 Bunk, D., and Eggers, C. (1993). Die Bedeutung beziehungsdynamischer Faktoren für die Psychopathogenese von im

Kindesalter Naziverfolgten [The significance of psychodynamic relationship factors for psychopathogenesis in persons persecuted by the Nazi regime in childhood]. *Fortschritte der Neurologie, Psychiatrie*, 61(2), 38-45.

257 Bures, Rudolf (1955). Fürsorge für die Invaliden der faschistischen Verfolgung in der Tschechoslowaskischen Republik [Care for the infirm survivors of fascist persecution in the Republic of Czechoslovakia]. In: Michel, Max (Ed.), *Gesundheitsschäden durch Verfolgung und Gefangenschaft und ihre Spätfolgen: Zusammenstellung der Referate und Ergebnisse der Internationalen Sozialmedizinischen Konferenz über die Pathologie der Ehemaligen Deportierten und Internierten, 5-7 Juni 1954 in Kopenhagen* [Health Damages Caused by Persecution and Internment and the Late Effects: Compilation of the Papers and Results of the International Conference of Social Medicine on the Pathology of Former Deported and Interned Persons, 5-7 June 1954 in Copenhagen]. Frankfurt am Main: Röderberg, pp. 240-245.

258 **Busch, Marcus (1978).** ***The legacy of affliction: An enquiry into the*** *intergenerational transmission of social pathology and its treatment amongst Nazi concentration camp survivors and their children.* Unpublished master's thesis, School of Social Work, University of British Columbia, Vancouver, Canada.

259 Buschbom, H. (1981). Die volkerrechtlichen und staatsrechtlichen Massnahmen zur Beseitigung des im Namen des Deutschen Reiches verübten nationalsozialistischen Unrechts [The measures undertaken according to international law and constitutional law in order to eliminate the National Socialist injustice caused in the name of the German Reich]. In: *Die Wiedergutmachung nationalsozialistischen Unrechts durch die Bundesrepublik Deutschland. Band 2: Das Bundesruckerstattungsgesetz* [The Compensation of National Socialism Crimes by the Federal Republic of Germany. Volume 2: The Federal Compensation Law]. München: Beck, pp. 1-73.

260 Bychowski, Gustav (1968). Permanent character changes as an aftereffect of persecution. In: Krystal, Henry (Ed.), *Massive Psychic Trauma*. New York: International Universities Press, pp. 75-86.

261 Byman, Beryl (1989). Bitterfruit: The legacy of Nazi medical experiments. *Minnesota Medicine*, 72(10), 580-586.

262 Cahill, Lisa S. (1994). Lessons we have learned? In: Michalczyk, John J. (Ed.), *Medicine, Ethics, and the Third Reich: Historical and Contemporary Issues*. Kansas City, MO: Sheed & Ward.

263 Cahn, Arlene (1988). *The capacity to acknowledge experience in Holocaust survivors and their children.* Unpublished doctoral dissertation, Adelphi University, The Institute of Advanced Psychological Studies, Garden City, New York, 305 pp. *Dissertation Abstracts International*, 49(4-B), p. 1381. (University Microfilms no. AAC 8810992).

264 Cahn, Theresa I. (1988). The diary of an adolescent girl in the ghetto: A study of age-specific reactions to the Holocaust. *Psychoanalytic Review*, 75(4), 589-617.

265 Canivet, F. (1955). Myokardschäden [Damages of the myocardium]. In: Michel, Max (Ed.), *Gesundheitsschäden durch Verfolgung und Gefangenschaft und ihre Spätfolgen: Zusammenstellung der Referate und Ergebnisse der Internationalen Sozialmedizinischen Konferenz über die Pathologie der Ehemaligen Deportierten und Internierten, 5-7 Juni 1954 in Kopenhagen* [Health Damages Caused by Persecution and Internment and the Late Effects: Compilation of the Papers and Results of the International Conference of Social Medicine on the Pathology of Former Deported and Interned Persons, 5-7 June 1954 in Copenhagen]. Frankfurt am Main: Röderberg, pp. 191.

266 Capińska, Krystyna, and Capiński, Tadeusz Z. (1969). Wyniki ambulatoryjnego badania dermatologicznego 150 byłych wiezniów Oświęcimia [The results of a dermatological investigation of 50 former prisoners of Auschwitz]. *Przegląd Lekarski*, 26, 31-31.

267 Capińska, Krystyna, and Capiński, Tadeusz Z. (1973). Ergebnisse der Ambulanten dermatologischen Untersuchung von 150 ehmaligen Auschwitz-Häftlingen 23 Jahre nach der Befreiung [Results of dermatological ambulatory examinations of 150 former Auschwitz inmates 23 years after liberation]. In: *Ermüdung und vorzeitiges Altern: Folge von Extrembelastungen* [Exhaustion and Premature Aging: Result of Extreme Stress]. Leipzig: Barth, pp. 158-163. [V. Internationaler Medizinischer Kongress der FIR. Paris, 21-24 September 1970].

268 Capińska, Krystyna; Capiński, Tadeusz Z.; and Piechocki, Marion (1978). Dalsze wyniki ogólnopolskich dermatologicznych badań byłych więźniów [Further results of an "All Poland" dermatological investigation of ex-prisoners]. *Przegląd Lekarski*, 35, 27-29.

269 Caplan, Arthur (1994). The relevance of the Holocaust to current biomedical issues. In: Michalczyk, John J. (Ed.), *Medicine, Ethics, and the Third Reich: Historical and Contemporary Issues*. Kansas City, MO: Sheed & Ward, pp. 3-12.

270 Carmelly, Felicia (1975). Guilt feelings in concentration camp survivors: comments of a "survivor." *Journal of Jewish Communal Services*, 52(2), 139-144.

271 Carmil, Devora, and Breznitz, Shlomo (1991). Personal trauma and world view: Are extremely stressful experiences related to political attitudes, religious beliefs, and future orientation? *Journal of Traumatic Stress*, 4(3), 393-405.

272 Carmil, Devora, and Carel, Rafael S. (1986). Emotional distress and satisfaction in life among Holocaust survivors: A community study of survivors and controls. *Psychological Medicine*, 16(1), 141-149.

273 Cath, Stanley H. (1981). The effects of the Holocaust on life-cycle experiences: The creation and recreation of families. *Journal of Geriatric Psychiatry*, 14(2), 155-163.

274 Cesa-Bianchi, M.; Devoto, Andrea; and Martini, Massimo (1978). Psychopathological consequences of internment in Nazi concentration camps. In: *Medizinische Untersuchungen der Spätfolgen des Krieges und des NS-Regimes bei Jugendlichen und Kindern von ehemaligen KZ-Häftlingen und Verfolgten* [Medical Research of the Late Effects of the War and National Socialism Regime on Youth and Children of Former Concentration Camp Inmates and Persecuted Persons]. Wien: Internationale Föderation der Widerstandskämpfer. [VI Internationaler Medizinischer Kongress der FIR. Prague, 1976].

275 Charny, Israel W. (1982). *How Can We Commit the Unthinkable?: Genocide, The Human Cancer*. Boulder, CO: Westview. 430 pp.

276 Charny, Israel W. (1988). Understanding the psychology of genocidal destructiveness. In: Charny, Israel W. (Ed.), *Genocide: A Critical Bibliographic Review*. New York: Facts on File and London: Mansell, pp. 191-208.

277 Charny, Israel W. (1990). To commit or not commit to human life: Children of victims and victimizers all. *Contemporary Family Therapy*, 12(5), 407-426.

278 Charny, Israel W., and Davidson, Shamai (Eds.) (1983). *The Book of the International Conference on the Holocaust and Genocide. Book One: The Conference Program and Crisis*. Tel Aviv: Institute of the International Conference on the Holocaust and Genocide. 348 pp.

279 Chayes, Michael (1987). *Holocaust survivors and their children: An intergenerational study of mourning, parenting and psychological* *adjustment*. Unpublished doctoral dissertation, Adelphi University, The Institute of Advanced Psychological Studies, Garden City, New York, 162 pp. *Dissertation Abstracts International*, 48(12-B), p. 3675. (University Microfilms no. AAC 8726548).

280 Chernick, Joseph I. (1990). *Living with death: Death anxiety and adaptation in old age among Auschwitz survivors and Jews who fled Nazi Germany*. Unpublished doctoral dissertation, California School of Professional Psychology, Berkeley/Alameda, 340 pp. *Dissertation Abstracts International*, 51(6-B), p. 3124. (University Microfilms no. AAC 9030500).

281 Chodoff, Paul (1963). Late effects of the concentration camp syndrome. *Archives of General Psychiatry*, 8, 323-333.

282 Chodoff, Paul (1966). Effects of extreme coercive and oppressive forces: Brainwashing and concentration camps. In: Arieti, Silvano (Ed.), *American Handbook of Psychiatry. Vol. 3*. New York: Basic Books, pp. 384-405.

283 Chodoff, Paul (1966). Nazi concentration camps survivors - still inmates. *Roche Report: Frontiers of Clinical Psychiatry*, 3(4).

284 Chodoff, Paul (1967). Depression and guilt in concentration camp survivors. *Psychotherapy and Psychosomatics*, 15(1), 11-12.

285 Chodoff, Paul (1968). The Nazi concentration camp and the American poverty ghetto: A comparison. *Journal of Contemporary Psychotherapy*, 1, 1-8.

286 Chodoff, Paul (1970). Depression and guilt among concentration camp survivors. *Existential Psychiatry*, 7, 78-87.

287 Chodoff, Paul (1970). The German concentration camp as a psychological stress. *Archives of General Psychiatry*, 22(1), 78-87.

288 Chodoff, Paul (1970). Psychological response to concentration camp survival. In: Abram, Harry S. (Ed.), *Psychological Aspects of Stress*. Springfield, IL: Thomas.

289 Chodoff, Paul (1975). Psychiatric aspects of the Nazi persecution. In: Arieti, Silvano (Ed.), *American Handbook of Psychiatry. Vol. 2. 2nd ed*. New York: Basic Books, pp. 932-946.

290 Chodoff, Paul (1980). Psychotherapy of the survivor. In: Dimsdale, Joel E. (Ed.), *Survivors, Victims and Perpetrators: Essays on the Nazi Holocaust*. Washington, D.C.: Hemisphere, pp. 205-216.

291 Chodoff, Paul (1981). Survivors of the Nazi Holocaust. *Children Today*, 10(5), 2-5.

292 Chodoff, Paul (1986). Survivors of the Nazi Holocaust. In: Moos, Rudolf H. (Ed.), *Coping with Life Crises: An Integrated Approach*. New York: Plenum, pp. 407-415.

293 Chung, M.C. (1995). Reviewing Frankl's "Will to Meaning" and its implications for psychotherapy dealing with post-traumatic stress disorder. *Medicine and War*, 11(1), 45-55.

294 Chylińska, Mieczysława (1984). W kręgu reakcji obronnych [Defense mechanisms]. *Przegląd Lekarski*, 41(1), 121-126.

295 Chylińska, Mieczysława (1984). Refleksje z obozu w Brzezince [Thoughts about the Birkenau concentration camp]. *Przegląd Lekarski*, 41(1), 115-120.

296 Chylińska, Mieczysława (1986). Działania SS w Brzezińce przeciw węzłom społeczno - emocjonalnym więźniów [Actions of SS personnel in Auschwitz-Birkenau against social and emotional bonds]. *Przegląd Lekarski*, 43(1), 145-161.

297 Chylińska, Mieczysława (1986). W kręgu przeżyć i doznań z obozowych apeli [Experiences and emotions during concentration camp roll calls]. *Przegląd Lekarski*, 43(1), 131-144.

298 Chylińska, Mieczysława (1987). Pod naporem beznadziejności w obozie [Under the pressure of hopelessness in the concentration camp]. *Przegląd Lekarski*, 44(1), 174-186.

299 Chylińska, Mieczysława (1988). Kobiety w Oświęcimiu-Brzezince [Women at the Auschwitz-Birkenau concentration camp]. *Przegląd Lekarski*, 45(1), 148-165.

300 Chylińska, Mieczysława (1989). Niektóre osobliwości bodźców obozowych [Some peculiarities of stimuli in concentration camps]. *Przegląd Lekarski*, 46(1), 57-66.

301 Chylińska, Mieczysława (1990). Z doznań więźniów po likwidacji obozów w Oświęcimiu-Brzezince [Experiences of the prisoners after liquidation of the Auschwitz-Birkenau concentration camp]. *Przegląd Lekarski* 47(1), 170-185.

302 Chylińska, Mieczysława (1995). Frauen in Auschwitz-Birkenau [Women in Auschwitz-Birkenau]. In: Hamburger Institut für

Sozialforschung (Eds.), *Die Auschwitz-Hefte. Ergänzungsband. Texte der polnischen Zeitschrift "Przegląd Lekarski" über historische, psychische und medizinische Aspekte des Lebens und Sterbens in Auschwitz.* [The Auschwitz Journal. Supplementary Volume. Text of the Polish Journal "Medical Review" on Historical, Psychic and Medical Aspects of Life and Death in Auschwitz]. Weinheim and Basel: Rogner and Bernhard, pp. 10-13.

303 Ciesławski, Marian (1981). Z przeżyć dzieci i matek-robotnic przymusowych na Pomorzu Zachodnim [Experiences of children and mothers invovlved in forced labor in West Pomerania]. *Przegląd Lekarski*, 38(1), 121-124.

304 Ciosińska, Irena (1987). W rewirach podobozów KL Ravensbrük i KL Sachsenhausen [At the hospitals of Ravensbrück and Sachsenhausen concentration camps]. *Przegląd Lekarski*, 44(1), 154-174.

305 Citrome, P. (1952). Conclusions d'une enquète sur le suicide dans les camps de concentration [Conclusions of a study on suicide in concentration camps]. *Cahiers d'Information Médicales, Sociales et Juridiques*, 12, 147-149.

306 Cohen, Betty B. (1991). Holocaust survivors and the crisis of aging. *Families in Society*, 72(4), 226-231.

307 Cohen, Elie A. (1952). *Het Duitse Concentratie-Kamp: Een Medische en Psychologische Studie* [The German Concentration Camp: A Medical and Psychological Study]. Amsterdam: H.J. Paris. 258 pp.

308 Cohen, Elie A. (1965). Reakcja początkowa na osadzenie w obozie koncentracyjnym [The primary reaction to imprisonment in concentration camps]. *Przegląd Lekarski*, 21, 28-31.

309 Cohen, Elie A. (1969). Het post-concentratiekampsyndroom [The post-concentration camp syndrome]. *Nederlands Tijdschrift voor Geneeskunde*, 113(46), 2049-2054.

310 Cohen, Elie A. (1972). The post-concentration camp syndrome. *Nederlands Tijdschrift voor Geneeskunde*, 116(38), 1680-1685.

311 Cohen, Elie A. (1972). W transporcie więźniów-Żydów z Holandii [On a transport of Jewish prisoners from Holland]. *Przegląd Lekarski*, 29, 120-132.

312 Cohen, Elie A. (1972). Uwagi o tzw KZ-syndromie [On the so-called KZ syndrome]. *Przegląd Lekarski*, 29(1), 21-27.

313 Cohen, Elie A. (1973). *The Abyss: A Confession*. New York: Norton. 111 pp.

314 Cohen, Elie A. (1979). *De Negentien Treinen Naar Sobibor* [The Nineteen Trains to Sobibor]. Brussels: Elsevier. 216 pp.

315 Cohen, Elie A. (1981). The post-concentration camp syndrome: A disaster syndrome. *Science and Public Policy*, 8(3), 239-246.

316 Cohen, Elie A. (1985). De tijd heelt niet alle wonden [Time does not heal all wounds]. *Nederlands Tijdschrift voor Geneeskunde*, 129(18), 826-827.

317 Cohen, Elie A. (1988). *Human Behavior in the Concentration Camp*. London: Free Association Books. 295 pp.

318 Cohen, Jonathan (1977). The impact of death and dying on concentration camp survivors. *Advances in Thanatology*, 4(1), 27-36.

319 Cohen, Jonathan (1985). Trauma and repression. *Psychoanalytic Inquiry*, 5(1), 163-189.

320 Cohen, Martin S. (1986). *An Enquiry on Needs for Psychosocial Help to Dutch Victims of World War II Living in Israel*. Ramat Gan, Israel: ELAH Foundation.

321 Cohen, Martin S. (1989). The rabbi and the Holocaust survivor. In: Marcus, Paul, and Rosenberg, Alan (Eds.), *Healing Their Wounds: Psychotherapy with Holocaust Survivors and Their Families*. New York: Praeger, pp. 167-179.

322 Cohen, Nava (1990). Medical experiments. In: Gutman, Israel (Ed.), *Encyclopedia of the Holocaust. Vol. 3*. New York: Macmillan, pp. 957-966.

323 Coke, L.R. (1961). Late effects of starvation. *Medical Services Journal of Canada*, 17, 313-324.

324 Collis, W.R.F. (1945). Belsen camp: A preliminary report. *British Medical Journal*, 814-816.

325 Conrad, Gertrude (1969). Casework with survivors of the Nazi persecution twenty years after liberation. *Journal of Jewish Communal Service*, 46(2), 170-175.

326 Cooper, R.H. (1979). Concentration camp survivors: A challenge for geriatric nursing. *Nursing Clinics of North America*, 14(4), 621-628.

327 Cooper-Hollander, Anne (1993). *Mashma'ut chavayat v'tafkid hasaba'ut b'kerev nitzoley hashoah* [The meaning of grandparenthood experience and role among Holocaust survivors]. Unpublished master's thesis, Department of Psychology, Tel Aviv University, Tel Aviv, Israel. 145 pp.

328 Coopmans, M. (1983). Tweede generatie vervolgingsslachtoffers 1940-1945 [Second generation victims of persecution 1940-1945]. *Voordrachtenreeks Nederlandse Vereniging voor Psychiatrie*, no. 4, pp. 56-95.

329 Copelman, L.S. (1961). Studien und Forschungen über die Pathogenese und die Behandlung des psycho-somatischen Syndroms der Deportierten [Studies and research of the pathogenesis and treatment of the psychosomatic syndromes of deportees]. In: *Die Behandlung der Asthenie und der vorzeutigen Vergreisung bei ehemaligen Widerstandskämpfern und KZ-Häftlingen* [Treatment of Asthenics and Premature Aging in Former Resistance Fighters and Concentration Camp Inmates]. Wien: Verlag der FIR, pp. 107-118. [III Internationale Medizinische Konferenz. Liege, 17-19 März 1961].

330 Copelman, L.S. (1973). Schizophrenia im Rahmen der Sozialpsychiatrie [Schizophrenia within the framework of social psychiatry]. In: *Ermüdung und vorzeitiges Altern: Folge von Extrembelastungen* [Exhaustion and Premature Aging: Result of Extreme Stress]. Leipzig: Barth, pp. 139-148. [V. Internationaler Medizinischer Kongress der FIR. Paris, 21-24 September 1970].

331 Copelman, L.S. (1973). Spät auftretende neuroendokrinologische Folgen der Konzentrationslager im Lichte von Stoffwechselstörungen [Delayed appearance of neuroendocrinological sequelae of concentration camps as reflected in metabolic disturbances]. In: *Ermüdung und vorzeitiges Altern: Folge von Extrembelastungen* [Exhaustion and Premature Aging: Result of Extreme Stress]. Leipzig: Barth, p. 288. [V. Internationaler Medizinischer Kongress der FIR. Paris, 21-24 September 1970].

332 Copelman, L.S. (1978). La délinquance juvenile chez l'enfant concentrationnaire [Juvenile delinquency of the concentration camp child]. In: *Medizinische Untersuchungen der Spätfolgen des Krieges und des NS-Regimes bei Jugendlichen und Kindern von ehemaligen KZ-Häftlingen und Verfolgten* [Medical Research of the Late Effects of the War and National Socialism Regime on Youth and Children of Former Concentration Camp Inmates and Persecuted Persons]. Wien: Internationale Föderation der Widerstandskämpfer. [VI Internationaler Medizinischer Kongress der FIR. Prague, 1976].

333 Copelman, L.S. (1978). L'état actuel de nos connaissances sur l'étiologie des sequelles de guerre [The contemporary state of our knowledge about the etiology of war sequelae]. In: *Medizinische Untersuchungen der Spätfolgen des Krieges und des NS-Regimes bei Jugendlichen und Kindern von ehemaligen KZ-Häftlingen und Verfolgten* [Medical Research of the Late Effects of the War and National Socialism Regime on Youth and Children of Former Concentration Camp Inmates and Persecuted Persons]. Wien: Internationale Föderation der Widerstandskämpfer. [VI Internationaler Medizinischer Kongress der FIR. Prague, 1976].

334 Corcoran, James F.T. (1982). The concentration camp syndrome and USAF Vietnam prisoners of war. *Psychiatric Annals*, 12(11), 991-994.

335 Cordell, Marta (1980). *Coping behavior of Nazi concentration camp survivors*. Unpublished doctoral dissertation, Pacific Graduate School of Psychology, 67 pp. *Dissertation Abstracts International*, 41(10-B), p. 3883. (University Microfilms no. AAC 8104648).

336 Corrado, Raymond R., and Tompkins, Eric (1989). A comparative model of the psychological effects on the victims of state and anti-state terrorism. *International Journal of Law and Psychiatry*, 12(4), 281-293.

337 Cremerius, J. (1960). Eine Kindertragödie. Psychose oder Neurose [A children's tragedy, psychosis or neurosis]. In: March, Hans (Ed.), *Verfolgung und Angst in ihren leib-seelischen Auswirkungen. Dokumente* [Persecution and Anxiety in Their Psychosomatic Forms of Expression. Documentation]. Stuttgart: Klett, pp. 28-33.

338 Cremerius, J. (1960). Schiksal und Neurose. Multiple leib-seelische Störungen nach KZ-häft [Fate and neurosis, multiple physical-mental disturbances after concentration camp imprisonment]. In: March, Hans (Ed.), *Verfolgung und Angst in ihren leib-seelischen Auswirkungen. Dokumente* [Persecution and Anxiety in Their Psychosomatic Forms of Expression. Documentation]. Stuttgart: Klett, pp. 34-40.

339 Cronstrom-Beskow, Solveig (1991). Coping strategies in death camps. *International Forum for Logotherapy*, 14(2), 92-96.

340 Cuica, A. (1978). La pathologie sequellaire (après l'age de 30 ans) des resistants [The pathological sequelae (after 30 years of age) in resistance fighters]. In: *Medizinische Untersuchungen der Spätfolgen des Krieges und des NS-Regimes bei Jugendlichen und Kindern von ehemaligen KZ-Häftlingen und Verfolgten* [Medical Research of the Late Effects of the War and National Socialism Regime on Youth and Children of Former Concentration Camp Inmates and Persecuted Persons]. Wien: Internationale Föderation der Widerstandskämpfer. [VI Internationaler Medizinischer Kongress der FIR. Prague, 1976].

341 Cycowicz, Giselle (1995). Working with survivors in homes for the aged. In: Lemberger, John (Ed.), *A Global Perspective on Working with Holocaust Survivors and the Second Generation*. Jerusalem: JDC-Brookdale Institute of Gerontology and Human Development, AMCHA, and JDC-Israel, pp. 269-275.

342 Dąbrowski, Stanisław; Schrammowa, Halina; and Zakowska-Dąbrowska, Teresa (1965). Trwałe zmiany psychiczne powstałe w wyniku pobytu w obozach koncentracyjnych I eksperymentów pseudolekarskich [Persistent psychological changes caused by incarceration in a concentration camp and by pseudomedical experiments]. *Przegląd Lekarski*, 21(1), 32-34.

343 Dadrian, Vahakn N. (1971). Factors of anger and aggression in genocide. *Journal of Human Relations*, 19(3), 396-417.

344 Dahl, H.K. (1995). Politisk fange i Norge og i Tyskland 1943-1945: En medsinstudents opplevelser [A political prisoner in Norway and Germany 1941-1945: Experiments of a medical student]. *Tidskrift for den Norske Laegeforening. Journal of the Norwegian Medical Association*, 115(11), 1397-1401.

345 Dahmer, H. (1979). Holocaust und die Amnesie [Holocaust and amnesia]. *Psyche: Zeitschrift für Psychoanalyse und ihre Anwendungen*, 33(11), 1039-1049.

346 Dahmer, H. (1990). Derealisierung und Wiederholung [Derealization and repetition]. *Psyche: Zeitschrift für Psychoanalyse und ihre Anwendungen*, 44(2), 133-143.

347 Dane, Jan (Ed.) (1984). *Keerzijde van de bevrijding: Opstellen over de maatschappelijke, psycho-sociale en medische aspekten van de problematiek van oorlogsgetroffenen* [The Other Side of Liberation: Essays on the Social, Psychosocial and Medical Aspects of the Problems of War Victims]. Deventer: Van Loghum Slaterus. 205 pp.

348 Dangel, Jan (1974). W "rewirach" obozów Oświęcim i Dachau [The Auschwitz and Dachau concentration camp medical centers]. *Przegląd Lekarski*, 31(1), 209-213.

349 Danieli, Yael (1980). Countertransference in the treatment and study of Nazi Holocaust survivors and their children. *Victimology*, 5(2-4), 355-367.

350 Danieli, Yael (1981). Differing adaptational styles in families of survivors of the Nazi Holocaust: Some implications for treatment. *Children Today*, 10((5), 6-10, 34-35.

351 Danieli, Yael (1981). The Group Project for Holocaust Survivors and their children. *Children Today*, 10(5), 11, 33.

352 Danieli, Yael (1981). Mit'am hahitarvut bedarcey hahistaglut hashonot shel mishpachot nitzoley hashoa [Fitting the intervention to different modes of adaptation in families of survivors]. *Masua*, 9, 169-178.

353 Danieli, Yael (1981). On the achievement of integration in aging survivors of the Nazi Holocaust. *Journal of Geriatric Psychiatry*, 14(2), 191-210.

354 Danieli, Yael (1981). *Therapists' difficulties in treating survivors of the Nazi Holocaust and their children.* Unpublished doctoral dissertation, New York University, 216 pp. *Dissertation Abstracts International*, 42(12-B), p. 4927. (University Microfilms no. AAC 8210968).

355 Danieli, Yael (1982). Families of survivors of the Nazi Holocaust: Some short- and long-term effects. In: Spielberger, Charles D.; Sarason, Irwin G.; and Milgram, Norman (Eds.), *Stress and Anxiety. Vol. 8.* Washington, D.C.: Hemisphere, pp. 405-421.

356 Danieli, Yael (1983). Psychotherapists' participation in the conspiracy of silence about the Holocaust. *Psychoanalytic Psychology*, 1(1), 23-43.

357 Danieli, Yael (1985). Odległe następstwa prześladowań hitlerowskich w rodzinach ocalałych ofiar [Remote sequelae of Hitler's persecutions in the families of survivors]. *Przegląd Lekarski*, 42(1), 34-41.

358 Danieli, Yael (1985). The treatment and prevention of long term effects and intergenerational transmission of victimization: A lesson from Holocaust survivors and their children. In: Figley, Charles R.

(Ed.), *Trauma and its Wake. Vol. 1: The Study and Treatment of Post-Traumatic Stress Disorder*. New York: Brunner/Mazel, pp. 295-313.

359 Danieli, Yael (1988). Confronting the unimaginable: Psychotherapists' reactions to victims of the Nazi Holocaust. In: Wilson, John P.; Harel, Zev; and Kahana, Boaz (Eds.), *Human Adaptation to Extreme Stress: From the Holocaust to Vietnam*. New York, Plenum, pp. 219-237.

360 Danieli, Yael (1988). The heterogeneity of post-war adaptation in families of Holocaust survivors. In: Braham, Randolph L. (Ed.), *The Psychological Perspectives of the Holocaust and of its Aftermath*. Boulder, CO: Social Sciences Monographs; and New York: Csengeri Institute for Holocaust Studies of the Graduate School and University Center of the City University of New York, p. 109-127.

361 Danieli, Yael (1988). On not confronting the Holocaust: Psychological reactions to victims/survivors and their children. In: *Remembering for the Future: Working Papers and Addenda. Vol. 2: The Impact of the Holocaust on the Contemporary World*. Oxford: Pergamon, pp. 1257-1271.

362 Danieli, Yael (1988). Treating survivors and children of survivors of the Nazi Holocaust. In: Ochberg, Frank M. (Ed.), *Post-Traumatic Therapy and Victims of Violence*. New York: Brunner/Mazel, pp. 278-294.

363 Danieli, Yael (1989). Mourning in survivors and children of the Nazi Holocaust: The role of group and community modalities. In: Dietrich, David R., and Shabad, Peter C. (Eds.), *The Problem of Loss and Mourning: Psychoanalytic Perspectives*. Madison, CT: International Universities Press, pp. 427-460.

364 Danieli, Yael (1993). Countertransference, trauma and training. In: Wilson, John P., and Lindy, Jacob D. (Eds.), *Countertransference in the Treatment of Post-Traumatic Stress Disorder*. New York: Guilford, pp. 368-388.

365 Danieli, Yael (1993). Diagnostic and therapeutic use of the multigenerational family tree in working with survivors and children of survivors of the Nazi Holocaust. In: Wilson, John P., and Raphael, Beverley (Eds.), *International Handbook of Traumatic Stress Syndromes*. New York: Plenum, pp. 889-898.

366 Danieli, Yael (1994). As survivors age. *PTSD [Post-Traumatic Stress Disorder] Research Quarterly*, 4(2), 20-24.

367 Danto, Bruce (1968). The role of "missed adolescence": In the etiology of the concentration camp survivor syndrome. In: Krystal, Henry (Ed.), *Massive Psychic Trauma*. New York: International Universities Press, pp. 248-259.

368 Dasberg, Haim (1987). Hachevra ha'yisraelit mul trauma meurgenet o hametapel mul hanitzol [Israeli society facing trauma (or: psychotherapists facing survivors)]. *Sihot: Israel Journal of Psychotherapy*, 1(2), 94-97.

369 Dasberg, Haim (1987). Psychological distress of Holocaust survivors and offspring in Israel, forty years later: A review. *Israel Journal of Psychiatry and Related Sciences*, 24(4), 243-256.

370 Dasberg, Haim (1991). Psychiatrische und psychosoziale Folgen der Holocaust: Epidemiologische Studien in Israel [Psychiatric and psychosocial consequences of the Holocaust: Epidemiologic studies in Israel]. In: Stoffels, Hans (Ed.), *Schicksale der Verfolgten: Psychische und somatische Auswirkungen von Terrorherschaft* [The Fate of Persecuted Persons: Psychic and Somatic Effects of Terror Reign]. Berlin: Springer.

371 Dasberg, Haim (1991). Why we were silent: An Israeli psychiatrist speaks to Germans on psychic pain and past persecution. *Israel Journal of Psychiatry and Related Sciences*, 28(2), 29-38.

372 Dasberg, Haim (1992). Child survivors of the Holocaust reach middle age: Psychotherapy of late grief reactions. *Journal of Social Work Policy in Israel*, 5-6, 71-83.

373 Dasberg, Haim (1992). The unfinished story of trauma as a paradigm for psychotherapists (a review and some empirical findings on paradigms and prejudices). *Israel Journal of Psychiatry and Related Sciences*, 29(1), 44-60.

374 Dasberg, Haim (1993). How psychotherapists cope with their patients' trauma. *Echoes of the Holocaust*, 2, 31-45. [Bulletin of the Jerusalem Center for Research into the Late Effects of the Holocaust, Talbieh Mental Health Center, Jerusalem, Israel].

375 Dasberg, Haim (1995). AMCHA: The National Israeli Center for Psychosocial Support of Holocaust Survivors and the Second Generation: Raisons d'être. In: Lemberger, John (Ed.), *A Global*

Perspective on Working with Holocaust Survivors and the Second Generation. Jerusalem: JDC-Brookdale Institute of Gerontology and Human Development, AMCHA, and JDC-Israel, pp. 1-11.

376 Dasberg, Haim, and Robinson, Shalom (1991). The impact of the Demjaniuk trial on the psychotherapeutic process in Israel. *Medicine and Law*, 10(4), 395-399.

377 Davidson, Shamai (1967). A clinical classification of the psychiatric disturbances of Holocaust survivors and their treatment. *Israel Annals of Psychiatry and Related Sciences*, 5, 96-98.

378 Davidson, Shamai (1973). The treatment of Holocaust survivors. In: Davidson, Shamai (Ed.), *Spheres of Psychotherapeutic Activity*. Kupat Cholim, pp. 77-87.

379 Davidson, Shamai (1979). Long-term psychosocial sequelae in Holocaust survivors and their families. In: *Israel-Netherlands Symposium on the Impact of Persecution. Jerusalem, 16-24 October 1977*. Rijswijk, The Netherlands: Ministry of Cultural Affairs, Recreation and Social Welfare, pp. 62-68.

380 Davidson, Shamai (1979). Massive trauma and social support. *Journal of Psychosomatic Research*, 23(6), 395-402.

381 Davidson, Shamai (1980). The clinical effects of massive psychic traumatization in families of Holocaust survivors. *Journal of Marital and Family Therapy*, 6(1), 11-21.

382 Davidson, Shamai (1980). Transgenerational transmission in the families of Holocaust survivors. *International Journal of Family Psychiatry*, 1(1), 95-112.

383 Davidson, Shamai (1981). Clinical and psychotherapeutic experience with survivors and their families. *Family Physician*, 10(2), 313-320.

384 Davidson, Shamai (1981). Psychosocial issues in the lives of survivors. *Journal of the '45 Aid Society*, 29-33.

385 Davidson, Shamai (1981). On relating to traumatized-persecuted people. In: *Israel-Netherlands Symposium on the Impact of Persecution. Dalfsen, Amsterdam, 14-18 April 1980*. Rijswijk, The Netherlands: Ministry of Cultural Affairs, Recreation and Social Welfare, pp. 55-63.

386 Davidson, Shamai (1981). Le syndrome des survivants: Revue générale [The survivor's syndrome: A general view]. *L'Evolution Psychiatrie*, 46(2), 319-331.

387 Davidson, Shamai (1983). Psychosocial aspects of Holocaust trauma in the life cycle of survivors: Refugees and their families. In: Baker, Ron (Ed.), *The Psychosocial Problems of Refugees*. London: British Refugee Council and the European Consultation on Refugees and Exiles, pp. 21-31.

388 Davidson, Shamai (1984). Human reciprocity among the Jewish prisoners. In: Gutman, Israel, and Saf, Avital (Eds.), *The Nazi Concentration Camps: Structure and Aims, the Image of the Prisoner, the Jews in the Camps. Proceedings of the Fourth Yad Vashem International Conference, Jerusalem, January 1980*. Jerusalem: Yad Vashem, pp. 555-572.

389 Davidson, Shamai (1985). Group formation and its significance in the Nazi concentration camps. *Israel Journal of Psychiatry and Related Sciences*, 22(1-2), 41-50.

390 Davidson, Shamai (1987). Trauma in the life cycle of the individual and the collective consciousness in relation to war and persecution. In: Dasberg, Haim; Davidson, Shamai; Durlacher, G.L.; Filet, B.C.; and de Wind, Eddy (Eds.), *Society and Trauma of War*. Assen/Maastricht, The Netherlands and Wolfeboro, NH: Van Gorcum, pp. 14-32.

391 Davidson, Shamai (1989). Avoidance and denial in the life cycle of Holocaust survivors. In: Edelstein, Eliezer L.; Nathanson, Donald L.; and Stone, Andrew M. (Eds.), *Denial: A Clarification of Concepts and Research*. New York: Plenum, pp. 309-320.

392 Davidson, Shamai (1992). *Holding on to Humanity: The Message of Holocaust Survivors. The Shamai Davidson Papers*. (Ed.: Charny, Israel W.) New York: New York University Press. 243 pp.

393 Davidson, Shamai; Bental, V.; and Winnik, Heinrich Z. (1967). Psychiatric disturbances of Holocaust ("Shoa") survivors. Symposium of the Israel Psychoanalytic Society [Held July 9th 1966, Tel Aviv]. *Israel Annals of Psychiatry and Related Disciplines*, 5(1), 91-100.

394 Davidson, Shamai; Bental, V.; and Winnik, Heinrich, Z. (1980). The survivor syndrome today: An overview. In: Garlans, C. (Ed.), *Group Analysis*. London: The Trust for Group Analysis, pp. 24-32.

395 Davis, Minna (1977). Breaking silence: Serving children of Holocaust survivors. *Journal of Jewish Communal Service*, 54, 294-302.

396 Dębicka-Małkowska, Danuta; Foersterling, Ewa; Kinal, Krystyna; and Lewandowska, Melita (1972). Wyniki bydgoskich badań byłych więźniów hitlerowskich obozów koncentracyjnych [The results of the investigations performed in the county of Bydgoszcz of former prisoners in Hitlerian concentration camps]. *Przegląd Lekarski*, 29, 23-34.

397 Degani, Yoav (1994). *Hatikva l'orech chayayhem shel nitzoley shoah: Hishtanut hatikvah ve hakesher beynah v'beyn matzavam haphysi v'hanapshi shel hanitzolim* [The hope of Holocaust survivors across the life span: The change of hope and the relationship between hope and the physical and mental condition of the survivors]. Unpublished master's thesis, Department of Psychology, Tel Aviv University, Tel Aviv, Israel. 192 pp.

398 de Graaf, Theo (1975). Pathological patterns of identification in families of survivors of the Holocaust. *Israel Annals of Psychiatry and Related Disciplines*, 13(4), 335-363.

399 de Jong, A.J. (1995). Personal therapy group-Berlin: Experiences with a closed group of Jewish, German psychotherapists. In: Lemberger, John (Ed.), *A Global Perspective on Working with Holocaust Survivors and the Second Generation*. Jerusalem: JDC-Brookdale Institute of Gerontology and Human Development, AMCHA, and JDC-Israel, pp. 305-317.

400 de Jong, A.J. (1995). The Sinai-Center: European Centre for Jewish Mental Services and Psychotrauma Treatment. In: Lemberger, John (Ed.), *A Global Perspective on Working with Holocaust Survivors and the Second Generation*. Jerusalem: JDC-Brookdale Institute of Gerontology and Human Development, AMCHA, and JDC-Israel, pp. 243-247.

401 de Koning, P. (1981). What psychotherapists have against working with people who were persecuted during World War II. In: *Israel-Netherlands Symposium on the Impact of Persecution. Dalfsen, Amsterdam, 14-18 April 1980*. Rijswijk, The Netherlands: Ministry of Cultural Affairs, Recreation and Social Welfare, pp. 49-54.

402 de Larebeyrette, J. (1961). Der Infarkt und andere Gefässtörungen vorhersehbar und daher vermeidbar [Cardiac infarct and other vascular diseases can be predicted and thus prevented]. In: *Die Behandlung der Asthenie und der vorzeitigen Vergreisung bei* *ehemaligen Widerstandskämpfern und KZ-Häftlingen* [Treatment of Asthenics and Premature Aging in Former Resistance Fighters and Concentration Camp Inmates]. Wien: Verlag der FIR, pp. 83-96. [III Internationale Medizinische Konferenz. Liege, 17-19 März 1961].

403 de Leeuw-Aalbers, A.J. (1947). Het kind als oorlogsslachtoffer [The child as war victim]. *Maandblad voor de Geestelijke Volksgezondheid*, 2(3), 3-15.

404 Delius, L. (1959). Pathogenese und Prognose vegetativer Regulationsstörungen [Pathogenesis and prognosis of disturbances in the vegetative regulation]. In: Schench, E.G., and Nathusius, W. von (Eds.), *Extrem Lebensverhaltnisse und ihre Folgen. Bericht über den 4. Ärtzekongress für Pathologie, Therapie und Begutachtung der Heimkehrenkrankheiten in Düsseldorf, 1959* [Extreme Life Conditions and Their Effects. Report on the 4th Physicians Conference on Pathology, Therapy and Survey of Returnees' Diseases in Dusseldorf, 1959]. Verband der Heimkehrer, pp. 54-57.

405 de Loos, W.S. (1987). Lichamelijke klachten en verschíjnselen anno 1987 en de oorzakelijke werking van oorlogsomstandigheden; wetenschappelijke argumenten en methodologische overwegingen [Physical complaints and symptoms around 1987 and the causative effects of war circumstances: Scientific arguments and methodologic considerations]. In: *Medical Causality and Late Consequences of War*. Utrecht: Stichting ICODO, pp. 43-57.

406 Denes, S. (1978). Premature aging and invalidity. In: *Medizinische Untersuchungen der Spätfolgen des Krieges und des NS-Regimes bei Jugendlichen und Kindern von ehemaligen KZ-Häftlingen und Verfolgten* [Medical Research of the Late Effects of the War and National Socialism Regime on Youth and Children of Former Concentration Camp Inmates and Persecuted Persons]. Wien: Internationale Föderation der Widerstandskämpfer. [VI Internationaler Medizinischer Kongress der FIR. Prague, 1976].

407 Desmonts, Théo (1955). Die Hautpigmentierung bei den KZ Insassen während und nach der Deportation [Pigmentation of the skin in concentration camp inmates during and after deportation]. In: Michel, Max (Ed.), *Gesundheitsschädendurch Verfolgung und Gefangenschaft und ihre Spätfolgen: Zusammenstellung der Referate und Ergebnisse der Internationalen Sozialmedizinischen Konferenz über die Pathologie der Ehemaligen Deportierten und Internierten, 5-7 Juni 1954 in Kopenhagen* [Health Damages Caused by Persecution and Internment and the Late Effects: Compilation of the Papers and

Results of the International Conference of Social Medicine on the Pathology of Former Deported and Interned Persons, 5-7 June 1954 in Copenhagen]. Frankfurt am Main: Röderberg, pp. 225.

408 Desmonts, Théo (1955). Puls, Blutdruck und Hungeroedem bei 196 politischen Deportierten [Pulse, bloodpressure and oedema due to famine in 196 political deportees]. In: Michel, Max (Ed.), *Gesundheitsschäden durch Verfolgung und Gefangenschaft und ihre Spätfolgen: Zusammenstellung der Referate und Ergebnisse der Internationalen Sozialmedizinischen Konferenz über die Pathologie der Ehemaligen Deportierten und Internierten, 5-7 Juni 1954 in Kopenhagen* [Health Damages Caused by Persecution and Internment and the Late Effects: Compilation of the Papers and Results of the International Conference of Social Medicine on the Pathology of Former Deported and Interned Persons, 5-7 June 1954 in Copenhagen]. Frankfurt am Main: Röderberg, pp. 192-194.

409 Desoille, Henri (1955). Berufliche Umschulung der kranken ehemaligen Deportierten in Frankreich [Vocational training of sick former deportees in France]. In: Michel, Max (Ed.), *Gesundheitsschäden durch Verfolgung und Gefangenschaft und ihre Spätfolgen: Zusammenstellung der Referate und Ergebnisse der Internationalen Sozialmedizinischen Konferenz über die Pathologie der Ehemaligen Deportierten und Internierten, 5-7 Juni 1954 in Kopenhagen* [Health Damages Caused by Persecution and Internment and the Late Effects: Compilation of the Papers and Results of the International Conference of Social Medicine on the Pathology of Former Deported and Interned Persons, 5-7 June 1954 in Copenhagen]. Frankfurt am Main: Röderberg, pp. 288-296.

410 Desoille, Henri (1960). Berufliche Umschulung der kranken ehemaligen Deportierten in Frankreich [Vocational training of sick former deportees in France]. In: Fichez, Louis F. (Ed.), *Andere Spätfolgen, auf Grund der Beobachtungen bei den ehemaligen Deportierten und Internierten der nazistischen Gefangnisse und Vernichtungslager* [Other Belated Consequences, Based on the Observations of Former Deportees and Internees of Nazi Prisons and Death Camps]. Wien: Verlag der FIR, pp. 219-227.

411 Desoille, Henri (1961). Hygiene und Diätetik für ehemalige Deportierte [Hygiene and diet for former deportees]. In: *Die Behandlung der Asthenie und der vorzeitigen Vergreisung bei ehemaligen Widerstandskämpfern und KZ-Häftlingen* [Treatment of Asthenics and Premature Aging in Former Resistance Fighters and Concentration Camp Inmates]. Wien: Verlag der FIR, pp. 241-244. [III Internationale Medizinisch Konferenz. Liege, 17-19 März 1961].

412 Des Pres, Terrence (1971). The survivors: On the ethos of survival in extremity. *Encounter*, 37(2), 3-19.

413 Des Pres, Terrence (1973). Survivors and the will to bear witness. *Social Research*, 40(4), 668-690.

414 Des Pres, Terrence (1976). *The Survivor: An Anatomy of Life in the Death Camps*. New York: Oxford University Press. 218 pp.

415 Des Pres, Terrence (1976). Victims and survivors. *Dissent*, 23(1), 49-56.

416 Des Pres, Terrence (1979). The Bettelheim problem. *Social Research*, 46(4), 619-647.

417 Des Pres, Terrence (1979). The lesson of Treblinka. *Quest*, 3, 15-18.

418 de Swaan, A. (1981). The survivor's syndrome: Private problems and social repression. In: *Israel-Netherlands Symposium on the Impact of Persecution. Dalfsen, Amsterdam, 14-18 April 1980*. Rijswijk, The Netherlands: Ministry of Cultural Affairs, Recreation and Social Welfare, pp. 85-94.

419 de Swaan, A. (1983). Het concentratiekampsyndroom als sociaal probleem [The concentration camp syndrome as a social problem]. In: de Swaan, A. (Ed.), *De Mens Is De Mens Een Zorg, Opstellen, 1971-1981* [The Human Being as a Caregiver, Summary, 1971-1981]. Amsterdam: Meulenhoff, pp. 140-150.

420 de Swaan, A. (1984). De maatschappelijke verwerking van oorlogsverledens [The social working through of war experiences]. In: Dane, Jan (Ed.), *Keerzijde van de bevrijding: Opstellen over de maatschappelijke, psycho-sociale en medische aspekten van de problematiek van oorlogsgetroffenen* [The Opposite Side of Liberation: Essays on the Social, Psychosocial and Medical Aspects of the Problems of War Victims]. Deventer: Van Loghum Slaterus, pp. 54-66.

421 Deutsch, Leon (1995). *The Survivor Syndrome: Medical and Psychological Consequences of the Holocaust*. Toronto, ECW.

422 Deveen, Walter (1955). Die rheumatischen Erkrankungen bei den ehemaligen Deportierten [Rheumatic illness in former deportees]. In: Michel, Max (Ed.), *Gesundheitsschäden durch Verfolgung und Gefangenschaft und ihre Spätfolgen: Zusammenstellung der Referate und Ergebnisse der Internationalen Sozialmedizinischen Konferenz* *über die Pathologie der Ehemaligen Deportierten und Internierten, 5-7 Juni 1954 in Kopenhagen* [Health Damages Caused by Persecution and Internment and the Late Effects: Compilation of the Papers and Results of the International Conference of Social Medicine on the Pathology of Former Deported and Interned Persons, 5-7 June 1954 in Copenhagen]. Frankfurt am Main: Röderberg, pp. 198-208.

423 Deveen, Walter (1961). Rheumatism and deportation. In: *International Conference on the Later Effects of Imprisonment and Deportation Organized by the World Veterans Federation. The Hague, November 20-25, 1961*. The Hague: World Veterans Federation, pp. 79-82.

424 Deveen, Walter (1964). Ätio-pathogenese und Therapie der Erschöpfung und vorzeitigen vergreisung [The aetiology and therapy due to exhaustion and premature aging]. In: *Ätio-Pathogenese und Therapie der Erschöpfung und vorzeitigen Vergreisung* [The Aetiology and Therapy Due to Exhaustion and Premature Aging]. Wien: Verlag der FIR, pp. 581-597. [IV Internationaler Medizinischer Kongress. Bucharest, 22-27 Juni 1964].

425 Devoto, Andrea; Buffulin, A.; and Martini, Massimo (1983). Ergebnisse einer psychologischen Analyse, durchgeführt an einer Gruppe ehemaliger Italienischer KZ-Häftlinge [Results of a psychological analysis of a group of former Italian concentration camp inmates]. *Cahiers d'Information Médicales, Sociales et Juridiques*, 19, 67-69.

426 Devoto, Andrea, and Martini, Massimo (1984). Aspetti psicologici e psicopatologici nei superstiti dei lager naziti [On the psychological and psychopathological effects on Nazi camp survivors]. *Rivista Sperimentale di Freniatria e Medicina Legale delle Alienazioni Mentali*, 108(2), 332-354.

427 de Vries, E.J. (1949). *The History of Resistance by Physicians in the Netherlands*. Haarlem, The Netherlands: Tjeenk Williuk.

428 de Vries, E.J. (1981). Social work in connection with "ways of relating to the traumatized-persecuted." In: *Israel-Netherlands Symposium on the Impact of Persecution. Dalfsen, Amsterdam, 14-18 April 1980*. Rijswijk, The Netherlands: Ministry of Cultural Affairs, Recreation and Social Welfare, pp. 72-76.

429 de Vries, E.J. (1984). Relatie tussen de materiele en immateriele aspekten bij de hulpverlening aan oorlogsgetruffenen [Relationship between material and intangible aspects of assistance to war victims]. *ICODO Info*, 1(1), 6-15.

430 de Wind, Eddy (1966). Directe en late gevolgen van extreme belastingssituaties: Het concentratiekamp [Direct and late sequelae of extreme stress: The concentration camp]. *Maandblad voor de Geestelijk Volksgezondheid*, 21, 287-300.

431 de Wind, Eddy (1968). Begegnung mit dem tod [Encounter with death]. *Psyche: Zeitschrift für Psychoanalyse und ihre Anwendungen*, 22, 423-441.

432 de Wind, Eddy (1968). The confrontation with death. *Psychoanalytic Quarterly*, 37(2), 322-324.

433 de Wind, Eddy (1971). Psychotherapy after traumatization caused by persecution. In: Krystal, Henry, and Niederland, William G. (Eds.), *Psychic Traumatization: Aftereffects in Individuals and Communities*. Boston, MA: Little, Brown, pp. 93-111.

434 de Wind, Eddy (1972). Persecution, aggression and therapy. *International Journal of Psycho-Analysis*, 53(2), 173-177.

435 de Wind, Eddy (1982). Psychoanalytische behandeling van ernstig getraumatiseerden (door vervolging en verzet) [Psychoanalytic treatment of patients severely traumatized by persecution and in the resistance]. *Tijdschrift Psychotherapie*, 8(3), 143-155.

436 de Wind, Eddy (1984). Some implications of former massive traumatization upon the actual analytic process. *International Review of Psycho-Analysis*, 65(3), 273-281.

437 de Wind, Eddy (1986). Psychische und soziale Faktoren der traumatisierung durch Krieg und Verfolgung [Psychic and social factors in traumatization through war and persecution]. *Psychosozial*, 9, 43-52.

438 de Wind, Eddy (1987). De tweede generatie: Stigma of psychische realiteit? [The second generation: Stigmatization or psychic reality?]. *Psychoanalytic Forum*, 5, 47-64.

439 de Wind, Eddy (1995). Encounter with death. In: Groen-Prakken, Han; Ladan, Antonie; and Stufkens, Antonius (Eds.), *The Dutch Annual of Psychoanalysis: 1995-1996. Vol. 2: Traumatisation and War*. Amsterdam: Swets & Zeitlinger, pp. 25-39.

440 Dickhaut, H.H. (1959). Zur Frage der Dauerschäden nach Fleckfieberenzephalitis [The problem of permanent damage after

typhus encephalitis]. *Fortschritte der Neurologie, Psychiatrie*, 27, 20-32.

441 Dickhaut, H.H. (1971). Dauerschäden nach Fleckfieber-Encephalitis [Permanent disturbances after typhus encephalitis]. In: Herberg, Hans-Joachim (Ed.), *Spätschäden nach Extrembelastungen* [Late Damage After Extreme Stress]. Herford: Nicolai, pp. 200-202. [II Internationalen Medizinisch-Juristischen Konferenz. Dusseldorf, 1969].

442 Dicks, Henry V. (1972). *Licensed Mass Murder: A Socio-Psychological Study of Some SS Killers*. New York: Basic Books. 283 pp.

443 Diem, R. (1988). Wspomnienia lekarza więźnia z Oświęcimia [Reminiscences of a physician-prisoner from Auschwitz]. *Przegląd Lekarski*, 45(1), 134-147.

444 Dietrich, David R., and Shabad, Peter C. (Eds.) (1989). *The Problem of Loss and Mourning: Psychoanalytic Perspectives*. Madison, CT: International Universities Press. 499 pp.

445 Dietrich, Donald (1994). Nazi eugenics: Adaptation and resistance among German Catholic intellectual leaders. In: Michalczyk, John J. (Ed.), *Medicine, Ethics, and the Third Reich: Historical and Contemporary Issues*. Kansas City, MO: Sheed & Ward, pp. 50-63.

446 Dietze, A. (1967). Begutachtung und Beurteilung von Leberschäden nach extremen Lebensverhaltnissen [Examination and evaluation of liver damage after extreme life situations]. In: Herberg, Hans-Joachim (Ed.), *Die Beurteilung von Gesundheitsschäden nach Gefangenschaft und Verfolgung* [The Assessment of Health Damages Following Internment and Persecution]. Herford: Nicolai, pp. 114-120. [Internationalen Medizinisch-Juristischen Symposiums in Köln].

447 Dietze, A. (1978). Katamnestische Untersuchungen bei Leberkrankheiten ehemaliger Gefangener [Catamnestic examinations in former prisoners with liver diseases]. In: *Medizinische Untersuchungen der Spätfolgen des Krieges und des NS-Regimes bei Jugendlichen und Kindern von ehemaligen KZ-Häftlingen und Verfolgten* [Medical Research of the Late Effects of the War and National Socialism Regime on Youth and Children of Former Concentration Camp Inmates and Persecuted Persons]. Wien: Internationale Föderation der Widerstandskämpfer. [VI Internationaler Medizinischer Kongress der FIR. Prague, 1976].

448 Dimant, Jiri (1965). Some comments on the psychology of life in the ghetto Terezin. In: Ehrmann, Frantisek (Ed.), *Terezin*. Prague: Council of Jewish Communities in the Czech Lands, pp. 125-139.

449 Dimsdale, Joel E. (1974). The coping behavior of Nazi concentration camp survivors. *American Journal of Psychiatry*, 131(7), 792-797.

450 Dimsdale, Joel E. (1978). Coping: Every man's war. *American Journal of Psychotherapy*, 32(3), 402-413.

451 Dimsdale, Joel E. (Ed.) (1980). *Survivors, Victims and Perpetrators: Essays on the Nazi Holocaust*. Washington, D.C.: Hemisphere. 474 pp.

452 Dimsdale, Joel E. (1980). The coping behavior of Nazi concentration camp survivors. In: Dimsdale, Joel E. (Ed.), *Survivors, Victims and Perpetrators: Essays on the Nazi Holocaust*. Washington, D.C.: Hemisphere, pp. 163-174.

453 Dobre, M.; Ciuca, A.; and Jordana, B. (1978). Les aspects psychologiques du vieillissement chez un groupe d'anciens combattants antifascistes [Psychological aspects of aging in a group of former antifascist fighters]. In: *Medizinische Untersuchungen der Spätfolgen des Krieges und des NS-Regimes bei Jugendlichen und Kindern von ehemaligen KZ-Häftlingen und Verfolgten* [Medical Research of the Late Effects of the War and National Socialism Regime on Youth and Children of Former Concentration Camp Inmates and Persecuted Persons]. Wien: Internationale Föderation der Widerstandskämpfer. [VI Internationaler Medizinischer Kongress der FIR. Prague, 1976].

454 Dobrowolski, L. (1978). Les résultats des examens médicaux de nombreux groupes d'anciens prisonniers Hitleriens [Results of medical examinations of numerous groups of former Hitler-prisoners]. In: *Medizinische Untersuchungen der Spätfolgen des Krieges und des NS-Regimes bei Jugendlichen und Kindern von ehemaligen KZ-Häftlingen und Verfolgten* [Medical Research of the Late Effects of the War and National Socialism Regime on Youth and Children of Former Concentration Camp Inmates and Persecuted Persons]. Wien: Internationale Föderation der Widerstandskämpfer. [VI Internationaler Medizinischer Kongress der FIR. Prague, 1976].

455 Dominik, Małgorzata (1967). Sytuacja zdrowotna I bytowa byłych więźniów oświecimskich w świetle ankiety [The health and social situation of ex-prisoners from Auschwitz - Results of a survey]. *Przegląd Lekarski*, 24(1), 102-104.

456 Dominik, Małgorzata (1971). Prisoners respond to the questionnaire. In: *Auschwitz Anthology. Vol. 3: It Did Not End in Forty-Five. Part 1*. Warsaw: International Auschwitz Committee, pp. 76-93.

457 Dominik, Małgorzata (1979). Potomstwo w niektórych rodzinach byłych wieźniów hitlerowskich obozów koncentracyjnych [The children of some families of former prisoners of Hitlerian concentration camps]. *Przegląd Lekarski*, 36(1), 25-38.

458 Dominik, Małgorzata (1987). Die Kinder von 50 ehemaliger KZ-Häftlinge [The children of 50 former concentration camp inmates]. In: Hamburger Institut für Sozialforschung (Eds.), *Die Auschwitz-Hefte. Texte der polnischen Zeitschrift "Przegląd Lekarski" über historische, psychische und medizinische Aspekte des Lebens und Sterbens in Auschwitz. Band 2* [The Auschwitz Journal. Text of the Polish Journal "Medical Review" on Historical, Psychic and Medical Aspects of Life and Death in Auschwitz. Volume 2]. Weinheim und Basel: Beltz, pp. 97-111.

459 Dominik, Małgorzata, and Teutsch, Aleksander (1978). Nerwice u potomstwa byłych więzniów obozów koncentracyjnych [Neuroses among the children of ex-concentration camp prisoners]. *Przegląd Lekarski*, 35(1), 16-20.

460 Dominik, Małgorzata, and Teutsch, Aleksander (1978). Neurosen bei der Nachkommenschaft ehemaliger Konzentrationslagerhäftlinge [Neuroses among the children of ex-concentration camp prisoners]. *Mitteilungen der FIR*, 15, 9-19.

461 Donnay, J.M.; Dethienne, F.; and Meyers, C. (1975). Incidence des facteurs traumatisants de la captivitée sur la morbidité somatique et psychiatrique de l'ancien prisonnier de guerre [The incidence of traumatizing factors during captivity on the somatic and psychiatric morbidity of ex-prisoners of war]. *Acta Psychiatrica Belgica*, 75, 33-48.

462 Doring, E. (1983). Die Bedeutung der gesellschaftlichen Verhältnisse für eine günstige Beeinflussung der Haftspätschäden [The meaning of social relations for a favorable influence on the sequelae of imprisonment]. *Cahiers d'Information Médicales, Sociales et Juridiques*, 19, 70-73.

463 Döring, Gerd K. (1963). Spezifische Spätschäden der weiblichen Psyche durch die politische Verfolgung [Specific late damage to the feminine psyche through political persecution]. In: Paul, Helmut, and Herberg, Hans-Joachim (Eds.), *Psychische Spätschäden nach*

Politischer Verfolgung [Psychological Late Damages Following Political Persecution]. Basel: Karger, pp. 155-168.

464 Dorner, Klaus (1983). Psychiatric management in the "Third Reich" and now. *Sozialpsychiatrische Informationen*, 13, 102-108.

465 Dor-Shav, Netta Kohn (1978). On the long range effects of concentration camp internment on Nazi victims: 25 years later. *Journal of Consulting and Clinical Psychology*, 46(1), 1-11.

466 Dreifuss, Gustav S. (1980). Psychotherapy of Nazi victims. *Psychotherapy and Psychosomatics*, 34(1), 40-44.

467 Dreifuss, Gustav S. (1981). Analisi dei superstiti dell'Olocausto [Analysis of Holocaust survivors]. *Rivista di Psicologia Analitica*, 12(23), 53-59.

468 Dreifuss, Gustav S. (1991). The analyst and the damaged victims of Nazi persecution. In: Samuels, Andrew (Ed.), *Psychopathology: Contemporary Jungian Perspectives*. New York: Guilford, pp. 309-326.

469 Dreyfus-Moreau, J. (1952). Étude structurale de deux cas de névrose concentrationnaire [Structural study of two cases of neurosis in concentration camp inmates]. *L'Evolution Psychiatrique*, 1, 201-220.

470 Drobniewski, Francis (1993). Why did Nazi doctors break their "Hippocratic" oaths? *Journal of the Royal Society of Medicine*, 86(9), 541-543.

471 Drohocki, Zenon (1975). Wstrząsy elektryczne w rewirze monowickim [Electroshock treatment in the Monowitz sick bay]. *Przegląd Lekarski*, 32(1), 162-166.

472 Dubiel, Antoni (1970). Ze wspomnień chorego więźnia Neu Sustrum i Gusen [Recollections of a sick prisoner of the Neu Sustrum and Gusen concentration camp]. *Przegląd Lekarski*, 26(1), 216-219.

473 Dubrow-Eichel, Linda (1993). *Marital relationships of children of Holocaust survivors*. Unpublished doctoral dissertation, University of Pennsylvania, Philadelphia, 251 pp. *Dissertation Abstracts International*, 53(11-A), p. 3800. (University Microfilms no. AAC 9227652).

474 Durst, Natan (1995). Child survivors: A child survivor ... and then what? In: Lemberger, John (Ed.), *A Global Perspective on Working* *with Holocaust Survivors and the Second Generation*. Jerusalem: JDC-Brookdale Institute of Gerontology and Human Development, AMCHA, and JDC-Israel, pp. 289-303.

475 Dux, Heinz (1983). A discussion on the legal aspects of Nazi psychiatry. *Sozialpsychiatrische Informationen*, 13, 81-90.

476 Dvorjetski, Marc (1953). Hameri harefui hayehudi v'harefua haposha'at hanatzit bitkufat hashoa [The Jewish medical rebellion and the criminal Nazi medicine during the Holocaust]. *Niv Harofeh*, 9-10, 1-15

477 Dvorjetski, Marc (1960). Tuberculosis among Jewish immigrants to Israel. In: *Experts Meeting on the Later Effects of Imprisonment and Deportation, Oslo*. Paris: World Veterans Federation, pp. 61-66.

478 Dvorjetski, Marc (1960). Biological and pathological problems of camp survivors in Israel. In: *Experts Meeting on the Later Effects of Imprisonment and Deportation, Oslo*. Paris: World Veterans Federation, pp. 89-97.

479 Dvorjetski, Marc (1960). Biological and sociological problems of camp survivor immigrants in Israel. In: *Experts Meeting on the Later Effects of Imprisonment and Deportation, Oslo*. Paris: World Veterans Federation, pp. 107-129.

480 Dvorjetski, Marc (1961). Cardiac pathology among Jewish internees in camps and ghettos and cardiac sequelae among Jewish survivors. In: *International Conference on the Later Effects of Imprisonment and Deportation Organized by the World Veterans Federation. The Hague, November 20-25, 1961*. The Hague: World Veterans Federation, pp. 39-52.

481 Dvorjetski, Marc (1961). Integration into the working population and vocational rehabilitation of former deportees in Israel. In: *International Conference on the Later Effects of Imprisonment and Deportation Organized by the World Veterans Federation. The Hague, November 20-25, 1961*. The Hague: World Veterans Federation, pp. 150-157.

482 Dwork, Deborah (1991). *Children with a Star: Jewish Youth in Nazi Europe*. New Haven, CT: Yale University Press. 354 pp.

483 Dyner, E. (1978). Specificité multisyndromique des maladies des anciens déportés [The specificity of multisyndrome diseases in formerly deported persons]. In: *Medizinische Untersuchungen der Spätfolgen des Krieges und des NS-Regimes bei Jugendlichen und Kindern von ehemaligen KZ-Häftlingen und Verfolgten* [Medical Research of the Late Effects of the War and National Socialism Regime on Youth and Children of Former Concentration Camp Inmates and Persecuted Persons]. Wien: Internationale Föderation der Widerstandskämpfer. [VI Internationaler Medizinischer Kongress der FIR. Prague, 1976].

484 Dyner, E., and Głowacki, Czesław (1978). Évaluation de l'état de santé actuel des anciens déportés, faite sur la base des examens medicaux poursuivis dans plusieurs milieux de Varsovie [Evaluation of the present state of health of former deportees on the basis of medical follow-up examinations in several districts of Warsaw]. In: *Medizinische Untersuchungen der Spätfolgen des Krieges und des NS-Regimes bei Jugendlichen und Kindern von ehemaligen KZ-Häftlingen und Verfolgten* [Medical Research of the Late Effects of the War and National Socialism Regime on Youth and Children of Former Concentration Camp Inmates and Persecuted Persons]. Wien: Internationale Föderation der Widerstandskämpfer. [VI Internationaler Medizinischer Kongress der FIR. Prague, 1976].

485 Dziaduś, Stanisław (1969). "Hirschberg" i "Treskau" podobozy Gross-Rosen. Urywki wspomnień ["Hirschberg" and "Treskau" branches of the Gross-Rosen concentration camp: Excerpts from the memoirs]. *Przegląd Lekarski*, 25(1), 138-145.

486 Dziaduś, Stanisław (1970). Z kompani karnej w Gross-Rosen [The penal company at the Gross-Rosen concentration camp]. *Przegląd Lekarski*, 26(1), 223-228.

487 Dziaduś, Stanisław (1975). W Saurer-Werke przed oswobodzeniem [The Saurer-Werke camp before liberation]. *PrzeglądLekarski*, 32(1), 178-182.

488 Eaton, William W.; Sigal, John J.; and Weinfeld, Morton (1982). Impairment in Holocaust survivors after 33 years: Data from an unbiased community sample. *American Journal of Psychiatry*, 139(6), 773-777.

489 Eaton, William W.; Sigal, John J.; and Weinfeld, Morton (1982). Psychiatric status of Holocaust survivors: Reply to Niederland. *American Journal of Psychiatry*, 139(6), 1647-1648.

490 Eckstaedt, Anita (1981). Eine klinische Studie zum Begriff der Traumareaktion, ein Kindheitsschicksal aus der Kriegszeit [A clinical study for the understanding of the reaction to trauma, a child's fate as a consequence of the war]. *Psyche: Zeitschrift für Psychoanalyse und ihre Anwendungen*, 35(7), 600-610.

491 Edel, E. (1973). Kausalitätsnachweis bei Begutachtung von Gesundheitsschäden infolge politischer Verfolgung [Probing causality in the evaluation of health damage as a result of political persecution]. In: *Ermüdung und vorzeitiges Altern: Folge von Extrembelastungen* [Exhaustion and Premature Aging: Result of Extreme Stress]. Leipzig: Barth, pp. 308-314. [V Internationaler Medizinischer Kongress der FIR. Paris, 21-24 September 1961].

492 Edel, E. (1978). Zur Problematik der Behandlungsfähigkeit der zweiten Generation [On the problems of treatment possibility in the second generation]. In: *Medizinische Untersuchungen der Spätfolgen des Krieges und des NS-Regimes bei Jugendlichen und Kindern von ehemaligen KZ-Häftlingen und Verfolgten* [Medical Research of the Late Effects of the War and National Socialism Regime on Youth and Children of Former Concentration Camp Inmates and Persecuted Persons]. Wien: Internationale Föderation der Widerstandskämpfer. [VI Internationaler Medizinischer Kongress der FIR. Prague, 1976].

493 Edelstein, Eliezer L. (1982). Reactivation of concentration camp experiences as a result of hospitalization. In: Spielberger, Charles D.; Sarason, Irwin G.; and Milgram, Norman (Eds.), *Stress and Anxiety. Vol. 8*. Washington, D.C.: Hemisphere, pp. 401-404.

494 Edwards, Richard W. (1989). The relation of the Holocaust to bioethics. *Wisconsin Medical Journal*, 88(11), 12-13.

495 Ehrlich, Phyllis (1988). Treatment issues in the psychotherapy of Holocaust survivors. In: Wilson, John P.; Harel, Zev; and Kahana, Boaz (Eds.), *Human Adaptation to Extreme Stress: From the Holocaust to Vietnam*. New York: Plenum, pp. 285-303.

496 Eickhoff, Friedrich-Willhelm (1986). Über das "entlehnte unbewusste Schuldgefuhl" als transgenerationellen Ubermittler missgluckter Trauer [A short note "on derived unconscious guilt feeling" as transgenerational transmitter of mismanaged grief]. *Sigmund Freud House Bulletin*, 10(2), 14-20.

497 Eickhoff, Friedrich-Willhelm (1989). On the "borrowed unconsciousness sense of guilt" and the palimpsestic structure of a symptom: Afterthoughts of the Hamburg Congress of the IPA. *International Review of Psycho-Analysis*, 16(3), 323-329.

498 Eisen, George (1988). *Children and Play in the Holocaust: Games Among the Shadows*. Amherst, MA: University of Massachusetts Press. 153 pp.

499 Eissler, Kurt R. (1960). Variationen in der psychoanalytischen Technique [Variations in psychoanalytic technique]. *Psychiatry*, 13, 609-624.

500 Eissler, Kurt R. (1963). Die Ermordung von wievielen seiner Kinder muss ein Mensch symptomfrei ertragen können, um eine normale Konstitution zu haben? [The murder of how many of his children must a person be able to endure symptom-free in order to have a normal constitution?]. *Psyche: Zeitschrift für Psychoanalyse und ihre Anwendungen*, 17, 241-291.

501 Eissler, Kurt R. (1967). Perverted psychiatry? *American Journal of Psychiatry*, 123(11), 1352-1358.

502 Eissler, Kurt R. (1968). Weitere Bemerkungen zum Problem der KZ Psychologie. Diskussion des Vortrages von Dr. Eddy de Wind [Additional comments on the problem of the concentration camp psychology. Discussion of the lecture by Dr. Eddie de Wind]. *Psyche: Zeitschrift für Psychoanalyse und ihre Anwendungen*, 22, 452-463.

503 Eitinger, Leo (1945). Sykehusbehandlingen i konsentrasjonsleiren Auschwitz [Hospital treatment in Auschwitz concentration camp]. *Tidsskrift for den Norske Laegeforening. Journal of the Norwegian Medical Association*, 65, 159-161.

504 Eitinger, Leo (1958). *Psykiatriske undersokelser blant flyktninger i Norge* [Psychiatric Investigations Among Refugees in Norway]. Oslo: Universitetsforlaget. 276 pp.

505 Eitinger, Leo (1960). A clinical and social psychiatric investigation of a "hard-core" refugee transport in Norway. *International Journal of Social Psychiatry*, 5(4), 261-275.

506 Eitinger, Leo (1960). Psychiatric delayed effects of internment in concentration camps. In: *Experts Meeting on the Late Effects of Imprisonment and Deportation, Oslo*. Paris: World Veterans Federation, pp. 55-66.

507 Eitinger, Leo (1960). The symptomatology of mental disease among refugees in Norway. *Journal of Mental Science*, 106, 947-966.

508 Eitinger, Leo (1961). Pathology of the concentration camp syndrome. *Archives of General Psychiatry*, 5, 371-379.

509 Eitinger, Leo (1961). Study of a group of former Norwegian deportees. Part 2: Psychiatric post-conditions in former concentration camp inmates. In: *International Conference on the Later Effects of Imprisonment and Deportation Organized by the World Veterans Federation. The Hague, November 20-25, 1961*. The Hague: World Veterans Federation, pp. 83-88.

510 Eitinger, Leo (1962). Concentration camp survivors in the post-war world. *American Journal of Orthopsychiatry*, 32(3), 367-375.

511 Eitinger, Leo (1962). Refugees and concentration camp survivors in Norway. *Israel Journal of Medical Sciences*, 21(1-2), 21-27.

512 Eitinger, Leo (1963). Preliminary notes on a study of concentration camp survivors in Norway. *Israel Annals of Psychiatry and Related Disciplines*, 1(1), 59-67.

513 Eitinger, Leo (1964). Tidligere konsentrasjonsleirfanger i Norge og i Israel [Former concentration camp inmates in Norway and Israel]. *Nordisk Medicin*, 72, 1207-1212.

514 Eitinger, Leo (1965). Der Parrallelismus zwischen dem KZ Syndrom und der chronischen Anorexia Nervosa [The parallelism of the concentration camp syndrome and chronic anorexia nervosa]. In: Meyer, Joachim-Ernst, and Feldmann, Harold (Eds.), *Anorexia Nervosa, Symposium am 24./25. April 1965 in Gottingen*. Stuttgart: Georg Thieme, pp. 118-122.

515 Eitinger, Leo (1966). Concentration camp survivors in Norway and Israel. In: David, Henry P. (Ed.), *Migration, Mental Health and Community Services: Proceedings of a Conference Convened By the American Joint Distribution Committee, Co-Sponsored By the World Federation for Mental Health, and Held in Geneva, Switzerland, November 28-30, 1966*. Geneva: American Joint Distribution Committee, pp. 14-22.

516 Eitinger, Leo (1966). The late effects of chronic excessive stress on two different population groups. In: Lopez Ibor, Juan J. (Ed.), *Proceedings. Fourth World Congress of Psychiatry, Madrid, 5-11 September 1966*. Amsterdam: Excerpta Medica Foundation, pp. 912-917.

517 Eitinger, Leo (1967). Schizophrenia among concentration camp survivors. *International Journal of Psychiatry in Medicine*, 3, 403-406.

518 Eitinger, Leo (1968). Attforingsproblemer hos tidliger konsentrasjonsleirfanger [Rehabilitation problems in ex-prisoners]. *Samtiden*, 53, 518-525.

519 Eitinger, Leo (1969). Anxiety in concentration camp survivors. *Australian and New Zealand Journal of Psychiatry*, 3, 348-351.

520 Eitinger, Leo (1969). Psychosomatic problems in concentration camp survivors. *Journal of Psychosomatic Research*, 13(2), 183-189.

521 Eitinger, Leo (1969). Rehabilitation of concentration camp survivors (following concentration camp trauma). *Psychotherapy and Psychosomatics*, 17, 42-49.

522 Eitinger, Leo (1970). Syndrom koncentračních taborů. Byvali norstí vězni německych koncentračnich taborů [The concentration camp syndrome - former Norwegian concentration camp prisoners]. *Ceskoslovenska Psychiatrie*, 66, 257-266.

523 Eitinger, Leo (1971). Acute and chronic psychiatric and psychosomatic reactions in concentration camp survivors. In: Levi, Lennart (Ed.), *Society, Stress and Disease. Vol. 1*. New York: Oxford University Press, pp. 219-230.

524 Eitinger, Leo (1971). Organic and psychosomatic aftereffects of concentration camp imprisonment. In: Krystal, Henry, and Niederland, William G. (Eds.), *Psychic Traumatization: Aftereffects in Individuals and Communities*. Boston, MA: Little, Brown, pp. 205-215.

525 Eitinger, Leo (1971). Psychiatrische Untersuchungsergebnisse bei KZ-überlebenden [Results of psychiatric examinations in survivors of concentration camps]. In: Herberg, Hans-Joachim (Ed.), *Spätschäden nach Extrembelastungen* [Late Damage After Extreme Stress]. Herford: Nicolai, pp. 144-152. [II Internationalen Medizinisch-Juristischen Konferenz. Dusseldorf, 1969].

526 Eitinger, Leo (1972). *Concentration Camp Survivors in Norway and Israel*. The Hague: Martinus Nijhoff. 199 pp.

527 Eitinger, Leo (1973). A follow-up study of the Norwegian concentration camp survivors' mortality and morbidity. *Israel Annals of Psychiatry and Related Disciplines*, 11(2), 199-209.

528 Eitinger, Leo (1973). Late effects of imprisonment in concentration camps during World War II. In: *Physical and Mental Consequences of Imprisonment and Torture: Lectures Presented at the Conference at Lysebu Near Oslo, October 5-7 1973*. London: Amnesty International, pp. 90-113.

529 Eitinger, Leo (1973). Umrtnost a nemocnost po excesivnim stressu [Mortality and morbidity after excessive stress]. *Ceskoslovenska Psychiatrie*, 69, 209-218.

530 Eitinger, Leo (1974). Coping with aggression. *Mental Health and Society*, 1, 297-301.

531 Eitinger, Leo (1975). Jewish concentration camp survivors in Norway. *Israel Annals of Psychiatry and Related Disciplines*, 13(4), 321-334.

532 Eitinger, Leo (1978). On being a psychiatrist and a survivor. In: Rosenfeld, Alvin H., and Greenberg, Irving (Eds.), *Confronting the Holocaust: The Impact of Elie Wiesel*. Bloomington, IN: Indiana University Press, pp. 186-230.

533 Eitinger, Leo (1980). The concentration camp syndrome and its late sequelae. In: Dimsdale, Joel E. (Ed.), *Survivors, Victims and Perpetrators: Essays on the Nazi Holocaust*. Washington, D.C.: Hemisphere, pp. 127-160.

534 Eitinger, Leo (1980). Jewish concentration camp survivors in the post-war world. *Danish Medical Bulletin*, 27(5), 224-228.

535 Eitinger, Leo (1981). Denial in concentration camps. *Nordisk Psykiatrisk Tidsskrift*, 5, 148-156.

536 Eitinger, Leo (1981). Studies on concentration camp survivors: The Norwegian and global contexts. *Journal of Psychology and Judaism*, 6(1), 23-32.

537 Eitinger, Leo (1982). Den medicinsk-psykiatrske litteraturen om "spätschäden" [The medical-psychiatric literature on compensation]. *Nordisk Judaistik. Scandinavian Jewish Studies*, 4, 2-10.

538 Eitinger, Leo (1983). Jewish concentration camp survivors. In: Ayalon, Ofra; Eitinger, Leo; Lansen, Johan; and Sunier, Armand; and others, *The Holocaust and its Perseverance: Stress, Coping and Disorder*. Assen, The Netherlands: Van Gorcum, pp. 4-16.

539 Eitinger, Leo (1984). Experiences in war and during catastrophes and their effects upon the human mind. *Journal of the Oslo City Hospital*, 34(9), 75-83.

540 Eitinger, Leo (1985). The concentration camp syndrome: An organic brain syndrome? *Integrative Psychiatry*, 3(2), 115-119.

541 Eitinger, Leo (1986). Posttraumatiske stresstilstander og medisinske erstatningssporsmal [Post-traumatic stress and medical questions related to compensation]. *Tiddskrift for den Norske Laegeforening. Journal of the Norwegian Medical Association*, 106(27), 2228-2239.

542 Eitinger, Leo (1990). KZ-Haft und psychische Traumatisierung [Concentration camp captivity and psychic traumatization]. *Psyche: Zeitschrift für Psychoanalyse und ihre Anwendungen*, 44(2), 118-132.

543 Eitinger, Leo (1990). Survivors of ghettos and camps. In: Gutman, Israel (Ed.), *Encyclopedia of the Holocaust. Vol. 4*. New York: Macmillan, pp. 1428-1431.

544 Eitinger, Leo (1990). World War II in Norwegian psychiatric literature. In: Lundeberg, Jan-Erik; Otto, Ulf; and Rubeck, Bo (Eds.), *Wartime Medical Services: Second International Conference. Stockholm, Sweden, 25-29 June 1990: Proceedings*. Stockholm, Sweden: Forsvarets forskningsanstalt, pp. 364-478.

545 Eitinger, Leo (1991). Psykiske senproblemer etter konsentrasjonsleir opphold [Late psychological problems after concentration camp incarceration]. *Nordisk Medicin*, 106(4), 132-136.

546 Eitinger, Leo (1992). Identification, treatment and care of the aging Holocaust survivor: A keynote address. In: Kenigsberg, Rositta E., and Lieblich, Cathy M. (Eds.), *The First National Conference on Identification, Treatment and Care of the Aging Holocaust Survivor, March 29-31, 1992: Selected Proceedings*. Miami, FL: Holocaust Documentation and Education Center and Southeast Florida Center on Aging, Florida International University, pp. 5-12.

547 Eitinger, Leo (1992). Aging Holocaust survivors and Alzheimer's Disease. In: Kenigsberg, Rositta E., and Lieblich, Cathy M. (Eds.), *The First National Conference on Identification, Treatment and Care of the Aging Holocaust Survivor, March 29-31, 1992: Selected Proceedings*. Miami, FL: Holocaust Documentation and Education Center and Southeast Florida Center on Aging, Florida International University, pp. 32-36.

548 Eitinger, Leo (1993). The aging Holocaust survivor. *Echoes of the Holocaust*, 2, 5-12. [Bulletin of the Jerusalem Center for Research into the Late Effects of the Holocaust. Talbieh Mental Health Center, Jerusalem, Israel].

549 Eitinger, Leo (1994). Auschwitz: A psychological perspective. In: Gutman, Israel and Berenbaum, Michael (Eds.), *Anatomy of the Auschwitz Death Camp*. Bloomington, IN: Indiana University Press, pp. 469-482.

550 Eitinger, Leo (1994). Manskliga rattigheter och lakares identitet. Paverka krolleger som handlar oetiskt [Human rights and physician's identity: Warn your colleagues who are acting unethically]. *Lakartidningen*, 91(22), 2251-2254.

551 Eitinger, Leo, and Askevold, Finn (1968). Psychiatric aspects. In: Strøm, Axel (Ed.), *Norwegian Concentration Camp Survivors*. Oslo, Universitetsforlaget, and New York: Humanities Press, pp. 45-84.

552 Eitinger, Leo, and Krell, Robert (1985). *The Psychological and Medical Effects of Concentration Camps and Related Persecutions on Survivors of the Holocaust: A Research Bibliography*. Vancouver, BC: University of British Columbia Press. 168 pp.

553 Eitinger, Leo, and Major, Ellinor F. (1993). Stress of the Holocaust. In: Goldberger, Leo, and Breznitz, Shlomo (Eds.), *Handbook of Stress: Theoretical and Clinical Aspects. 2nd ed.* New York: Free Press, pp. 617-640.

554 Eitinger, Leo, and Rieck, Miriam (1981). *Bibliographical Collection of Literature Concerning Medical and Psychological Sequelae to Concentration Camp Imprisonment*. Haifa, Israel: Haifa University, Ray D. Wolfe Centre for Study of Psychological Stress.

555 Eitinger, Leo, and Strøm, Axel (1973). *Mortality and Morbidity after Excessive Stress: A Follow-Up Investigation of Norwegian Concentration Camp Survivors*. Oslo: Universitetsforlaget, and New York: Humanities Press. 153 pp.

556 Eitinger, Leo, and Strøm, Axel (1981). New investigations on the mortality and morbidity of Norwegian ex-concentration camp prisoners. *Israel Journal of Psychiatry and Related Sciences*, 18(3), 173-195.

557 Eizenberg, Krina (1982). *Olamom hachevrati shel banim l'horim nitzoley shoah arachim v'emunot b'tfisat yachasim beyn ish'im* [The social world of the second generation of Holocaust survivor's values and beliefs about interpersonal relations]. Unpublished master's thesis, Department of Psychology, Tel Aviv University, Tel Aviv, Israel. 78 pp.

558 Eliasberg, W.G. (1964). Theory and practice in the psychiatric evaluation of restitution cases. *Israel Annals of Psychiatry and Related Disciplines*, 2(1), 81-92.

559 Eliasberg, W.G. (1967). Older and recent psychiatric views on the victims of Nazi persecution. *Harefuah*, 72, 347-348.

560 Ellenbogen, Raphael (1961). Frequency and gravity of the various diseases and disabilities among survivors of concentration camps. In: *International Conference on the Later Effects of Imprisonment and Deportation Organized by the World Veterans Federation. The Hague, November 20-25, 1961*. The Hague: World Veterans Federation, pp. 115-121.

561 Ellenbogen, Raphael (1967). Die Beurteilung der Folgen von Internierung und Deportation in Frankreich [The evaluation of the sequels of internment and deportation in France]. In: Herberg, Hans-Joachim (Ed.), *Die Beurteilung von Gesundheitsschäden nach Gefangenschaft und Verfolgung* [The Assessment of Health Damages Following Internment and Persecution]. Herford: Nicolai, pp. 34-43. [Internationalen Medizinisch-Juristischen Symposiums in Köln].

562 Engdahl, Brian E., and Eberly, Raina E. (1990). The effects of torture and other maltreatment: Implications for psychology. In: Suedfeld, Peter (Ed.), *Psychology and Torture*. New York: Hemisphere, pp. 31-47.

563 Engel, Werner H. (1962). Reflections on the psychiatric consequences of persecution. An evaluation of restitution claimants. *American Journal of Psychotherapy*, 16, 191-203.

564 Engels, Dinah E. (1982). *Uit naam van, een literatuurstudie naar de kinderen van overlevenden van de tweede wereldoorlog* [In the name of, a study of literature of children of survivors of the Second World War]. Unpublished doctoral dissertation, University of Groningen, The Netherlands.

565 Engels, Dinah E. (1983). Het postconcentratiekampsyndroom [The post-concentration camp syndrome]. *Tijdschrift voor Psychotherapie*, 9(5), 215-229.

566 Engeset, Arne (1961). Luftencefalografiske funn hos tidligere konsentrasjonsleirfanger [Pneumoencephalographic findings in ex-prisoners]. *Tidsskrift for den Norske Laegeforening. Journal of the Norwegian Medical Association*, 81, 810-811.

567 Engeset, Arne (1961). Study of a group of former Norwegian deportees. Part 4: Pneumoencephalographic findings in ex-concentration camp inmates. In: *International Conference on the Later Effects of Imprisonment and Deportation Organized by the World Veterans Federation. The Hague, November 20-25, 1961*. The Hague: World Veterans, pp. 93-95.

568 Engeset, Arne (1968). Pneumoencephalographical examinations. In: Strøm, Axel (Ed.), *Norwegian Concentration Camp Survivors*. Oslo: Universitetsforlaget, and New York: Humanities Press, pp. 124-131.

569 Enriguez, Micheline (1988). L'enveloppe de mémoire et ses trous [The envelope of memory and its holes]. *Topfique Revue Freudienne*, 18(42), 185-205.

570 Epstein, Arthur W. (1982). Mental phenomena across generations: The Holocaust. *Journal of the American Academy of Psychoanalysis*, 10(4), 565-570.

571 Epstein, Beth Broder (1975). Meeting in Tel Aviv. In: Steinitz, Lucy Y., and Szonyi, David M. (Eds.), *Living After the Holocaust: Reflections by the Post-War Generation in America*. New York: Bloch, pp. 93-100.

572 Epstein, Helen (1976). Children of the Holocaust: Searching for a past - and a future. *Present Tense*, 3, 21-25.

573 Epstein, Helen (1977, June 19). Heirs of the Holocaust: The lingering legacy for children of survivors. *New York Times Magazine*, 12-15+.

574 Epstein, Helen (1988). *Children of the Holocaust: Conversations with Sons and Daughters of Survivors*. New York: Penguin. 355 pp.

575 Erdreich, Marius (1984). A traumata-oriented psychotherapy. *Dynamische Psychiatrie*, 17(5-6), 419-431.

576 Erel, Dalia (1989). *Interactziat hanisuim etzel yaldei nitzoley hashoah: Haavarah beyn dorit b'tifkud hazugi shel habanim al reka post-traumati (Mechkar geshush shel hamisha zugot shepanu l'yi'ootz)* [Marital interaction of children and Holocaust survivors:

The intergenerational transmission of post-traumatic impacts on marital functioning (An exploratory study of five couples in marital therapy)]. Unpublished master's thesis, Bob Shapell School of Social Work, Tel Aviv University, Tel Aviv, Israel. 2 parts, 342 pp.

577 Erlich, Shelia (1990). *The relationship of Holocaust reference group involvement, Jewish identification, Holocaust identification and self-esteem in survivors of the Holocaust.* Unpublished doctoral dissertation, New York University, 139 pp. *Dissertation Abstracts International*, 51(9-B), p. 4586. (University Microfilms no. AAC 9102614).

578 Ernst, Edzard (1995). A leading medical school seriously damaged: Vienna 1938. *Annals of Internal Medicine*, 122(10), 789-792.

579 Ertel, Rachel (1985). Jeux et enjeux de la mémoire et de l'histoire [Stakes in the games of memory and history]. *Revue Française de Psychanalyse*, 49(4), 1029-1952.

580 Eskin, Vivian (1995). The impact of parental communication of Holocaust-related trauma on children of Holocaust survivors. In: Lemberger, John (Ed.), *A Global Perspective on Working with Holocaust Survivors and the Second Generation*. Jerusalem: JDC-Brookdale Institute of Gerontology and Human Development, AMCHA, and JDC-Israel, pp. 377-390.

581 Ewalt, Jack R. (1985). "The concentration camp syndrome: An organic brain syndrome?": Commentary. *Integrative Psychiatry*, 3(2), 119-120.

582 Fabowska-Grzeżułko, Zofia (1970). Ewakuacja z Wattenstedt podobozu Ravensbrük [Evacuation from the Ravensbrück-Wattenstedt concentration camp]. *Przegląd Lekarski*, 26(1), 172-173.

583 Factor, Haim (1995). The need for long-term care services among elderly Holocaust survivors living in Israel. In: Lemberger, John (Ed.), *A Global Perspective on Working with Holocaust Survivors and the Second Generation*. Jerusalem: JDC-Brookdale Institute of Gerontology and Human Development, AMCHA, and JDC-Israel, pp. 13-23.

584 Fajgenblat, Szymon (1979). Ocular disturbances in hunger disease. In: Winick, Myron (Ed.) *Hunger Disease: Studies by the Jewish Physicians in the Warsaw Ghetto*. New York: John Wiley & Sons, pp. 197-202.

585 Falgowski, Józef (1970). Esesówska służba zdrowia w obozie na Majdanku [Health facilities provided by the SS at Majdanek concentration camp]. *Przegląd Lekarski*, 26(1), 172-173.

586 Falk, Bunny; Hersen, Michel; and Van-Hasselt, Vincent B. (1994). Assessment of post-traumatic stress disorder in older adults: A critical review. *Clinical Psychology Review*, 14(5), 383-415.

587 Faust, C. (1952). Hirnatrophie nach Hungerdystrophie [Atrophy of the brain after malnutrition]. *Nervenarzt*, 23, 406.

588 Faust, C. (1983). Chronische reaktive Depression. Krankheiten nach Gefangenschaft und Verfolgung [Chronic reactive depression. Disorders following imprisonment and persecution]. *Fortschritte der Medizin*, 101(9), 372-376.

589 Faust, C. (1983). Psychosoziale Aspekte im dritten Lebensalter [Psychosocial aspects in the third stage of life]. *Fortschritte der Medizin*, 101(18), 819-823.

590 Federn, Ernst (1948). Terror as a system: The concentration camp, Buchenwald as it was. *Psychiatric Quarterly*, 22(1), 52-86.

591 Federn, Ernst (1951). The endurance of torture. *Complex*, 4, 34-41.

592 Federn, Ernst (1960). Some clinical remarks on the psychopathology of genocide. *Psychiatric Quarterly*, 34, 538-549.

593 Federn, Ernst (1995). Psychoanalyse in Buchenwald [Psychoanalysis in Buchenwald]. *Zeitschrift für Individualpsychologie*, 20(2), 88-91.

594 Federowicza, Tadeusz (1970). Z wspomnień o postawie lekarzy w obozach [Attitude of the concentration camp physicians]. *Przegląd Lekarski*, 26(1), 238-242.

595 Feenstra, W. (1994). De psychische gezondheid van naoorlogse kinderen van oorlogsgettroffenen: Resultaten van een onderzoek [The psychologic health of post-war children of war victims: Results of an investigation]. *Maandblad voor de Geestelijke Volksgezondheid*, 49, 541-553.

596 Fejkeil, Władysław (1958). Typhus exanthematicus at Auschwitz concentration camp from 1941-1945. *Rozpravy Wydzialu Manknud*, 3, 5-50.

597 Fejkiel, Władysław (1971). Health service in the Auschwitz I concentration camp, main camp. In: *Auschwitz Anthology. Vol. 2: In Hell They Preserved Human Dignity. Part 2*. Warsaw: International Auschwitz Committee, pp. 4-37.

598 Fejkiel, Władysław (1973). Bewertung des Gesundheitszustandes ehemaliger Auschwitz-Häftlinge an denen verbrecherische Experimente vorgenommen worden sind [Evaluation of the state of health of former Auschwitz prisoners who underwent criminal experimentation]. In: *Ermüdung und vorzeitiges Altern: Folge von Extrembelastungen* [Exhaustion and Premature Aging: Result of Extreme Stress]. Leipzig: Barth, pp. 315-320. [V Internationaler Medizinischer Kongress der FIR. Paris, 21-24 September 1970].

599 Fejkiel, Władysław (1975). Przełrwałe uszkodzenia i zmiany ustroju w następsłwie przebyłego duru wysypkowego [Lasting defects and changes in the system following epidemic typhus]. *Przegląd Lekarski*, 32(8), 668-671.

600 Fejkiel, Władysław (1978). Dauerschäden und pathologische Veranderungen im organismus als Folge des Fleckfiebers [Permanent damage and pathological modifications in the organism as sequelae of typhus]. In: *Medizinische Untersuchungen der Spätfolgen des Krieges und des NS-Regimes bei Jugendlichen und Kindern von ehemaligen KZ-Häftlingen und Verfolgten* [Medical Research of the Late Effects of the War and National Socialism Regime on Youth and Children of Former Concentration Camp Inmates and Persecuted Persons]. Wien: Internationale Föderation der Widerstandskämpfer. [VI Internationaler Medizinischer Kongress der FIR. Prague, 1976].

601 Fejkiel, Władysław (1978). Das Infektionskrankheitsbild und dessen Epidemien in kunstlich gebildeter Gemeinschaft in Konzentrationslager Auschwitz [The infectious disease syndrome and its epidemics in artificially created groups in the concentration camp Auschwitz]. In: *Medizinische Untersuchungen der Spätfolgen des Krieges und des NS-Regimes bei Jugendlichen und Kindern von ehemaligen KZ-Häftlingen und Verfolgten* [Medical Research of the Late Effects of the War and National Socialism Regime on Youth and Children of Former Concentration Camp Inmates and Persecuted Persons]. Wien: Internationale Föderation der Widerstandskämpfer. [VI Internationaler Medizinischer Kongress der FIR. Prague, 1976].

602 Felman, Shoshana, and Laub, Dori (1992). *Testimony: Crises of Witnessing in Literature, Psychoanalysis, and History*. New York: Routledge. 294 pp.

603 Felson, Irit, and Ehrlich, H. Shmuel (1990). Identification patterns of offspring of Holocaust survivors and their parents. *American Journal of Orthopsychiatry*, 60(4), 506-520.

604 Felstiner, John (1986). Paul Celan's "Todesfuge." *Holocaust and Genocide Studies*, 1(2), 249-264.

605 Fenig, Shmuel, and Levav, Itzhak (1991). Demoralization and social supports among Holocaust survivors. *Journal of Nervous and Mental Disease*, 179(3), 167-172.

606 Fenig, Shmuel; Levav, Itzhak; Kohn, Robert; and Yelin, Nava (1993). Telephone versus face to face interviewing in a community psychiatric survey. *American Journal of Public Health*, 83(6), 896-898.

607 Feuerstein, Chester W. (1980). Working with the Holocaust victims psychologically: Some vital cautions. In: Quaytman, Wilfred (Ed.), *Holocaust Survivors: Psychological and Social Sequelae*. New York: Human Sciences Press, pp. 70-78. [Published as a special issue of *Journal of Contemporary Psychotherapy*, 11(1)].

608 Fichez, Louis F. (1955). Einige Schlussfolgerungen aus den Forschungsergebnissen über Verfolgten-Krankheiten [Some conclusions regarding the research results on diseases of persecuted people]. In: Michel, Max (Ed.), *Gesundheitsschäden durch Verfolgung und Gefangenschaft und ihre Spätfolgen: Zusammenstellung der Referate und Ergebnisse der Internationalen Sozialmedizinischen Konferenz über die Pathologie der Ehemaligen Deportierten und Internierten, 5-7 Juni 1954 in Kopenhagen* [Health Damages Caused by Persecution and Internment and the Late Effects: Compilation of the Papers and Results of the International Conference of Social Medicine on the Pathology of Former Deported and Interned Persons, 5-7 June 1954 in Copenhagen]. Frankfurt am Main: Röderberg, pp. 338-341.

609 Fichez, Louis F. (Ed.) (1960). *Andere Spätfolgen, auf Grund der Beobachtungen bei den ehemaligen Deportierten und Internierten der nazistischen Gefangnisse und Vernichtungslager* [Other Belated Consequences, Based on the Observations of Former Deportees and Internees of Nazi Prisons and Death Camps]. Wien: Verlag der FIR. 226 pp.

610 Fichez, Louis F. (Ed.) (1960). *Die chronische progressive Asthenie, auf Grund von Beobachtungen an ehemaligen Deportierten und Gefangenen der Nazigefängnisse und Vernichtungslager* [Chronic

Progressive Asthenia, Based on Observations of Former Deportees and Prisoners of Nazi Prisons and Death Camps]. Wien: Verlag der FIR. 80 pp. [Materialien der Internationalen Konferenz von Kopenhagen und Miskau, zusammengestellt vom ärztlichen Sekretariat der internationalen Föderation der Widerstandskämpfer].

611 Fichez, Louis F. (1964). *L'etio-pathogénie et la thérapeutique de l'asthenie et de la senescence premature* [The Etio-Pathology and the Treatment of Asthenia and Premature Aging]. Bucharest.

612 Fichez, Louis F. (1973). Eröffnungsansprache [Opening speech]. In: *Ermüdung und vorzeitiges Altern: Folge von Extrembelastungen* [Exhaustion and Premature Aging: Result of Extreme Stress]. Leipzig: Barth, pp. 20-25. [V Internationaler Medizinischer Kongress der FIR. Paris 21-24 September 1970].

613 Fichez, Louis F. (1975). Stoffwechselstörungen als folge des Hungers und psycho-physiologische Probleme der Ermüdung und vorzeitigen Vergreisung [Metabolic disturbances as a result of hunger and psychophysiological problems of fatigue and premature aging]. *Mitteilungen der FIR*, 1-9.

614 Fichez, Louis F. (1983). Etúde de morbidité a long terme chez les anciens deportés des camps d'extermination Nazis [Study of the long term morbidity of former deportees from Nazi extermination camps]. *Cahiers d'Informations Médicales, Sociales et Juridiques*, 19, 104-106.

615 Fichez, Louis F. (1983). Premiers résultats de l'étude du bilan lipidique des anciens deportés hommes et femmes hospitalisés dans un centre specialisé [First results of the study of the lipid balance of former deported men and women hospitalized in a specialized center]. *Cahiers d'Informations Médicales, Sociales et Juridiques*, 19, 117-121.

616 Fichez, Louis F., and Kotz, Alexander (1961). *Die vorzeitige Vergreisung und ihre Behandlung: An Hand von Beobachtungen an ehemaligen Deportierten und KZ-Häftlingen* [Premature Aging and its Treatment According to the Observations of Former Deportees and Concentration Camp Prisoners]. Wien: Verlag der FIR. 174 pp.

617 Fichez, Louis F., and Landau, A. (1964). Schlaftherapie bei chronischer Asthenie und vorzeitiger Seneszenz ehemaliger Deportierter und Konzentrationslagerinsassen [Sleep therapy of chronic asthenia and premature aging in former deportees and concentration camp inmates]. In: *Ätio-Pathogenese und Therapie der Erschöpfung und vorzeitigen Vergreisung* [The Aetiology,

Pathogenesis and Therapy of Exhaustion and Premature Aging]. Wien: Verlag der FIR, pp. 421-426. [IV Internationaler Medizinischer Kongress. Bucharest. 22-27 Juni 1964].

618 Fichez, Louis F., and Weinstein, S. (1960). Die Tuberkulose bei den franzosischen Überlebenden der Nazistischen Gefängnisse und Vernichtungslager [Tuberculosis in French survivors of the Nazi prisons and extermination camps]. In: Fichez, Louis F. (Ed.), *Andere Spätfolgen, auf Grund der Beobachtungen bei den ehemaligen Deportierten und Internierten der nazistischen Gefangnisse und Vernichtungslager* [Other Belated Consequences, Based on the Observations of Former Deportees and Internees of Nazi Prisons and Death Camps]. Wien: Verlag der FIR, pp. 77-88.

619 Finer-Greenberg, Rosalie (1987). *Factors contributing to the degree of psychopathology in first and second-generation Holocaust survivors*. Unpublished doctoral dissertation, California School of Professional Psychology, Los Angeles, 160 pp. *Dissertation Abstracts International*, 49(5-B), p. 1939. (University Microfilms no. AAC 8801241).

620 Fink, Hans F. (1968). Developmental arrest as a result of Nazi persecution during adolescence. *International Journal of Psycho-Analysis*, 49(2-3), 327-329.

621 Fink, Klaus P. (1979). Victims of political-racial persecution. *Nursing Times*, 75(12), 496-499.

622 Finzen, Asmus (1983). Mass murder and guilt feelings: Observations on the psychopathology of conscience. *Sozialpsychiatrische Informationen*, 13, 91-101.

623 Fisch, Robert Z. (1989). Alexithymia, masked depression and loss in a Holocaust survivor. *British Journal of Psychiatry*, 154, 708-710.

624 Fischer, H. (1988). Arztliche Versorgung, sanitare Verhaltnisse und Human versuche im Frauen Konzentrationlager Ravensbrük [Medical management, health conditions and human experimentation at the Ravensbrück female concentration camp]. *Gesnerus*, 45(1), 49-66.

625 Fischer, Josey G. (1991). *The Persistence of Youth: Oral Testimonies of the Holocaust*. Westport, CT: Greenwood. 171 pp.

626 Fischer, O. (1967). Die Bedeutung der amoebenruhr als Versorgungs und Verfolgungsleiden [The importance of amoebic dysentery as a disease caused by persecution and entitled to compensation]. In: *Die*

Beurteilung von Gesundheitsschäden nach Gefangenschaft und Verfolgung [The Assessment of Health Damages Following Internment and Persecution]. Herford: Nicolai, pp. 102-107. [Internationalen Medizinisch-Juristischen Symposiums in Köln].

627 Fishbane, Mona D. (1979). *Children of survivors of the Nazi Holocaust: A psychological inquiry*. Unpublished doctoral dissertation, University of Massachusetts, Amherst, 210 pp. *Dissertation Abstracts International*, 40(1-B), p. 449. (University Microfilms no. AAC 7912680).

628 Fisher, S.H. (1960). Psychiatric symptomatology and later effects in war imprisonment. In: *Experts Meeting on the Later Effects of Imprisonment and Deportation, Oslo*. Paris: World Veterans Federation, pp. 67-78.

629 Fishman, J.S. (1973/1974). Jewish war orphans in the Netherlands: The Guardianship issue 1945-1950. *The Wiener Library Bulletin*, 27(30-31), 31.

630 Fitzek, Josef M., and Herberg, Hans-Joachim (1963). Auslesegesichtspunkte und allgemeine Erfahrungen bei den Untersuchungen des Köllner Arbeitkreises [Points of view in selection and general experiences of the investigations done by the working group of Cologne]. In: Paul, Helmut, and Herberg, Hans-Joachim (Eds.), *Psychische Spätsschäden nach politischer Verfolgung* [Psychological Late Damages Following Political Persecution]. Basel: Karger, pp. 169-178.

631 Fliederbaum, Julian (1979). Clinical aspects of hunger disease in adults. In: Winick, Myron (Ed.), *Hunger Disease: Studies by the Jewish Physicians in the Warsaw Ghetto*. New York: John Wiley & Sons, pp. 11-43.

632 Fliederbaum, Julian (1979). Metabolic changes in hunger disease. In: Winick, Myron (Ed.), *Hunger Disease: Studies by the Jewish Physicians in the Warsaw Ghetto*. New York: John Wiley & Sons, pp. 69-123.

633 Flountzis, A. (1964). Besonderheiten des Problems der Asthenie und des vorzeitigen Alterns der grieschischen antifaschistischen Deportierten und Häftlinge [Peculiarities of the problem of asthenia and premature aging of Greek antifascist deportees and prisoners]. In: *Ätio-Pathogenese und Therapie der Erschöpfung und vorzeitigen Vergreisung* [The Aetiology, Pathogenesis and Therapy of Exhaustion and Premature Aging]. Wien: Verlag der FIR, pp. 337-343. [IV

Internationaler Medizinischer Kongress. Bucharest, 22-27 Juni 1964].

634 Fodor, R. (1957). The impact of Nazi occupation of Poland on the Jewish mother-child relationship. *YIVO Annual of Jewish Social Sciences*, 11.

635 Fogelman, Eva (1979). *Survivors and Their Children: Psychosocial Impact of the Holocaust*. New York: Zachor. 17 pp. [A bibliography for the First International Conference on Children of Holocaust Survivors, November 4-5, 1979, New York City].

636 Fogelman, Eva (1987). *The rescuers: A sociopsychological study of altruistic behavior during the Nazi era*. Unpublished doctoral dissertation, City University of New York, 336 pp. *Dissertation Abstracts International*, 48(12-B), p. 3715. (University Microfilms no. AAC 8801711).

637 Fogelman, Eva (1988). Intergenerational group therapy: Child survivors of the Holocaust and offspring of survivors. *Psychoanalytic Review*, 75(4), 619-640.

638 Fogelman, Eva (1988). Therapeutic alternatives for Holocaust survivors and second generation. In: Braham, Randolph L. (Ed.), *The Psychological Perspectives of the Holocaust and of its Aftermath*. Boulder, CO: Social Science Monographs; and New York: Csengeri Institute for Holocaust Studies of the Graduate School and University Center of the City University of New York, pp. 79-108.

639 Fogelman, Eva (1989). Group treatment as a therapeutic modality for generations of the Holocaust. In: Marcus, Paul, and Rosenberg, Alan (Eds.), *Healing Their Wounds: Psychotherapy with Holocaust Survivors and Their Families*. New York: Praeger, pp. 119-133.

640 Fogelman, Eva (1990). Second generation of survivors. In: Gutman, Israel (Ed.), *Encyclopedia of the Holocaust. Vol. 4*. New York: Macmillan, pp. 1434-1435.

641 Fogelman, Eva (1991). From mourning to creativity: The second generation of survivors in Israel and the United States. *Midstream*, 38(3), 31-33.

642 Fogelman, Eva (1991). Survivor victims of war and Holocaust. In: Leviton, Daniel (Ed.), *Horrendous Death and Health: Toward Action*. New York: Hemisphere, pp. 37-45.

643 Fogelman, Eva (1992). Intergenerational group therapy: Child survivors of the Holocaust and offspring of survivors. *Psychiatria Hungarica*, 7(3), 255-269.

644 Fogelman, Eva (1994). *Conscience and Courage: Rescuers of Jews during the Holocaust*. New York: Anchor/Doubleday. 393 pp.

645 Fogelman, Eva (1994). Effects of interviews with rescued child survivors. In: Kestenberg, Judith S., and Fogelman, Eva (Eds.), *Children during the Nazi Reign: Psychological Perspectives on the Interview Process*. Westport, CT: Praeger, pp. 81-89.

646 Fogelman, Eva, and Hogman, Flora (1994). A follow-up study: Child survivors of the Nazi Holocaust reflect on being interviewed. In: Kestenberg, Judith S., and Fogelman, Eva (Eds.), *Children during the Nazi Reign: Psychological Perspectives on the Interview Process*. Westport, CT: Praeger, pp. 73-80.

647 Fogelman, Eva, and Savran, Bella (1979). Therapeutic groups for children of Holocaust survivors. *International Journal of Group Psychotherapy*, 29(2), 211-235.

648 Fogelman, Eva, and Savran, Bella (1980). Brief group therapy with offspring of Holocaust survivors: Leaders' reactions. *American Journal of Orthopsychiatry*, 50(1), 96-108.

649 Forbert, Adolf (1980). W Oświęcimiu po oswobodzeniu obozu [In Auschwitz after liberation]. *Przegląd Lekarski*, 37(1), 182-184.

650 Fox, John F. (1983). The Holocaust and today's generation. *Patterns of Prejudice*, 17(1), 3-24.

651 Frąckowski, Kazimierz (1970). Żydzi i księża w obozie koncentracyjnym Sachsenhausen Oranienburg [Jews and priests at the Sachsenhausen-Orianienburg concentration camp]. *PrzeglądLekarski*, 26(1), 159-164.

652 Franaszek, Ewa; Chlebowska, Maria; and Hoehne, Teresa (1977). Stan jamy ustnej więźniów w obozach koncentracyjnych (w świetle badań ankietowych) [The oral and dental status in the concentration camps (a questionnaire investigation)]. *Przegląd Lekarski*, 34(1), 25-28.

653 Frančić, Vilim (1970). Organizacja wręźniów-profesorów w obozie Sachsenhausen [An organization of university professors, inmates of the Sachsenhausen concentration camp]. *Przegląd Lekarski*, 26(1), 150-158.

654 Frankl, Viktor E. (1954). Group therapeutic experiences in a concentration camp. *Group Psychotherapy*, 7, 81-90.

655 Frankl, Viktor E. (1959). *From Death Camp to Existentialism: A Psychiatrist's Path to a New Therapy*. Boston, MA: Beacon. 111 p.

656 Frankl, Viktor E. (1961). Psychologie und Psychiatrie des Konzentrationslagers [The psychology and psychiatry of the concentration camps]. In: Gruhle, Hans W. (Ed.), *Psychiatrie der Gegenwart: Forschung und Praxis. Band 3: Soziale und angewandte Psychiatrie* [Psychiatry in the Present: Research and Practice. Vol. 3: Social and Applied Psychiatry]. Berlin: Springer, pp. 743-759.

657 Frankl, Viktor E. (1965). Higiena psychiczna w sytuacji przymusowej: Doswiadczenia z zakresu psychoterapii w obozie koncentracyjnym [Mental hygiene in an extreme situation: A psychotherapeutic experience from the concentration camp]. *Przegląd Lekarski*, 21(1), 24-28.

658 Frankl, Viktor E. (1965). On the psychology of the concentration camp. In: *The Doctor and the Soul: From Psychotherapy to Logotherapy*. New York: Knopf, pp. 93-104.

659 Frankl, Viktor E. (1979). *Trotzdem Ja zum Leben sagen: Ein Psychologe erlebt das Konzentrationslager* [Say Yes to Life In Spite of Everything: A Psychologist Experiences the Concentration Camp]. München: Kosel. 198 pp.

660 Frankl, Viktor E. (1986). *The Doctor and the Soul: From Psychotherapy to Logotherapy*. New York: Vintage. 318 pp.

661 Frankl, Viktor E. (1992). *Man's Search for Meaning: An Introduction to Logotherapy*. Boston, MA: Beacon. 196 pp.

662 Frankle, Helene (1978). The survivor as a parent. *Journal of Jewish Communal Service*, 55, 241-246.

663 Franzblau, Michael J. (1994). Relevance of the Nazi medical behavior to the health profession today. In: Michalczyk, John J. (Ed.), *Medicine, Ethics, and the Third Reich: Historical and Contemporary Issues*. Kansas City, MO: Sheed & Ward, pp. 197-198.

664 Fresco, Nadine (1981). La diaspora des cendres [The diaspora of ashes]. *Nouvelle Revue de Psychanalyse*, 24, 205-220.

665 Fresco, Nadine (1984). Remembering the unknown. *International Review of Psycho-Analysis*, 11(4), 417-427.

666 Freud, Anna, and Dann, Sophie (1951). An experiment in group upbringing. In: Eissler, Ruth S.; Freud, Anna; Hartmann, Heinz; and Kris, Ernst (Eds.), *Psychoanalytic Study of the Child. Vol. 6*. New York: International Universities Press, pp. 127-168.

667 Freyberg, Joan T. (1980). Difficulties in separation-individuation as experienced by offspring of Nazi Holocaust survivors. *American Journal of Orthopsychiatry*, 50(1), 87-95.

668 Freyberg, Joan T. (1989). The emerging self in the survivor family. In: Marcus, Paul, and Rosenberg, Alan (Eds.), *Healing Their Wounds: Psychotherapy with Holocaust Survivors and Their Families*. New York: Praeger, pp. 85-104.

669 Fried, Hedi (1995). Cafe 84: Social daycare center for survivors and their children. In: Lemberger, John (Ed.), *A Global Perspective on Working with Holocaust Survivors and the Second Generation*. Jerusalem: JDC-Brookdale Institute of Gerontology and Human Development, AMCHA, and JDC-Israel, pp. 81-91.

670 Fried, Hedi, and Waxman, Howard M. (1987). Cafe 84: Dagcenterver ksamhet for judiska overlevande [Cafe 84: A day center activity for Jewish survivors]. *Psykisk Haelsa*, 28(1), 19-23.

671 Fried, Hedi, and Waxman, Howard M. (1988). Stockholm's Cafe 84: A unique day program for Jewish survivors of concentration camps. *Gerontologist*, 28(2), 253-255.

672 Friedlander, Saul (1979). *When Memory Comes*. New York: Farrar, Straus, Giroux. 185 pp.

673 Friedler, Ya'acov (1984). German doctor at seminar "Holocaust hardest subject of all." *Dynamische Psychiatrie*, 17(5-6), 416-418.

674 Friedman, Paul (1948). The effects of imprisonment. *Acta Medica Orientalia*, 7, 163-167.

675 Friedman, Paul (1948). The road back for the DP's: Healing the psychological scars of Nazism. *Commentary*, 6(6), 502-510.

676 Friedman, Paul (1949). Some aspects of concentration camp psychology. *American Journal of Psychiatry*, 105, 601-605.

677 Friedman, Paul (1990). Some aspects of concentration camp psychology. *Psyche: Zeitschrift für Psychoanalyse und ihre Anwendungen*, 4(2), 164-172.

678 Fromm, Erika (1987). Post-traumatic stress in the second generation: The children of survivors of the Holocaust. *ICODO Info*, 1, 5-25.

679 Fuchs, G. (1950). Zur Läge der durch den Nationalsozialismus geschädigten Arzte [On the condition of physicians damaged by National Socialism]. *Osterreichische Arztezeitung*, 6, 285-289.

680 Fully, G. (1964). Abhandlung über die Pathogenese der Wirbelschäden auf Grund anatomischer Festellungen die an Skeletten von Deportierten, welche in den deutschen Konzentrationslagern verstorben sind, gemacht wurden [Report about the pathogenesis of damage to the vertebrae, based on anatomical findings, which were established on the skeletons of those who died in German concentration camps]. In: *Ätio-Pathogenese und Therapie der Erschöpfung und vorzeitigen Vergreisung* [The Aetiology, Pathogenesis and Therapy of Exhaustion and Premature Aging]. Wien: Verlag der FIR, pp. 291-295. [IV Internationaler Medizinischer Kongress. Bucharest, 22-27 Juni 1964].

681 Furman, Erna (1973). The impact of the Nazi concentration camps on the children of survivors. In: Anthony, E. James, and Koupernik, Cyrille (Eds.), *The Child in His Family. Vol. 2: The Impact of Disease and Death*. New York: John Wiley & Sons, pp. 379-384.

682 Furshpan, Mark (1985). *Family dynamics as perceived by the second generation of Holocaust survivors*. Unpublished doctoral dissertation, State University of New York at Buffalo, 165 pp. *Dissertation Abstracts International*, 47(3-B), p. 1271. (University Microfilm no. AAC 8609110).

683 Furst, Sidney S. (1978). The stimulus barrier and the pathogenicity of trauma. *International Journal of Psycho-Analysis*, 59(2-3), 345-352.

684 Gallagher, Hugh G. (1990). *By Trust Betrayed: Patients, Physicians, and the License to Kill in the Third Reich*. New York: Henry Holt. 342 pp.

685 Gampel, Yolanda (1982). A daughter of silence. In: Bergmann, Martin S., and Jucovy, Milton E. (Eds.), *Generations of the Holocaust*. New York: Basic Books, pp. 120-136.

686 Gampel, Yolanda (1986). L'effrayant et le menaçant: De la transmission á la répetition [The frightening and the menacing: From transmission to repetition]. *Psychanalyse a l'Université*, 11(41), 87-102.

687 Gampel, Yolanda (1987). Heibetim shel ha'avara bein dorit [Aspects of intergenerational transmission]. *Sihot: Israel Journal of Psychotherapy*, 2(1), 27-31.

688 Gampel, Yolanda (1988). Facing war, murder, torture, and death in latency. *Psychoanalytic Review*, 75(4), 499-509.

689 Gampel, Yolanda (1990). I am a Holocaust child, now I am fifty. In: Wilson, Arnold (Ed.), *The Holocaust Survivor and the Family*. New York: Praeger.

690 Gampel, Yolanda (1992). I was a Shoah child. *British Journal of Psychotherapy*, 8(4), 390-400.

691 Gampel, Yolanda (1992). Psychoanalysis, ethics, and actuality. *Psychoanalytic Inquiry*, 12(4), 526-550.

692 Gampel, Yolanda (1994). The effects of interviews on children survivors and the interviewers in Israel. In: Kestenberg, Judith S., and Fogelman, Eva (Eds), *Children during the Nazi Reign: Psychological Perspectives on the Interview Process*. Westport, CT: Praeger, pp. 161-174.

693 Gampel, Yolanda (1994). Identifizierung, Identitat und generationsubergreif ende Trandmission [Identification, identity and transgenerational transmission]. *Zeitschrift für Psychoanalytische Theorie und Praxis*, 9(3), 301-319.

694 Garfunkel, Gloria (1995). Lifeline. In: Sussman, Michael B. (Ed.), *A Perilous Calling: The Hazards of Psychotherapy Practice*. New York: John Wiley, pp. 148-159.

695 Garland, Caroline (1993). The lasting trauma of the concentration camps. *British Medical Journal*, 307(6896), 77-78.

696 Garmada, Ludwik (1978). Reminiscencje z tzw obozo janowskiego [Reminiscences from the Janow concentration camp]. *Przegląd Lekarski*, 35(1), 166-170.

697 Garmada, Ludwik (1990). Pamiętny apel w obozie "Janowskim" we Lwowie [The memorable roll call in the Janowska camp in Lwow]. *Przegląd Lekarski*, 47(1), 160-163.

698 Garmezy, Norman, and Master, Ann (1990). The adaptation of children to a stressful world: Mastery of fear. In: Arnold, L. Eugene (Ed.), *Childhood Stress*. New York: John Wiley & Sons, pp. 460-473.

699 Garstka, Stanley M. (1974). Hitlerowski obóz koncentracyjny we Flossenbürgu [The Nazi concentration camp in Flossenberg]. *Przegląd Lekarski*, 31(1), 191-195.

700 Gassler, Karin (1995). Wunden, die nicht vergehen: Extremtraumatisiering in der Pubertät [Wounds that won't heal: Extreme traumatization in puberty]. *Psyche: Zeitschrift für Psychoanalyse und ihre Anwendungen*, 49(1), 41-68.

701 Gątarski, Julian (1966). Badania elektroencefalograficzne u osób urodzonych lub przebywających w dziecinstwie w hitlerowskich obozach koncentracyjnych [Electroencephalographic findings in persons who either were born in concentration camps or spent their early life there]. *Przegląd Lekarski*, 23, 37-38.

702 Gątarski, Julian (1971). Electroencephalographic examinations of people born in camps or who had stayed in their childhood in Nazi concentration camps. In: *Auschwitz Anthology. Vol. 2: In Hell They Preserved Human Dignity. Part 3*. Warsaw: International Auschwitz Committee, pp. 133-142.

703 Gątarski, Julian; Orwid, Maria; and Małgorzata, Dominik (1978). Wyniki badania psychiatryczego i elektroencefalograficznego 130 byłych więźniów Oswięcimia-Brzezinki [Results of psychiatric and electroencephalographic investigations of ex-prisoners from Auschwitz-Birkenau]. *Przegląd Lekarski*, 35, 29-32.

704 Gawalewicz, Adolf (1971). A number gets back its name. In: *Auschwitz Anthology. Vol. 3: It Did Not End in Forty-Five. Part 1*. Warsaw: International Auschwitz Committee, pp. 4-66.

705 Gawalewicz, Adolf (1971). Waiting room to the gas. In: *Auschwitz Anthology. Vol. 2: In Hell They Preserved Human Dignity. Part 1*. Warsaw: International Auschwitz Committee, pp. 107-149.

706 Gawalewicz, Adolf (1987). Problemy interpretacji faktografii oświecimskiej [Problem of interpretation of Auschwitz factography]. *Przegląd Lekarski*, 44(1), 95-102.

707 Gawalewicz, Adolf (1995). Wie die Fakten über Auschwitz interpretiert werden [How the facts about Auschwitz are interpreted].

In: Hamburger Institut für Sozialforschung (Eds.), *Die Auschwitz-Hefte. Ergänzungsband. Texte der polnischen Zeitschrift "Przegląd Lekarski" über historische, psychische und medizinische Aspekte des Lebens und Sterbens in Auschwitz* [The Auschwitz Journal. Supplementary Volume. Text of the Polish Journal "Medical Review" on Historical, Psychic and Medical Aspects of Life and Death in Auschwitz]. Weinheim und Basel: Rogner and Bernhard, pp. 3-9.

708 Gawalewicz, J., and Jaceqicz, W. (1978). Wymieralność w latach 1945-1976 bylych wiezniów Dachau duchownych rzymskokatolickich [The mortality during the years 1945-1976 of Roman Catholic priests who have been prisoners in Dachau]. *Przegląd Lekarski*, 35, 29-32.

709 Gawryluk, Franciszek (1975). Wspomnienia z obozu we Flossenbürgu [Reminiscences from the Flossenberg camp]. *Przegląd Lekarski*, 35(1), 171-178.

710 Gay, Miriam (1972). Children of ex-concentration camp inmates. In: Miller, Louis (Ed.), *Mental Health in Rapid Social Change*. Jerusalem: Academic Press, pp. 337-338.

711 Gay, Miriam (1982). The adjustment of parents to wartime bereavement. In: Spielberger, Charles D.; Sarason, Irwin G.; and Milgram, Norman (Eds.), *Stress and Anxiety. Vol. 8*. Washington, D.C.: Hemisphere, pp. 243-247.

712 Gay, Miriam; Fuchs, Jonah; and Blittner, Mordechai (1974). Characteristics of the offspring of Holocaust survivors in Israel. *Mental Health and Society*, 1(5-6), 302-312.

713 Gay, Miriam, and Shulman, Shmuel (1978). Comparison of children of Holocaust survivors with children of the general population in Israel. *Mental Health and Society*, 5(5-6), 252-256.

714 Gelles, Jeremiah M. (1995). Medicine and the Holocaust. *Annals of Internal Medicine*, 123(12), 964-965.

715 Gerber, Jean M. (1989). *Trauma and rebirth: Intergenerational effects of the Holocaust*. Unpublished master's thesis, University of British Columbia, Vancouver, Canada. [Available on microfiche from the National Library of Canada, Ottawa. Order no. LE 3B76 A8 G47].

716 Gershon, Karen (Ed.) (1966). *We Came as Children: A Collective Autobiography*. London: Gollancz. 176 pp.

717 Gertler, Ray J. (1986). *A study of interpersonal adjustment in children of Holocaust survivors*. Unpublished doctoral dissertation, Pacific Graduate School of Psychology, 191 pp. *Dissertation Abstracts International*, 47(10-B), p. 4298. (University Microfilms no. AAC 8623648).

718 Gertz, Kerri R. (1986). *Psychosocial characteristics of children whose parent(s) survived the Nazi Holocaust and children whose parents were not in the Nazi Holocaust and implications for counseling children of survivors*. Unpublished doctoral dissertation, University of California, Los Angeles, 248 pp. *Dissertation Abstracts International*, 47(9-A), p. 3312. (University Microfilms no. AAC 8629889).

719 Gerwood, Joseph B. (1994). Meaning and love in Viktor Frankl's writing: Reports from the Holocaust. *Psychological Reports*, 75(3,1) 1075-1081.

720 Giberovitch, Myra (1992). Establishing trusting relationships with clients. In: Kenigsberg, Rositta E., and Lieblich, Cathy M. (Eds.), *The First National Conference on Identification, Treatment and Care of the Aging Holocaust Survivor, March 29-31, 1992: Selected Proceedings*. Miami, FL: Holocaust Documentation and Education Center and Southeast Florida Center on Aging, Florida International University, pp. 42-57.

721 Giberovitch, Myra (1992). Decisions, issues and innovative responses concerning families of survivors. In: Kenigsberg, Rositta E., and Lieblich, Cathy M. (Eds.), *The First National Conference on Identification, Treatment and Care of the Aging Holocaust Survivor, March 29-31, 1992: Selected Proceedings*. Miami, FL: Holocaust Documentation and Education Center and Southeast Florida Center on Aging, Florida International University, pp. 64-74.

722 Giberovitch, Myra (1995). Formulating an agenda to meet the needs of elderly Holocaust survivors. In: Lemberger, John (Ed.), *A Global Perspective on Working with Holocaust Survivors and the Second Generation*. Jerusalem: JDC-Brookdale Institute of Gerontology and Human Development, AMCHA, and JDC-Israel, pp. 135-144.

723 Giberovitch, Myra (1995). Social work practice with aging survivors. In: Lemberger, John (Ed.), *A Global Perspective on Working with Holocaust Survivors and the Second Generation*. Jerusalem: JDC-Brookdale Institute of Gerontology and Human Development, AMCHA, and JDC-Israel, pp. 277-288.

724 Gigliotti, E.J.W. (1995). Psychological aspects of concentration camp survival. *Proteus*, 12(2), 21-25.

725 Gilbert, Martin (1986). *The Holocaust: The Jewish Tragedy*. London: Collins. 959 pp.

726 Gilbert-Dreyfuss, H. (1960). Die funktionelle Nebennierenschwäche der ehemaligen Häftlinge [The functional weakness of the adrenals in former internees]. In: Fichez, Louis F. (Ed.), *Andere Spätfolgen, auf Grund der Beobachtungen bei den ehemaligen Deportierten und Internierten der nazistischen Gefangnisse und Vernichtungslager* [Other Belated Consequences, Based on the Observations of Former Deportees and Internees of Nazi Prisons and Death Camps]. Wien: Verlag der FIR, pp. 33-40.

727 Gilbert-Dreyfuss, H.; Fichez, Louis F.; and Franck, L.J. (1955). Günstige Wirkungen der Schlafkur bei ehemaligen Deportierten mit asthenischer Abmagerung auch zusammen mit Lungentuberkulose [Beneficial effects of sleep therapy with former deportees being asthenically thin, also with lung tuberculosis]. In: Michel, Max (Ed.), *Gesundheitsschäden durch Verfolgung und Gefangenschaft und ihre Spätfolgen: Zusammenstellung der Referate und Ergebnisse der Internationalen Sozialmedizinischen Konferenz über die Pathologie der Ehemaligen Deportierten und Internierten, 5-7 Juni 1954 in Kopenhagen* [Health Damages Caused by Persecution and Internment and the Late Effects: Compilation of the Papers and Results of the International Conference of Social Medicine on the Pathology of Former Deported and Interned Persons, 5-7 June 1954 in Copenhagen]. Frankfurt am Main: Röderberg, pp. 317-323.

728 Gilbert-Dreyfuss, H., and Franck, L.J. (1955). Die Ernährungsstörungen bei den Deportierten [Nutritional disturbances in deportees]. In: Michel, Max (Ed.), *Gesundheitsschäden durch Verfolgung und Gefangenschaft und ihre Spätfolgen: Zusammenstellung der Referate und Ergebnisse der Internationalen Sozialmedizinischen Konferenz über die Pathologie der Ehemaligen Deportierten und Internierten, 5-7 Juni 1954 in Kopenhagen* [Health Damages Caused by Persecution and Internment and the Late Effects: Compilation of the Papers and Results of the International Conference of Social Medicine on the Pathology of Former Deported and Interned Persons, 5-7 June 1954 in Copenhagen]. Frankfurt am Main: Röderberg, pp. 107-126.

729 Gilbert-Dreyfuss, H.; Sebaoun, J.; and Zara, M. (1961). Thyroid disorders following concentration camp internment. In: *International Conference on the Later Effects of Imprisonment and Deportation*

Organized by the World Veterans Federation. The Hague, November 20-25, 1961. The Hague: World Veterans, pp. 69-72.

730 Gill, Anton (1988). *The Journey Back from Hell: Memoirs of Concentration Camps Survivors*. New York: William Morrow. 494 pp.

731 Giza, Jerzy S. (1975). Die Lager problematik in den Untersuchungen Amerikanischer Psychiater [Problems of inmates of concentration camps in examinations by American psychiatrists]. *Mitteilungen der FIR*, 9, 15-20.

732 Giza, Jerzy S., and Morasiewicz, Wiesław (1973). Z zagadnień popędów w obozach koncentracyjnych. Przyczynek do analizy tzw. KZ syndromu [Problems of impulsiveness in concentration camps. Analysis of the concentration camp syndrome]. *Przegląd Lekarski*, 30(1), 29-41.

733 Giza, Jerzy S., and Morasiewicz, Wiesław (1974). Poobozowe zaburzenia seksualne u kobiet jako element tzw. KZ syndromu [Post-concentration camp sexual disturbances among women as an element of the so-called concentration camp syndrome]. *Przegląd Lekarski*, 31, 65-75.

734 Glas-Larsson, Margarete; Botz, Gerhard; and Pollak, Michael (1982). Survivre dans un camp de concentration [Surviving a concentration camp]. *Actes de la recherche en sciences sociales*, 41, 3-28.

735 Glassman-Simons, G.R. (1984). *The child of survivors: A literature study of the child of survivors compared with the Jewish child in recent and contemporary history*. Unpublished master's thesis, University of Amsterdam, Netherlands.

736 Gleitman, Benny (1982). *Bitoo'ee aggressiah v'asham b'banim v'banot shel nitzoley hashoah* [Patterns of expressing aggression and guilt in sons and daughters of Holocaust survivors]. Unpublished master's thesis, Department of Psychology, Tel Aviv University, Tel Aviv, Israel. 26 pp.

737 Glick, David (1995). Reflections of the Holocaust. *Pastoral Psychology*, 44(1), 13-27.

738 Glicksman, W. (1953). Social differentiation in the German concentration camp. *YIVO Annual Jewish Social Science*, 8, 123-150.

739 Głogowski, Leon (1971). From "guinea pig" in Auschwitz to the post of head of the hospital in Birkenau. In: *Auschwitz Anthology. Vol. 2:*

In Hell They Preserved Human Dignity. Part 1. Warsaw: International Auschwitz Committee, pp. 150-183.

740 Głowacki, Czesław (1973). Pathologic precocious senility in women, former inmates of concentration camps during World War II. *Ginekologia Polska*, 44(3), 315-318.

741 Głowacki, Czesław (1973). Zmiany patologiczive narzadu rodnego u kobiet bylych więźniarek obozów koncentrcyjnch [Gynecological pathological changes in female concentration camp ex-prisoners]. *Ginekologia Polska*, 44, 901-906.

742 Głowacki, Czesław (1976). Brak miesiączki u kobiet byłych więźniów obozów koncentracyjnych [Amenorrhea in female concentration camp ex-prisoners]. *Ginekologia Polska*, 47, 1403-1408.

743 Głowacki, Czesław (1978). Die biologischen Auswirkungen von Spätfolgen einer in frühen Jugend durchgemachten Hungerdystrophie bei Frauen, die im Konzentrationslager Auschwitz-Birkenau festgehalten wurden. II Ausbleiben der Menstruation nach der Lagerhäft [Biological aspects of late sequelae of hunger dystrophy undergone in early childhood in women that were imprisoned in concentration camp Auschwitz-Birkenau. Omission of menstruation after camp internment]. In: *Medizinische Untersuchungen der Spätfolgen des Krieges und des NS-Regimes bei Jugendlichen und Kindern von ehemaligen KZ-Häftlingen und Verfolgten* [Medical Research of the Late Effects of the War and National Socialism Regime on Youth and Children of Former Concentration Camp Inmates and Persecuted Persons]. Wien: Internationale Föderation der Widerstandskämpfer. [VI Internationaler Medizinischer Kongress der FIR. Prague, 1976].

744 Goder, Liora (1981). *Haify'unim haishiutim shel dor sheyni l'nitzoley shoah b'yisrael* [Personality characteristics of the offspring of Nazi Holocaust survivors in Israel]. Unpublished master's thesis, Department of Psychology, Tel Aviv University, Tel Aviv, Israel. 113 pp.

745 Goderez, Bruce I. (1987). The survivor syndrome: Massive psychic trauma and post-traumatic stress disorder. *Bulletin of the Menninger Clinic*, 51(1), 96-113.

746 Godorowski, Kazimierz (1985). Problematyka psychologiczno-medyczna hitlerowskich obozów koncentracyjnych w piśmienictwie włoskim [Psychologico-medical problems of Hitler's concentration camps in Italian literature]. *Przegląd Lekarski*, 42(1), 191-196.

747 Godorowski, Kazimierz (1986). Antypsychoterapia i antypedagogika: Wzórce totalitarny sociotechniki [Antipsychotherapy and anti-pedagogics: Examples of totalitarian sociotechniques]. *Przegląd Lekarski*, 43(1), 17-20.

748 Gogołowska, Stanisława (1975). Służba zdrowia w obozie janowskim [Health services at the Janowska camp]. *Przegląd Lekarski*, 32(1), 89-96.

749 Goldburg, Jay B. (1983). *The transmittal of the trauma of the Holocaust to survivor children and American Jewish children.* Unpublished doctoral dissertation, Drake University, Des Moines, Iowa, 154 pp. *Dissertation Abstracts International*, 44(3-B), p. 953. (University Microfilms no. AAC 8316265).

750 Goldman, Brian (1994). Medicine in the Terezin Ghetto: Commitment to care amidst a concentration camp's horrors. *Canadian Psychiatric Association Journal*, 150(1), 62-63.

751 Goldschmidt, E.P. (1946). Over de joodsche oorlogspleegkinderen [Concerning Jewish war orphans in foster families]. *Maandblad voor de Geestelijke Volksgezondheid*, 12, 310-311.

752 Goldsmith, Marilynn (1985). *Family patterns across three generations of Holocaust survivor families*. Unpublished doctoral dissertation, University of Pittsburgh, Pennsylvania, 204 pp. *Dissertation Abstracts International*, 47(5-B), p. 2195. (University Microfilms no. AAC 8617235

753 Goldstein, Jacob; Lukoff, Irving F.; and Strauss, Herbert A. (1951). A case history of a concentration camp survivor. *American O.S.E. Review*, 8, 11-28.

754 Goldstein, Jacob; Lukoff, Irving F.; and Strauss, Herbert A. (1991). *Individuelles und kollektives Verhalten im Nazi Konzentrationslagern: Soziologische und psychologische Studien zu Berichten ungarisch-jüdischer Überlebender* [Individual and Collective Accounts in Nazi Concentration Camps: Sociological and Psychological Studies and Reports on Hungarian Jewish Survivors]. Frankfurt am Main and New York: Campus. 198 pp.

755 Goldwasser, Norman (1986). Effects of the Holocaust on survivors and their families. In: Auerbach, Stephen M., and Stolberg, Arnold L. (Eds.), *Crisis Intervention with Children and Families*. Washington, D.C.: Hemisphere, pp. 227-242.

756 Goodman, Jeffrey S. (1979). *The transmission of parental trauma: Second generation effects of Nazi concentration camp survival.* Unpublished doctoral dissertation, California School of Professional Psychology, Fresno, 121 pp. *Dissertation Abstracts International*, 39(8-B), p. 4031. (University Microfilms no. AAC 7901805).

757 Gordon, Arlene C. (1990). Self-disclosure in Holocaust survivors: Effects on the next generation. In: Stricker, George, and Fisher, Martin (Eds.), *Self-Disclosure in the Therapeutic Relationship*. New York: Plenum, pp. 227-245.

758 Gottesfeld, Johanna; Van der Hal, Elisheva; and Tauber, Yvonne (1995). An alternative model of group work with second generation Holocaust survivors. In: Lemberger, John (Ed.), *A Global Perspective on Working with Holocaust Survivors and the Second Generation*. Jerusalem: JDC-Brookdale Institute of Gerontology and Human Development, AMCHA, and JDC-Israel, pp. 391-399.

759 Gottschick, Johann (1963). *Psychiatrie der Kriegsgefangenschaft dargestellt auf Grund von Beobachtungen in dem USA an deutschen Kriegsgefangenen aus dem letzten Weltkrieg* [Psychiatry of War Internment Based on Observations Made on German Prisoners of War of the Last World War in the USA]. Stuttgart: Gustav Fischer. 269 pp.

760 Goudsmit, W. (1972). Leven na een oorlog... of: Over oorlogsslachtoffers [Life after a war... or: About war victims]. *Maandblad voor de Geestelijke Volksgezondheid*, 9, 412-416.

761 Goukassian, H. (1959). Hungerdystrophie [Hunger dystrophy]. In: Michel, Max (Ed.), *Gesundheitsschäden durch Verfolgung und Gefangenschaft und ihre Spätfolgen: Zusammenstellung der Referate und Ergebnisse der Internationalen Sozialmedizinischen Konferenz über die Pathologie der Ehemaligen Deportierten und Internierten, 5-7 Juni 1954 in Kopenhagen* [Health Damages Caused by Persecution and Internment and the Late Effects: Compilation of the Papers and Results of the International Conference of Social Medicine on the Pathology of Former Deported and Interned Persons, 5-7 June 1954 in Copenhagen]. Frankfurt am Main: Röderberg, pp. 127-134.

762 Grauer, H. (1969). Psychodynamics of the survivor syndrome. *Canadian Psychiatric Association Journal*, 14(6), 617-622.

763 Greenblatt, Steven (1978). The influence of survival guilt on chronic family crises. *Journal of Psychology and Judaism*, 2(2), 19-28.

764 Greenfeld, Howard (1993). *The Hidden Children*. New York: Ticknor & Fields Books for Young Readers. 118 pp.

765 Greenspan, Henry (1986). *Who can retell? On the recounting of life history by Holocaust survivors*. Unpublished doctoral dissertation, Brandeis University, Waltham, Massachusetts, 383 pp. *Dissertation Abstracts International*, 47(1-A), p. 322. (University Microfilms no. AAC 8606421).

766 Greenspan, Henry (1992). Lives as texts: Symptoms as modes of recounting in the life histories of Holocaust survivors. In: Rosenwald, George C., and Ochberg, Richard L. (Eds.), *Storied Lives: The Cultural Politics of Self-Understanding*. New Haven, CT: Yale Universities Press.

767 Greve, W. (1963). Die Rückgliederung von Verfolgten: Ihre Begutachtung [The rehabilitation of persecutees: Evaluation]. *Therapiewoche*, 22, 1-4.

768 Greve, W., and Ruffin, H. (1963). Erfahrungen bei der begutachtung von verfolgten [Experiences in the evaluation of persecutees]. *Jahrbuch für Psychologie und Psychotherapie*, 11, 66-81.

769 Grobin, W. (1965). Medical assessment of late effects of National Socialist persecution. *Canadian Medical Association Journal*, 92, 911-917.

770 Grobman, Alex (1993). *Rekindling the Flame: American Jewish Chaplains and the Survivors of European Jewry, 1944-1948*. Detroit, MI: Wayne State University Press. 259 pp.

771 Grodin, Michael A. (1994). Historical origins of the Nuremberg code. Jewish doctors in Germany. In: Michalczyk, John J. (Ed.), *Medicine, Ethics, and the Third Reich: Historical and Contemporary Issues*. Kansas City, MO: Sheed & Ward, pp. 169-194.

772 Grodin, Michael A.; Annas, George J.; and Glantz, Leonard (1994). Medicine and human rights: A proposal for international action. In: Michalczyk, John J. (Ed.), *Medicine, Ethics, and the Third Reich: Historical and Contemporary Issues*. Kansas City, MO: Sheed & Ward.

773 Groen, J. (1947). Psychogenesis and psychotherapy of ulcerative colitis. *Psychosomatic Medicine*, 9, 151.

774 Grønvik, Odd, and Lønnum, Arve (1961). Neurologiske folgetilstander hos tidligere konsentrasjonsleirfanger [Neurological sequelae in concentration camp ex-prisoners]. *Tidsskrift for den Norske Laegeforening. Journal of the Norwegian Medical Association*, 81, 810-816.

775 Grønvik, Odd, and Lønnum, Arve (1961). Study of a group of former Norwegian deportees. Part 3: The neurological condition of ex-prisoners from concentration camps. In: *International Conference on the Later Effects of Imprisonment and Deportation Organized by the World Veterans Federation. The Hague, November 20-25, 1961.* The Hague: World Veterans Federation, pp. 89-92.

776 Grønvik, Odd, and Lønnum, Arve (1962). Neurological conditions in former concentration camp inmates. *Journal of Neuropsychiatry*, 4, 51-54.

777 Gross, Shlomit (1988). The relationship of severity of the Holocaust condition to survivors' child-rearing abilities and their offsprings' mental health. *Family Therapy*, 15(3), 211-222.

778 Grossman, Frances G. (1981). Creativity as a means of coping with anxiety. *The Arts in Psychotherapy*, 8(3-4), 185-192.

779 Grossman, Frances G. (1984). A psychological study of gentiles who saved the lives of Jews during the Holocaust. In: Charny, Israel W. (Ed.), *Towards the Understanding and Prevention of Genocide: Proceedings of the International Conference on the Holocaust and Genocide*. Boulder, CO: Westview, pp. 202-216.

780 Grossman, Frances G. (1989). The art of the children of Terezin: A psychological study. *Holocaust and Genocide Studies*, 4(2), 213-229.

781 Grubrich-Simitis, Ilse (1979). Extreme traumatization as cumulative trauma: Psychoanalytic investigations of the effects of concentration camp experience in survivors and their children. *Psyche: Zeitschrift für Psychoanalyse und ihre Anwendungen*, 33(11), 991-1023.

782 Grubrich-Simitis, Ilse (1981). Extreme traumatization as cumulative trauma: Psychoanalytic investigations of the effects of concentration camp experience in survivors and their children. In: Solnit, Albert J.; Eissler, Ruth S.; Freud, Anna; Kris, Marianne, and Neubauer, Peter B. (Eds.), *Psychoanalytic Study of the Child. Vol. 36*. New Haven, CT: Yale University Press, pp. 415-450.

783 Grubrich-Simitis, Ilse (1984). Vom Konkretismus zur Metaphorik. Gedanken zur psychoanalytischen Arbeit mit Nachkommen der Holocaust Generationanlasslich einer Neuerscheinung [From concretism to metaphor: Psychoanalytic work with descendants of the Holocaust generation]. *Psyche: Zeitschrift für Psychoanalyse und ihre Anwendungen*, 38(1), 1-27.

784 Grunberg, Kurt (1987). Folgen nationalsozialistischer Verfolgung bei judischen Nachkommen Uberlebender in der Bundesrepublik Deutschland [Consequences of Nazi persecution among Jewish descendents of survivors in the Federal Republic of Germany]. *Psyche: Zeitschrift für Psychoanalyse und ihre Anwendungen*, 41(6), 492-507.

785 Grunberger, B. (1963). Der Antisemit und der Oedipuskomplex [The anti-Semite and the oedipus complex]. *Psyche: Zeitschrift für Psychoanalyse und ihre Anwendungen*, 16, 255.

786 Grygier, Tadeusz (1973). *Oppression: A Study in Social and Criminal Psychology*. Westport, CT: Greenwood. 362 pp.

787 Guterman, S.S. (1975). Alternative theories in the study of slavery, the concentration camp, and personality. *British Journal of Sociology*, 186, 186-202.

788 Gutman, Israel, and Berenbaum, Michael (Eds.) (1994). *Anatomy of the Auschwitz Death Camp*. Bloomington, IN: Indiana University Press. 638 pp.

789 Gutt, Romuald W. (1971). Remarks on the subject of ethics of Nazi physicians. In: *Auschwitz Anthology. Vol. 1: Inhuman Medicine. Part* 2. Warsaw: International Auschwitz Committee, pp. 205-221.

790 Guttmann, David (1995). Meaningful aging: Establishing a club for survivors of the Holocaust in Hungary. In: Lemberger, John (Ed.), *A Global Perspective on Working with Holocaust Survivors and the Second Generation*. Jerusalem: JDC-Brookdale Institute of Gerontology and Human Development, AMCHA, and JDC-Israel, pp. 259-267.

791 Guy, Helen; Charny, Israel W.; Rahav, Giora; and Shaked, Ami (1996). *Intimacy, happiness and sexual satisfaction among second generation Holocaust survivors* [Paper presented at the Second World Conference of the International Society for Traumatic Stress Studies, Jerusalem, July].

792 Haans, T. (1981). Een maatschappelijke benadering van het KZ-syndroom [A social approach to the concentration camp syndrome]. In: Boutellier, H., and Wouda, L. (Eds.), *Progressieve Ontwikkelingen in de Psychologie* [Progressive Developments in Psychology]. Amsterdam: SUA, pp. 93-100.

793 Haans, T. (1983). Oorlogsoverlevende of psychiatriese patient, de maatschappelijke achtergronden van het KZ-syndroom [Survivor of the war or psychiatric patient, the social backgrounds of the concentration camp syndrome]. *Psychologie & Maatschappij*, 2, 2.

794 Haans, T. (1984). Oorlogsoverlevenden: teruggekeerden of slachtoffers? [Survivors of the war: returned people or victims?]. In: Dane, Jan (Ed.), *Keerzijde van de bevrijding: Opstellen over de maatschappelijke, psycho-sociale en medische aspekten van de problematiek van oorlogsgetroffenen* [The Other Side of Liberation: Essays on the Social, Psychosocial and Medical Aspects of the Problems of War Victims]. Deventer: Van Loghum Slaterus, pp. 36-55.

795 Haans, T. (1988). Group psychotherapy with survivors of World War II persecution. *Group Analysis*, 21, 267-280.

796 Haas, Peter J. (1994). The healing-killing paradox. In: Michalczyk, John J. (Ed.), *Medicine, Ethics, and the Third Reich: Historical and Contemporary Issues*. Kansas City, MO: Sheed & Ward, pp. 19-23.

797 Haber, Calvin H. (1988). The analysis of a latency age survivor of the Holocaust. *Psychoanalytic Review*, 75(4), 641-651.

798 Hackenbroch, M. (1971). Die Beurteilung degenerativer Erkrankungen des Stutzsystems bei ehemaligen Kriegsgefangenen und Verfolgten [The evaluation of degenerative diseases of the support-system in former prisoners of war and in persecutees]. In: Herberg, Hans-Joachim (Ed.), *Spätschäden nach Extrembelastungen* [Late Damage After Extreme Stress]. Herford: Nicolai, pp. 127-133. [II Internationalen Medizinisch-Juristischen Konferenz. Dusseldorf, 1969].

799 Hadar, Y. (1991). Existentielle erfahrung oder Krankheitssyndrom? Über legungen zum Begrift der "Zweiten Generation" [Existential experience or sickness syndrome? Reflections on understanding the second generation]. In: Stoffels, Hans (Ed.), *Schiksale der Verfolgten: Psychische und somatische Auswirkungen von Terrorherrschaft* [The Fate of Persecuted Persons: Psychic and Somatic Effects of Terror Reign]. Berlin: Springer, pp. 160-172.

800 Hadda, Janet R. (1989). Mourning the Yiddish language and some implications for treatment. In: Marcus, Paul, and Rosenberg, Alan (Eds.), *Healing Their Wounds: Psychotherapy with Holocaust Survivors and Their Families*. New York: Praeger, pp. 257-270.

801 Hadju, G. (1967). About the Hungarian aspects of the medical expert's assessment concerning decrease of working ability in persons submitted to "pseudoscientific medical experiments" in the Nazi concentration camps. *Acta Medicinae Legalis et Socialis*, 20(2), 297-302.

802 Haesler, Ludwig (1994). Survivors and their offspring in post-war Germany. *Echoes of the Holocaust,* 3, 1-8. [Bulletin of the Jerusalem Center for Research into the Late Effects of the Holocaust. Talbieh Mental Health Center, Jerusalem, Israel].

803 Häfner, Heinz (1968). Psychological disturbances following prolonged persecution. *Social Psychiatry*, 3(3), 79-88.

804 Häfner, Heinz (1969). Psychosocial changes following racial and political persecution. *Social Psychiatry*, 4(7), 101-117.

805 Hagen, Gunnar (1954). Evaluation, du point de vue assurance, de quelques suites de la maladie de famine chez d'anciens déportés Danois en camps de concentration [Assessment, from the point of view of social insurance, of some of the effects of hunger disease on Danish deportees in the concentration camps]. In: Thygesen, Paul (Ed.), *La Déportation dans les Camps de Concentration Allemands et ses Séquelles: Une Analyse médicale et sociale* [Deportation in the German Concentration Camps and its Consequences: A Medical and Social Analysis]. Copenhague: Edité par la Croix Rouge Danoise, pp. 78-80.

806 Hagen, Gunnar (1955). Einschätzung einiger Folgeerscheinungen der Hungerkrankheit bei dänischen Opfern des Naziterrors vom Standpunkt der Sozialversicherung [Assessment of some of the effects of hunger disease on Danish victims of Nazi terror from the point of view of social insurance]. In: Michel, Max (Ed.), *Gesundheitsschäden durch Verfolgung und Gefangenschaft und ihre Spätfolgen: Zusammenstellung der Referate und Ergebnisse der internationalen Sozialmedizinischen Konferenz über die Pathologie der Ehemaligen Deportierten und Internierten, 5-7 Juni 1954 in Kopenhagen* [Health Damages Caused by Persecution and Internment and the Late Effects: Compilation of the Papers and Results of the International Conference of Social Medicine on the Pathology of

Former Deported and Interned Persons, 5-7 June 1954 in Copenhagen]. Frankfurt am Main: Röderberg, pp. 268-273.

807 Hagen, W. (1973). Krieg, Hunger und Pestilenz in Warschau, 1939-1943 [War, hunger, and pestilence in Warsaw, 1939-1943]. *Gesundheitswesen und Desinfektion*, 8, 115-128.

808 Hahn, Susanne (1994). Nursing issues during the Third Reich. In: Michalczyk, John J. (Ed.), *Medicine, Ethics, and the Third Reich: Historical and Contemporary Issues*. Kansas City, MO: Sheed & Ward, pp. 143-152.

809 Haine, J.C. (1974). Evaluation des séquelles invalidantes tardives de la captivité trente ans après le conflict de 1940-1945 [Evaluation of late disabling sequelae of captivity 30 years after the war of 1940-1945]. *Revue Médicale de Bruxelles*, 54, 639-653.

810 Halberstadt-Freud, Hendrika C. (1995). Fünfzig jahre nach Anne Frank: Reaktivierung einer transgenerationellen traumatisierung in der Überstragung [Fifty years after Anne Frank. Reactivation of transgenerational traumatization in transference]. *Psyche: Zeitschrift für Psychoanalyse und ihre Anwendungen*, 49(1), 1-17.

811 Hałgas, Kazimierz (1967). Z obozu koncentracyjnego w Gross-Rosen (Wspomnienia lekarza) [From the concentration camp in Gross-Rosen (a physician's memoirs)]. *Przegląd Lekarski*, 23(1), 197-203.

812 Hałgas, Kazimierz (1975). Epidemia jaglicy w obozie Gross-Rosen w r. 1943 [Trachoma at the Gross-Rosen concentration camp in 1943]. *Przegląd Lekarski*, 32(1), 167-171.

813 Hałgas, Kazimierz (1977). Zagadnienia sanitarne komanda Dyhernfurth II [Sanitary conditions at the Dyhernfurth command]. *Przegląd Lekarski*, 34(1), 122-130.

814 Hałgas, Kazimierz (1980). Z pracy w tzw. rewirach dla jeńców radzieckich w Oświęcimiu i w Gross-Rosen [Section for Soviet prisoners-of-war in the Auschwitz-Birkenau concentration camp]. *Przegląd Lekarski*, 37(1), 162-171.

815 Hałgas, Kazimierz (1987). Die Arbeit im "Revier" für sowjetische Kriegsgefangene in Auschwitz. Ein Bericht [Work in the "ward" for Soviet prisoners of war in the Auschwitz-Birkenau concentration camp]. In: Hamburger Institut für Sozialforschung (Eds.), *Die Auschwitz-Hefte. Texte der polnischen Zeitschrift "Przegląd Lekarski" über historische, psychische und medizinische Aspekte des Lebens* *und Sterbens in Auschwitz. Band 1* [The Auschwitz Journal. Text of the Polish Journal "Medical Review" on Historical, Psychic and Medical Aspects of Life and Death in Auschwitz. Volume 1]. Weinheim und Basel: Beltz, pp. 167-172.

816 Halik, Vicki; Rosenthal, Doreen A.; and Pattison, Philippa E. (1990). Intergenerational effects of the Holocaust: Patterns of engagement in the mother-daughter relationship. *Family Process*, 29(3), 325-339.

817 Hałlof-Mikołajewska, Z. (1989). Koniec gehenny obozowej [The end of the concentration camp gehenna]. *Przegląd Lekarski*, 46(1), 164-167.

818 Hamburger Institut für Sozialforschung (Eds.) (1987). *Die Auschwitz-Hefte. Texte der polnischen Zeitschrift "Przegląd Lekarski" über historische, psychische und medizinische Aspekte des Lebens und Sterbens in Auschwitz. Band 1* [The Auschwitz Journal. Text of the Polish Journal "Medical Review" on Historical, Psychic and Medical Aspects of Life and Death in Auschwitz. Volume 1]. Weinheim und Basel: Beltz. 328 pp.

819 Hamburger Institut für Sozialforschung (Eds.) (1987). *Die Auschwitz-Hefte. Texte der polnischen Zeitschrift "Przegląd Lekarski" über historische, psychische und medizinische Aspekte des Lebens und Sterbens in Auschwitz. Band* 2 [The Auschwitz Journal. Text of the Polish Journal "Medical Review" on Historical, Psychic and Medical Aspects of Life and Death in Auschwitz. Volume 2]. Weinheim und Basel: Beltz. 329 pp.

820 Hammerman, Sylvia I. (1980). *Historical awareness and identity development in young adult offspring of Holocaust survivors*. Unpublished doctoral dissertation, Boston University, School of Education, 226 pp. *Dissertation Abstracts International*, 41(5-B), p. 1941. (University Microfilms no. AAC 8024105).

821 Hanauske-Abel, and Hartmut M. (1986). From Nazi Holocaust to nuclear Holocaust: A lesson to learn? *Lancet*, 2(8501), 271-273.

822 Hanke, Edward (1968). Refleksje więźnia obozu koncentracyjnego w Dachau, Wincentego Spaltensteina [Memoirs of Wincenty Spaltenstein, prisoner of the concentration camp in Dachau]. *Przegląd Lekarski*, 24(1), 110-115.

823 Hano, J. (1989). "Oddzial naukowy" w Dachau [The "Scientific Department" in Dachau]. *Przegląd Lekarski*, 46(1), 171-179.

824 Hanover, Lawrence A. (1981). *Parent-child relationships in children of survivors of the Nazi Holocaust*. Unpublished doctoral dissertation, United States International University, San Diego, California, 196 p. *Dissertation Abstracts International*, 42(2-B), p. 770. University Microfilms no. AAC 8114741).

825 Hantman, Shira; Solomon, Zahava; and Prager, Edward (1994). How the Gulf War affected aged Holocaust survivors. In: Brink, Terry L. (Ed.), *Holocaust Survivors' Mental Health*. New York: Haworth, pp. 27-37. [Published as a special issue of *Clinical Gerontologist*, 14(3).]

826 Harari, Edwin (1995). The longest shadow: A clinical commentary on Moshe Lange's "Silence: Therapy with Holocaust survivors and their families." *Australian and New Zealand Journal of Family Therapy*, 16(1), 11-13.

827 Harel, Zev (1983). Hitmodedut im matzavei lachatz v'histaglut: Rishuma aroch hatevach shel hashoah al hanitzolim [Coping with stress and adaptation: The long range impact of the Holocaust on survivors]. *Society and Welfare*, 5(3), 221-230.

828 Harel, Zev (1995). Serving Holocaust survivors and survivor families. *Marriage and Family Review*, 21(1-2), 29-49.

829 Harel, Zev; Kahana, Boaz; and Kahana, Eva F. (1984). The effects of the Holocaust: Psychiatric, behavioral, and survivor perspectives. *Journal of Sociology and Social Welfare*, 11(4), 915-929.

830 Harel, Zev; Kahana, Boaz; and Kahana, Eva F. (1988). Psychological well being among Holocaust survivors and immigrants in Israel. *Journal of Traumatic Stress*, 1(4), 413-429.

831 Harel, Zev; Kahana, Boaz; and Kahana, Eva F. (1993). Social resources and the mental health of aging Nazi Holocaust survivors and immigrants in Section A: Trauma and the aging process: Studies related to World War II. In: Wilson, John P., and Raphael, Beverley (Eds.), *International Handbook of Traumatic Stress Syndromes*. New York: Plenum, pp. 219-274.

832 Harmat, Paul (1989). The Holocaust of Hungary's psychoanalysts. *Journal of the American Academy of Psychoanalysis*, 17(2), 313-319.

833 Harris, Jaki R. (1992). *Children of the Holocaust: Coping with death*. Unpublished master's thesis, Sarah Lawrence College, Bronxville,

New York, 163 pp. *Masters Abstracts International*, 30(4), p. 1491. (University Microfilms no. AAC 1347918).

834 Hass, Aaron (1990). *In the Shadow of the Holocaust: The Second Generation*. Ithaca, NY: Cornell University Press. 178 pp.

835 Hass, Aaron (1995). *The Aftermath: Living with the Holocaust*. Cambridge: Cambridge University Press. 213 pp.

836 Hass, Aaron (1995). Survivor guilt in Holocaust survivors and their children. In: Lemberger, John (Ed.), *A Global Perspective on Working with Holocaust Survivors and the Second Generation*. Jerusalem: JDC-Brookdale Institute of Gerontology and Human Development, AMCHA, and JDC-Israel, pp. 163-184.

837 Hassan, Judith (1995). Furthering the work of professionals serving Holocaust survivors. In: Lemberger, John (Ed.), *A Global Perspective on Working with Holocaust Survivors and the Second Generation*. Jerusalem: JDC-Brookdale Institute of Gerontology and Human Development, AMCHA, and JDC-Israel, pp. 145-150.

838 Hassan, Judith (1995). Individual counselling techniques with Holocaust survivors. In: Lemberger, John (Ed.), *A Global Perspective on Working with Holocaust Survivors and the Second Generation*. Jerusalem: JDC-Brookdale Institute of Gerontology and Human Development, AMCHA, and JDC-Israel, pp. 185-203.

839 Hassan, Judith (1995). Helping elderly Holocaust survivors cope with aging. In: Lemberger, John (Ed.), *A Global Perspective on Working with Holocaust Survivors and the Second Generation*. Jerusalem: JDC-Brookdale Institute of Gerontology and Human Development, AMCHA, and JDC-Israel, pp. 249-258.

840 Hau, T.F. (1972). Vergleichende Untersuchungen an psychosomatisch erkrankten Jugendlichen der Geburtsjährgange der Vorkrieg-, Kriegsund und Nachkriegszeit [Comparison studies on psychosomatically ill youngsters born before, during and after the war]. *Praxis der Kinderpsychologie und Kinderpsychiatrie*, 6, 193-200.

841 Haver, Dali (1993). *Ikveyyato v'ya'ilito shel signon hitmodedut ishi l'orech tvach hachayim shel nitzoley hashoah* [Life span consistency and efficiency of personal coping style in Holocaust survivors]. Unpublished master's thesis, Department of Psychology, Tel Aviv University, Tel Aviv, Israel. 81 pp.

842 Hays, David, and Danieli, Yael (1976). Intentional groups with a specific problem orientation focus. In: Rosenbaum, Max, and Snadowsky, Alvin (Eds.), *The Intensive Group Experience*. New York: Free Press, pp. 111-145.

843 Hazan, Yoram (1987). "Dor sheni l'shoah" - musag be'safek ["The second generation of the Holocaust": A questionable concept]. *Sihot: Israel Journal of Psychotherapy*, 1, 104-108.

844 Heftler, N. (1979). Étude sur l'état actuel, psycho-sociologique, des enfants nés après le retour de déportation de leurs parents (père, mère, ou les deux) [Investigation of the present state of children, born after the deportation and liberation of their parents (father, mother or both)]. *Medizinisch Untersuchungen FIR*, 21-26.

845 Heger, W. (1969). *Om Norske Konsentrasjonsleir-fangers Stilling Idad. Ettervirkninger og Sosiale Problemer* [The Situation of the Norwegian Concentration Camp Ex-Prisoners Today: Late Sequels and Social Problems]. Hoston: Norske Kvinners Masjonalrads Sosialskole.

846 Heller, David (1982). Themes of culture and ancestry among children of concentration camp survivors. *Psychiatry*, 45(3), 247-261.

847 Heller, Joseph (1955). Folgeerscheinungen am Herzen und an den Gefässen [Late effects in the heart and vascular systems]. In: Michel, Max (Ed.), *Gesundheitsschädendurch Verfolgung und Gefangenschaft und ihre Spätfolgen: Zusammenstellung der Referate und Ergebnisse der Internationalen Sozialmedizinischen Konferenz über die Pathologie der Ehemaligen Deportierten und Internierten, 5-7 Juni 1954 in Kopenhagen* [Health Damages Caused by Persecution and Internment and the Late Effects: Compilation of the Papers and Results of the International Conference of Social Medicine on the Pathology of Former Deported and Interned Persons, 5-7 June 1954 in Copenhagen]. Frankfurt am Main: Röderberg, pp. 195-197.

848 Heller, Joseph (1960). Betrachtungen über die wichtigsten Herz und Gefässerkrankungen bei ehemaligen Deportierten und Internierten. Die Aussichten ihrer Behandlung [Remarks about the most important cardiovascular diseases in former deportees and internees. The chances of their treatment]. In: Fichez, Louis F. (Ed.), *Andere Spätfolgen, auf Grund der Beobachtungen bei den ehemaligen Deportierten und Internierten der nazistischen Gefangnisse und Vernichtungslager* [Other Belated Consequences, Based on the Observations of Former Deportees and Internees of Nazi Prisons and Death Camps]. Wien: Verlag der FIR, pp. 99-129.

849 Helmreich, William B. (1975). How Jewish students view the Holocaust: A preliminary appraisal. In: Steinitz, Lucy Y., and Szonyi, David M. (Eds.), *Living After the Holocaust: Reflections of the Post-War Generation in America*. New York: Bloch, pp. 101-114.

850 Helmreich, William B. (1987). Post-war adaptation of Holocaust survivors in the United States. *Holocaust and Genocide Studies*, 2(2), 307-315.

851 Helmreich, William B. (1990). Counselling: Whether or not war crimes trials go ahead in Britain the debate will ensure that Holocaust survivors are haunted by their memories. *Social Work Today*, 21(39), 17.

852 Helmreich, William B. (1990). The impact of Holocaust survivors on American society: A socio-cultural portrait. *Judaism*, 39(1), 14-27.

853 Helmreich, William B. (1992). *Against All Odds: Holocaust Survivors and the Successful Lives They Made in America*. New York: Simon & Schuster. 370 pp.

854 Helweg-Larsen, Per (1955). Tuberkulose-Spätfolgen [Tuberculosis-late sequelae]. In: Michel, Max (Ed.), *Gesundheitsschäden durch Verfolgung und Gefangenschaft und ihre Spätfolgen: Zusammenstellung der Referate und Ergebnisse der Internationalen Sozialmedizinischen Konferenz über die Pathologie der Ehemaligen Deportierten und Internierten, 5-7 Juni 1954 in Kopenhagen* [Health Damages Caused by Persecution and Internment and the Late Effects: Compilation of the Papers and Results of the International Conference of Social Medicine on the Pathology of Former Deported and Interned Persons, 5-7 June 1954 in Copenhagen]. Frankfurt am Main: Röderberg, pp. 101-106.

855 Helweg-Larsen, Per; Hoffmeyer, Henrik; Kieler, Jørgen; Hess Thaysen, Eigil; Hess Thaysen, Jørn; Thygesen, Paul; and Hertle Wulff, Munke (1952). *Famine Disease in German Concentration Camps, Complications and Sequelae: With Special Reference to Tuberculosis, Mental Disorders and Social Consequences*. Copenhagen: Ejnar Munksgaard. 460 pp. [Also published as *Acta Psychiatrica et Neurologica Scandinavica*, Supplementum 83.]

856 Helweg-Larsen, Per; Hoffmeyer, Henrik; Kieler, Jørgen; Hess Thaysen, Eigil; Hess Thaysen, Jørn; Thygesen, Paul; and Hertle Wulff, Munke (1954). La maladie de famine dans les camps de concentration allemands ses séquelles. Chapitre spécial pour: la tuberculose, les troubles psychiques et leurs conséquences sociales [Hunger disease in the German concentration camps and its aftereffects. Special chapter: Tuberculosis, psychic problems and their social consequences. In: Thygesen, Paul (Ed.), *La Déportation dans les Camps de Concentration Allemands et ses Séquelles: Une Analyse médicale et sociale* [Deportation in the German Concentration Camps and its Consequences: A Medical and Social Analysis]. Copenhague: Edité par la Croix Rouge Danoise, pp. 11-55.

857 Helweg-Larsen, Per; Hoffmeyer, Henrik; Kieler, Jørgen; Hess Thaysen, Eigil; Hess Thaysen, Jørn; Thygesen, Paul; and Hertle Wulff, Munke (1955). Die Hungerkrankheit in den deutschen Konzentrationslagern [Hunger disease in German concentration camps]. In: Michel, Max (Ed.), *Gesundheitsschäden durch Verfolgung und Gefangenschaft und ihre Spätfolgen: Zusammenstellung der Referate und Ergebnisse der Internationalen Sozialmedizinischen Konferenz über die Pathologie der Ehemaligen Deportierten und Internierten, 5-7 Juni 1954 in Kopenhagen* [Health Damages Caused by Persecution and Internment and the Late Effects: Compilation of the Papers and Results of the International Conference of Social Medicine on the Pathology of Former Deported and Interned Persons, 5-7 June 1954 in Copenhagen]. Frankfurt am Main: Röderberg, pp. 148-171.

858 Helweg-Larsen, Per; Hoffmeyer, Henrik; Kieler, Jørgen; Hess Thaysen, Eigil; Hess Thaysen, Jørn; Thygesen, Paul; and Hertle Wulff, Munke (1955). Herz und Gefäss-symptome der Hungerdystrophie [Cardiovascular symptoms in hunger dystrophy]. In: Michel, Max (Ed.), *Gesundheitsschäden durch Verfolgung und Gefangenschaft und ihre Spätfolgen: Zusammenstellung der Referate und Ergebnisse der Internationalen Sozialmedizinischen Konferenz über die Pathologie der Ehemaligen Deportierten und Internierten, 5-7 Juni 1954 in Kopenhagen* [Health Damages Caused by Persecution and Internment and the Late Effects: Compilation of the Papers and Results of the International Conference of Social Medicine on the Pathology of Former Deported and Interned Persons, 5-7 June 1954 in Copenhagen]. Frankfurt am Main: Röderberg, pp. 181-190.

859 Helweg-Larsen, Per; Hoffmeyer, Henrik; Kieler, Jørgen; Hess Thaysen, Eigil; Thygesen, Paul; and Hertle Wulff, Munke (1949). Sultsygdommen og dens folgetilstande hos koncentrationslejrfanger [The starvation disease and its sequelae in concentration camp prisoners]. *Ugeskrift for Laeger*, 111, 1-65.

860 Hemmendinger, Judith (1980). Readjustment of young concentration camp survivors through a surrogate family experience. *Interaction*, 3(3), 127-134.

861 Hemmendinger, Judith (1981). A la sortie des camps de la mort: Reinsertion dans la vie [Coming out of the camps: Return to life]. *Israel Journal of Psychiatry and Related Sciences*, 18(4), 331-334.

862 Hemmendinger, Judith (1984). *Les Enfants de Buchenwald: Que sont Devenus les 1000 Enfants Juifs Sauves en 1945?* [The Children of Buchenwald: What Became of the 1000 Jewish Children Saved in 1945?]. Lausanne: Favre. 203 pp.

863 Hemmendinger, Judith (1985). *De Kinderen van Buchenwald: Wat is er geworden van de duizend joodse Kinderen die in 1945 werden bevrijd?* [The Children of Buchenwald: What Became of the 1000 Jewish Children Saved in 1945?]. Baarn: Mingus. 159 pp.

864 Hemmendinger, Judith (1986). *Survivors: Children of the Holocaust*. Bethesda, MD: National Press. 149 pp.

865 Hemmendinger, Judith (1994). The children of Buchenwald: After liberation and now. *Echoes of the Holocaust*, 3, 40-51. [Bulletin of the Jerusalem Center for Research into the Late Effects of the Holocaust. Talbieh Mental Health Center, Jerusalem, Israel].

866 Hendin, Herbert (1985). "The concentration camp syndrome: An organic brain syndrome?": Commentary. *Integrative Psychiatry*, 3(2), 123-125.

867 Hendriks, G. (1975). Het KZ-syndroom en de sociale omgeving, een korte vergelijkende analyse over de psychische nawerkingen van de tweede wereld oorlog bij vervolgden in Polen en Nederland [The concentration camp syndrome and the social surroundings, a brief comparative analysis on the psychic sequelae of World War II in persecuted people in Poland and Holland]. *Maatschappelijk Welzijn*, 3, 62-68.

868 Henseler, H. (1965). Zum gegenwärtigen Stand der beurteilung Erlebnisdedingter Spätschäden nach Verfolgung [The present state of the evaluation of compensation experiences after persecution]. *Nervenarzt*, 36, 333-338.

869 Hentoff, Nat (1994). Contested terrain: The Nazi analogy in bioethics. In: Michalczyk, John J. (Ed.), *Medicine, Ethics, and the Third Reich: Historical and Contemporary Issues*. Kansas City, MO: Sheed & Ward, pp. 16-18.

870 Herberg, Hans-Joachim (1961). The cardiovascular sequelae of detention. In: *International Conference on the Later Effects of*

Imprisonment and Deportation Organized by the World Veterans Federation. The Hague, November 20-25, 1961. The Hague: World Veterans Federation, pp. 53-56.

871 Herberg, Hans-Joachim (1963). Die ärztliche Beurteilung Verfolgter im Entschädigungserfahren [The medical evaluation of persecuted people in the work of indemnification]. In: Paul, Helmut, and Herberg, Hans-Joachim (Eds.), *Psychische Spätschäden nach politischer Verfolgung* [Psychological Late Damages Following Political Persecution]. Basel: Karger, pp. 239-252.

872 Herberg, Hans-Joachim (1963). Psychische Belastungen und erlebnisreaktive Störungen in der Pathogenes innerer Krankheiten [Psychic stress and experiential disturbances in the pathogenesis of internal diseases]. In: Paul, Helmut, and Herberg, Hans-Joachim (Eds.), *Psychische Spätschäden nach politischer Verfolgung* [Psychological Late Damages Following Political Persecution]. Basel: Karger, pp. 257-280.

873 Herberg, Hans-Joachim (Ed.) (1967). *Die Beurteilung von Gesundheitsschäden nach Gefangenschaft und Verfolgung* [The Assessment of Health Damage Following Internment and Persecution]. Herford: Nicolai. 126 pp. [Internationalen Medizinisch-Juristischen Symposiums in Köln].

874 Herberg, Hans-Joachim (1967). Der gegenwärtige Stand der Beurteilung von Gesundheitsschäden nach Gefangenschaft und Verfolgung in der Bundesrepublik Deutschland [The present state of the evaluation of health damage after imprisonment and persecution in the German Federal Republic]. In: *Die Beurteilung von Gesundheitsschäden nach Gefangenschaft und Verfolgung* [The Assessment of Health Damages Following Internment and Persecution]. Herford: Nicolai, pp. 12-20. [Internationalen Medizinisch-Juristischen Symposiums in Köln].

875 Herberg, Hans-Joachim (Ed.) (1971). *Spätschäden nach Extrembelastungen* [Late Damage After Extreme Stress]. Herford: Nicolai. 338 pp. [II Internationalen Medizinische-Juristischen Konferenz. Dusseldorf, 1969].

876 Herman, David (1991). "Ruinboys" or rainbows?: Survivors of the Holocaust and their children. *Jewish Quarterly*, 38(2), 21-26.

877 Herman, Judith L. (1992). Complex PTSD: A syndrome in survivors of prolonged and repeated trauma. *Journal of Traumatic Stress*, 5(3), 377-391.

878 Herman, S. (1980). The meaning of death: Experience with survivors in Holland. In: Garlans, C. (Ed.), *Group Analysis*. London: The Trust for Group Analysis, pp. 33-42.

879 Hermann, Knud (1955). Die psychischen Symptomen des KZ Syndroms Versuch einer pathogenetischen Schätzung [The psychic symptoms of the concentration camp syndrome: An attempt at a psychopathogenic evaluation]. In: Michel, Max (Ed.), *Gesundheitsschäden durch Verfolgung und Gefangenschaft und ihre Spätfolgen: Zusammenstellung der Referate und Ergebnisse der Internationalen Sozialmedizinischen Konferenz über die Pathologie der Ehemaligen Deportierten und Internierten, 5-7 Juni 1954 in Kopenhagen* [Health Damages Caused by Persecution and Internment and the Late Effects: Compilation of the Papers and Results of the International Conference of Social Medicine on the Pathology of Former Deported and Interned Persons, 5-7 June 1954 in Copenhagen]. Frankfurt am Main: Röderberg, pp. 41-47.

880 Hermann, Knud (1955). Das Problem der Konzentrationslager Zehn Jahre nach der Befreiung (Enquête 1951-1953) [The problem of the concentration camps ten years after liberation (Inquiry: 1951-1953)]. In: Michel, Max (Ed.), *Gesundheitsschäden durch Verfolgung und Gefangenschaft und ihre Spätfolgen: Zusammenstellung der Referate und Ergebnisse der Internationalen Sozialmedizinischen Konferenz über die Pathologie der Ehemaligen Deportierten und Internierten, 5-7 Juni 1954 in Kopenhagen* [Health Damages Caused by Persecution and Internment and the Late Effects: Compilation of the Papers and Results of the International Conference of Social Medicine on the Pathology of Former Deported and Interned Persons, 5-7 June 1954 in Copenhagen]. Frankfurt am Main: Röderberg, pp. 59-72.

881 Hermann, Knud, and Thygesen, Paul (1954). KZ-syndromet hungerdystrofiends fölgetilstand 8 ar efter [The concentration camp syndrome. The sequelae of hunger dystrophy eight years later]. *Ugeskrift for Laeger*, 116, 825-836.

882 Hermann, Knud, and Thygesen, Paul (1954). Le syndrome des camps de concentration 8 ans après la libération [The concentration camp syndrome eight years after liberation]. In: Thygesen, Paul (Ed.), *La Déportation dans les Camps de Concentration Allemands et ses Séquelles: Une Analyse médicale et sociale* [Deportation in the German Concentration Camps and its Consequences: A Medical and Social Analysis]. Copenhague: Edité par la Croix Rouge Danoise, pp. 56-69.

883 Hers, J.F. (1988). The pathophysiology of imprisonment, deportation and resistance. In: Hers, J.F., and Terpstra, Johan L. (Eds.), *Stress: Medical and Legal Analysis of Late Effects of World War II Suffering in the Netherlands*. Leiden: Kooyker, pp. 75-82.

884 Hers, J.F., and Terpstra, Johan L. (Eds.) (1988). *Stress: Medical and Legal Analysis of Late Effects of World War II Suffering in the Netherlands*. Leiden: Kooyker. 186 pp.

885 Hers, J.F., and Terpstra, Johan L. (1988). Late effects of imprisonment, deportation, resistance and miltary action: A cause of premature aging? In: Hers, J.F., and Terpstra, Johan L. (Eds.), *Stress: Medical and Legal Analysis of Late Effects of World War II Suffering in the Netherlands*. Leiden: Kooyker, pp. 83-104.

886 Herskovic, Steven A. (1990). *A comparative study of stress and coping strategies of adult children of Holocaust survivors and adult children of non-Holocaust survivors*. Unpublished doctoral dissertation, United States International University, San Diego, California, 174 pp. *Dissertation Abstracts International*, 51(2-B), p. 1029. (University Microfilms no. AAC 9012957).

887 Hertz, Dan G. (1990). Trauma and nostalgia: New aspects on the coping of aging Holocaust survivors. *Israel Journal of Psychiatry and Related Sciences*, 27(4), 189-198.

888 Hertz, Dan G. (1993). Heinrich Zvi Winnik: Profile of a pioneer Israeli researcher of the Holocaust. *Echoes of the Holocaust*, 2, 1-4. [Bulletin of the Jerusalem Center for Research into the Late Effects of the Holocaust. Talbieh Mental Health Center, Jerusalem, Israel].

889 Hertz, Dan G., and Freyberger, Hellmuth (1982). Factors influencing the evaluation of psychological and psychosomatic reactions in survivors of the Nazi persecution. *Journal of Psychosomatic Research*, 26(1), 83-89.

890 Herzka, Heinz S.; Von Schumacher, A.; and Tyrangiel, S. (1989). Children of the persecuted: The offspring of the Nazi victims and refugee's children today. *Praxis der Kinderpsychologie und Kinderpsychiatrie*, 29, 154.

891 Herzog, James M. (1981). Father hurt and father hunger: The effect of a survivor father's waning years on his son. *Journal of Geriatric Psychiatry*, 14(2), 211-223.

892 Herzog, James M. (1982). World beyond metaphor: Thoughts on the transmission of trauma. In: Bergmann, Martin S., and Jucovy, Milton E. (Eds.), *Generations of the Holocaust.* New York: Basic Books, pp. 103-119.

893 Hes, Jozef Ph. (1983). Some remarks on the case of specificity in the administration of psychiatric help. In: Ayalon, Ofra; Eitinger, Leo; Lansen, Johan; Sunier, Armand; and others, *The Holocaust and its Perseverance: Stress, Coping and Disorder.* Assen, The Netherlands: Van Gorcum, pp. 49-51.

894 Hess Thaysen, Eigil, and Hess Thaysen, Jørn (1954). *Les Problèmes Médicaux Chez les Anciens Deportés* [The Medical Problems of Elderly Deportees]. Copenhagen: Congresverslag.

895 Hess Thaysen, Eigil, and Hess Thaysen, Jørn (1955). Medizinische Probleme bei früheren, in deutsche Konzentrationslager Deportierten [Medical problems in former concentration camp internees]. In: Michel, Max (Ed.), *Gesundheitsschäden durch Verfolgung und Gefangenschaft und ihre Spätfolgen: Zusammenstellung der Referate und Ergebnisse der Internationalen Sozialmedizinischen Konferenz über die Pathologie der Ehemaligen Deportierten und Internierten, 5-7 Juni 1954 in Kopenhagen* [Health Damages Caused by Persecution and Internment and the Late Effects: Compilation of the Papers and Results of the International Conference of Social Medicine on the Pathology of Former Deported and Interned Persons, 5-7 June 1954 in Copenhagen]. Frankfurt am Main: Röderberg, pp. 172-180.

896 Heymont, Irving (1982). *Among the Survivors of the Holocaust, 1945: The Landsberg Letters of Major Irving Heymont, United States Army.* Cincinnati, OH: American Jewish Archives. 111 pp.

897 Hicklin, Margot (1946). War-damaged children: Some aspects of recovery. *British Association of Psychiatric Social Workers*, May-July.

898 Hilberg, Raoul (1980). The nature of the process: The perpetrators - The victims. In: Dimsdale, Joel E. (Ed.), *Survivors, Victims, and Perpetrators: Essays on the Nazi Holocaust.* Washington, D.C.: Hemisphere, pp. 5-54.

899 Hilderiuk-Wagner, L. (1989). *Psycho-sociaalse problematiek van de tweede generatie oorlogsslachtoffers* [Psychosocial problems of the second generation war victims]. Unpublished doctoral dissertation, Catholic University, Nijmegen, Netherlands.

900 Hirschfield, Miriam J. (1977). Care of the aging Holocaust survivor. *American Journal of Nursing*, 77(7), 1187-1189.

901 Hirschler, P. (1951). Over oorlogneuroses [Concerning war neuroses]. *Nederlands Tijdschrift voor Geneeskunde*, 6, 159.

902 Hochheimer, W. (1963). Vorurteilsminderung in der Erziehung und die Prophylaxe des Antisemitismus [Decreasing prejudice through education and the prevention of antisemitism]. *Psyche: Zeitschrift für Psychoanalyse und ihre Anwendungen*, 16, 285.

903 Hochman, John (1978). On the analysis of a child of Holocaust survivors with some notes on countertransference problems. *Bulletin of the Southern California Psychoanalytic Institute and Society*, 33.

904 Hocking, F. (1965). Human reactions to extreme environmental stress. *Medical Journal of Australia*, 52, 477-482.

905 Hocking, F. (1970). Psychiatric aspects of extreme environmental stress. *Diseases of the Nervous System*, 31(8), 324-326.

906 Hodgkins, Benjamin J., and Douglass, Richard L. (1984). Research issues surrounding Holocaust survivors: Adaptability and aging. *Journal of Sociology and Social Welfare*, 11(4), 894-914.

907 Hoefer, Carl H. (1983). Die Konzentrationslager Haft im Lichte einer Phanomenologie der Entfremdung [The concentration camp experience in light of the phenomenology of alienation]. *Zeitschrift für Klinische Psychologie, Psychopathologie und Psychotherapie*, 31(4), 333-351.

908 Hoff, H. (1971). Die Klinik psychischer Verfolgungschäden [The hospital for psychic persecution]. In: Herberg, Hans-Joachim (Ed.), *Spätschäden nach Extrembelastungen* [Late Damage After Extreme Stress]. Herford: Nicolai, pp. 285-289. [II Internationalen Medizinische-Juristischen Konferenz. Dusseldorf, 1969].

909 Hoffman, T. (1967). Verfolgungsschaden Haftungsgrenze und Stellenwert psychischer Schäden unter Beruecksichtigung der Sonderrelungen und Beweiserleichterungen im BEG [The importance, limits and evaluation of psychological damages as practised according to the newer German restitution law's (BEG) special regulations]. In: Herberg, Hans-Joachim (Ed.), *Die Beurteilung von Gesundheittsschäden nach Gefangenschaft und Verfolgung* [The Assessment of Health Damages Following Internment and Persecution]. Herford: Nicolai, pp. 58-65. [Internationalen Medizinisch-Juristischen Symposiums in Köln].

910 Hoffmeyer, Henrik (1954). Principes therapeutiques [Therapeutic principles]. In: Thygesen, Paul (Ed.), *La Déportation dans les Camps de Concentration Allemands et ses Séquelles: Une Analyse médicale et sociale* [Deportation in the German Concentration Camps and its Consequences: A Medical and Social Analysis]. Copenhague: Edité par la Croix Rouge Danoise, pp. 73-77.

911 Hoffmeyer, Henrik (1955). Soziale und therapeutische Aspekte der Spätfolgen [Social and therapeutic aspects of late sequelae]. In: Michel, Max (Ed.), *Gesundheitsschäden durch Verfolgung und Gefangenschaft und ihre Spätfolgen: Zusammenstellung der Referate und Ergebnisse der Internationalen Sozialmedizinischen Konferenz über die Pathologie der Ehemaligen Deportierten und Internierten, 5-7 Juni 1954 in Kopenhagen* [Health Damages Caused by Persecution and Internment and the Late Effects: Compilation of the Papers and Results of the International Conference of Social Medicine on the Pathology of Former Deported and Interned Persons, 5-7 June 1954 in Copenhagen]. Frankfurt am Main: Röderberg, pp. 251-255.

912 Hofrichter, Rita (1992). Enhancing communications: Triggers, words and resources. In: Kenigsberg, Rositta E., and Lieblich, Cathy M. (Eds.), *The First National Conference on Identification, Treatment and Care of the Aging Holocaust Survivor, March 29-31, 1992: Selected Proceedings*. Miami, FL: Holocaust Documentation and Education Center and Southeast Florida Center on Aging, Florida International University, pp. 58-63.

913 Hogman, Flora (1983). Displaced Jewish children during World War II: How they coped. *Journal of Humanistic Psychology*, 23(1), 51-66.

914 Hogman, Flora (1985). Role of memories in lives of World War II orphans. *Journal of the American Academy of Child Psychiatry*, 24(4), 390-396.

915 Hogman, Flora (1988). The experience of Catholicism for Jewish children during World War II. *Psychoanalytic Review*, 75(4), 511-532.

916 Hogman, Flora (1995). Memory of the Holocaust. *Echoes of the Holocaust*, 4, 36-49. [Bulletin of the Jerusalem Center for Research into the Late Effects of the Holocaust. Talbieh Mental Health Center, Jerusalem, Israel].

917 Holtzer, G. (1987). Medische causaliteit by oorlogs-getroffenen 1940-1945: Het nare van het literatuuronderzoek van Schudel en Pepplinkhuizen [Medical effects on war victims: The problem with the literature reviews of Schudel and Pepplinkhuizen]. *Medisch Contact*, 42, 970-972.

918 Honingman, C.R. (1979). Concentration camp survivors: A challenge for psychiatric nursing. *Nursing Clinics of North America*, 4, 621-628.

919 Hoppe, Klaus (1962). Persecution, depression and aggression. *Bulletin of the Menninger Clinic*, 26, 195-203.

920 Hoppe, Klaus (1964). Über den Einfluss der Ubergangsobjekte und Phänomene auf die Behandlungssituation [Concerning the influence of transitional objects and phenomena in symptom formation]. In: Scheunert, G. (Ed.), *Jahrbuch der Psychoanalyse. Vol. 4*. Bern and Stuttgart: Huber.

921 Hoppe, Klaus (1965). Persecution and conscience. *Psychoanalysis Review*, 52, 106-116.

922 Hoppe, Klaus (1965). Psychotherapie bei Konzentrationslageropfern [Psychotherapy of concentration camp victims]. *Psyche: Zeitschrift für Psychoanalyse und ihre Anwendungen*, 19(5), 290-319.

923 Hoppe, Klaus (1966). The psychodynamics of concentration camp victims. *Psychoanalytic Forum*, 1(1), 76-85.

924 Hoppe, Klaus (1966). Zum gegenwärtigen Stand der Beurteilung erlebnisbedingter Spätschäden nach Verfolgung [On the present status of compensation and evaluation experiences following persecution]. *Nervenarzt*, 37, 124.

925 Hoppe, Klaus (1968). Psychosomatische Reaktionen und Erkrankungen bei Überlebenden schwerer Verfolgung [Psychosomatic reactions and disorders in survivors of severe persecution]. *Psyche: Zeitschrift für Psychoanalyse und ihre Anwendungen*, 22(6), 464-477.

926 Hoppe, Klaus (1968). Psychotherapy with survivors of Nazi persecution. In: Krystal, Henry (Ed.), *Massive Psychic Trauma*. New York: International Universities Press, pp. 204-219.

927 Hoppe, Klaus (1968). Resomatization of affects in survivors of persecution. *International Journal of Psycho-Analysis*, 49(2-3), 324-326.

928 Hoppe, Klaus (1968). Symposium on psychological problems after severe mental stress. In: Lopez Ibor, Juan J. (Ed.), *Proceedings.*

Fourth World Congress of Psychiatry, Madrid 5-11 September 1966. Vol. 2. New York: Excerpta Medica Foundation.

929 Hoppe, Klaus (1971). The aftermath of Nazi persecution reflected in recent psychiatric literature. *International Psychiatry Clinics*, 8, 169-204.

930 Hoppe, Klaus (1971). Chronic reactive aggression in survivors of extreme persecution. *Comprehensive Psychiatry*, 12(3), 230-237.

931 Hoppe, Klaus (1984). Differing views of survivorship: Severed ties. In: Luel, Steven A., and Marcus, Paul (Eds.), *Psychoanalytic Reflections on the Holocaust: Selected Essays*. New York: Ktav, pp. 95-112.

932 Hopper, Earl, and Kreeger, Lionel (1980). The survivor syndrome workshop. In: Garlans, C. (Ed.), *Group Analysis*. London: The Trust for Group Analysis, pp. 67-81.

933 Hormuth, Stefan E., and Stephan, Walter G. (1981). Effects of viewing "Holocaust" on Germans and Americans: A just-world analysis. *Journal of Applied Social Psychology*, 11(3), 240-251.

934 Horwitz, Gilit (1991). *Tguvot m'rayanim b'rayonot im nitzoley shoah: Hamifgash im hanitzol v'zichronotav* [Interviews with Holocaust survivors: Interviewers' responses viv-a-vis the survivor and his memories]. Unpublished master's thesis, Department of Psychology, Tel Aviv University, Tel Aviv, Israel. 139 pp.

935 Hottinger, Adolf; Gsell, O.; Uehlinger, E.; Salzman, C.; and Labhart, A. (1948). *Hungerkrankheit Hungerödem, Hungertuberkulose: Historische klinische, pathophysiologische und pathologisch anatomische Studien und Beobachtungen an ehemaligen Insassen aus Konzentrationslagern* [Hunger Disease, Hunger Edema, Hunger Tuberculosis: Historical, Clinical, Pathophysiological and Pathological Anatomical Studies and Observations of Former Inmates of Concentration Camps]. Basel: Benno Schwabe. 297 p.

936 Hovens, J.E.; Op den Velde, Wybrand; Falger, P.R.; Schouten, E.G.; de Groen, J.H.; and Van Duijn, H. (1992). Anxiety, depression and anger in Dutch resistance veterans from World War II. *Psychotherapy and Psychosomatics*, 57(4), 172-179.

937 Hübschmann, H. (1959). Tuberkulose und Wiedergutmachung [Tuberculosis and indemnification]. *Beiträge zur Klinik der Tuberkulose*, 120, 305-314.

938 Hübschmann, H. (1963). Terror und Krankheit [Terror and disease]. *Advances in Psychosomatic Medicine*, 3, 28-34.

939 Hübschmann, H. (1973). Politische Verfolgung als Ursache der "Alterskrankheiten" Bluthochdruck und Arteriosklerose [Political persecution as the cause of geriatric diseases: High blood pressure and arteriosclerosis]. In: *Ermüdung und vorzeitiges Altern: Folge von Extrembelastungen* [Exhaustion and Premature Aging: Result of Extreme Stress]. Leipzig: Barth, pp. 167-171. [V Internationaler Medizinischer Kongress der FIR. Paris, 21-24 September 1970].

940 Hübschmann, H. (1978). Die Bedeutung der Latenz für die Beurteilung von Verfolgungsbedingten Gesundheitsschäden [The meaning of the latency for the evaluation of health damage caused by persecution]. In: *Medizinische Untersuchungen der Spätfolgen des Krieges und des NS-Regimes bei Jugendlichen und Kindern von ehemaligen KZ-Häftlingen und Verfolgten* [Medical Research of the Late Effects of the War and National Socialism Regime on Youth and Children of Former Concentration Camp Inmates and Persecuted Persons]. Wien: Internationale Föderation der Widerstandskämpfer. [VI Internationaler Medizinischer Kongress der FIR. Prague, 1976].

941 Hugenholtz, P. (1947). Psychologische opmerkingen over den na-oorlogschen mens [Psychological observations on the post-war person]. *Nederlands Tijdschrift voor Geneeskunde*, 1, 20.

942 Huk, Benedikt (1955). Reihenuntersuchung ehemaliger KZ-ler [Social examinations of concentration camp ex-prisoners]. In: Michel, Max (Ed.), *Gesundheitsschäden durch Verfolgung und Gefangenschaft und ihre Spätfolgen: Zusammenstellung der Referate und Ergebnisse der Internationalen Sozialmedizinischen Konferenz über die Pathologie der Ehemaligen Deportierten und Internierten, 5-7 Juni 1954 in Kopenhagen* [Health Damages Caused by Persecution and Internment and the Late Effects: Compilation of the Papers and Results of the International Conference of Social Medicine on the Pathology of Former Deported and Interned Persons, 5-7 June 1954 in Copenhagen]. Frankfurt am Main: Röderberg, pp. 82-83.

943 Hunt, R. (1978). Entering the future looking backwards (Holocaust and Nazi experience). *Hastings Center Report*, 8(3), 5-6.

944 Hunter, Ernest (1993). The snake on the caduceus: Dimensions of medical and psychiatric responsibility in the Third Reich. *Australian and New Zealand Journal of Psychiatry*, 27(1), 149-156.

945 Huppert, Elisabeth (1988). Jewish according to Hitler. *Patio*, 11, 115-118.

946 Hustinx, A. (1973). Het existentieel emotioneel stressyndroom [The existential emotional stress syndrome]. *Maandblad voor de Geestelijke Volksgezondheid*, 5, 197-206.

947 Iliescu, C.C., and Kleinermann, L. (1964). Die Herz- und Gefässtörungen unter den Bedingungen des Häftlingslebens und der Unterernährung [Cardio-vascular disturbances in conditions of imprisonment and malnutrition]. In: *Ätio-Pathogenese und Therapie der Erschöpfung und vorzeitigen Vergreisung* [The Aetiology, Pathogenesis and Therapy of Exhaustion and Premature Aging]. Wien: Verlag der FIR, pp. 296-301. [IV International Medizinischer Kongress. Bucharest, 22-27 Juni 1964].

948 Inbona, Jean-Marie (1961). Contribution to the study of cardiovascular symptoms among former deportees liberated from German concentration camps. In: *International Conference on the Later Effects of Imprisonment and Deportation Organized by the World Veterans Federation. The Hague, November 20-25, 1961*. The Hague: World Veterans Federation, pp. 57-60.

949 Inbona, Jean-Marie (1963). Contribution a l'étude des symptomes cardiovasculaires chez les anciens deportés libérés des camps de concentration allemands [Contributions to the study of the cardiovascular symptoms in former deportees who were liberated from German concentration camps]. *Semaine Médicale Professionnelle et Medico-Sociale*, 839, 87-89.

950 International Auschwitz Committee (1970). *Auschwitz Anthology. Vol. 1: Inhuman Medicine. Part 1*. Warsaw: International Auschwitz Committee. 274 pp.

951 International Auschwitz Committee (1971). *Auschwitz Anthology. Vol. 1: Inhuman Medicine. Part 2*. Warsaw: International Auschwitz Committee. 261 pp.

952 International Auschwitz Committee (1971). *Auschwitz Anthology. Vol. 2: In Hell They Preserved Human Dignity. Part 1*. Warsaw: International Auschwitz Committee. 212 pp.

953 International Auschwitz Committee (1971). *Auschwitz Anthology. Vol. 2: In Hell They Preserved Human Dignity. Part 2*. Warsaw: International Auschwitz Committee. 227 pp.

954 International Auschwitz Committee (1971). *Auschwitz Anthology. Vol. 2: In Hell They Preserved Human Dignity. Part 3*. Warsaw: International Auschwitz Committee. 222 pp.

955 International Auschwitz Committee (1972). *Auschwitz Anthology. Vol. 3: It Did Not End in Forty-Five. Part 1.* Warsaw: International Auschwitz Committee. 211 pp.

956 International Auschwitz Committee (1972). *Auschwitz Anthology. Vol. 3: It Did Not End in Forty-Five. Part 2.* Warsaw: International Auschwitz Committee. 262 pp.

957 Ironside, Wallace (1980). Conservation-withdrawal and action-engagement: On a theory of survivor behavior. *Psychosomatic Medicine*, 42(1), 163-175.

958 Ivy, Andrew (1949). Nazi medical crimes of a medical nature. *Journal of the American Medical Association*, 139, 131-138.

959 Iwaszko, T., and Kłodziński, Stanisław (1977). Bunt skazancow 28 x 1942 r. w oswiecimskim bloku nr 11. Kpt. dr. Henryk Suchnicki [Rebellion of inmates condemned to death at Barracks 11 of the Auschwitz concentration camp on 28th October 1942 under the leadership of Capt. Dr. Henryk Suchnicki]. *Przegląd Lekarski*, 34(1), 118-122.

960 Izaks, Julia (1984). *Effects of the Holocaust on Dutch Jewish victims, residents of Israel: 30 years afterwards*. Unpublished master's thesis, School of Social Work, Bar Ilan University, Ramat Gan, Israel. 162 pp.

961 Jabłoński, Cezary (1980). Wymieralność w getcie Brzezinach [Mortality in the Brzeziny ghetto]. *Przegląd Lekarski*, 37(1), 40-43.

962 Jackman, Norman R. (1958). Survival in the concentration camp. *Human Organization*, 17(2), 23-26.

963 Jacob, Wolfgang (1961). Gesellschaftliche Voraussetzungen zur Überwindung der KZ-schäden [Social preconditions for overcoming concentration camp damage]. *Nervenarzt*, 32, 542-545.

964 Jacob, Wolfgang (1967). Zur Beurteilung der Zusammenhangfrage körperllicher und seelischer Verfolgungsschäden in der gutachtlichen Praxis des Entschädigungsverfahrens [Evaluation of the question of connection between somatic and psychic damages due to persecution in the indemnification practice]. In: Herberg, Hans-Joachim (Ed.), *Die Beurteilung von Gesundheitsschäden nach Gefangenschaft und Verfolgung* [The Assessment of Health Damages Following Internment and Persecution]. Herford: Nicolai, pp. 66-72. [Internationalen Medizinisch-Juristischen Symposiums in Köln].

965 Jacob, Wolfgang (1971). Erb-und Welteinflüsse bei "Anlageleiden" [Heredity and environmental influences in "endogenous" diseases]. In: Herberg, Hans-Joachim (Ed.), *Spätschäden nach Extrembelastungen* [Late Damage After Extreme Stress]. Herford: Nicolai, pp. 29-35. [II Internationalen Medizinisch-Juristischen Konferenz. Dusseldorf, 1969].

966 Jacobs, Alan (1991). Aspects of survival: Triumph over death and loneliness. *Transactional Analysis Journal*, 21(1), 4-11.

967 Jacobsen, E. (1955). Luftencephalogrammet ved KZ syndromet [The pneumoencephalogram in the concentration camp syndrome]. *Ugeskrift for Laeger*, 117, 809-812.

968 Jacobson, Kenneth (1994). *Embattled Selves: An Investigation into the Nature of Identity Through Oral Histories of Holocaust Survivors*. New York: Atlantic Monthly Press. 358 p.

969 Jacobs-Stam, C.M. (1981). *Oorlog, een breuk in het bestaan, achtergrond en problemen van door de oorlog getroffenen* [War, a Rupture in the Existence, Background and Problems of Victims of the War]. Deventer: Van Loghum Slaterus. 106 pp.

970 Jaffe, Ruth (1962). Hahistaglut hanafshit shel nitsolei hamishtar hanatzi aharei aliyatam leyisrael [Emotional adaptation of Nazi regime survivors after their immigration to Israel]. *Dapim Refuiim*, 21(2), 127-130.

971 Jaffe, Ruth (1963). Group activity as a defence method in concentration camps. *Israel Annals of Psychiatry and Related Disciplines*, 1(2), 235-243.

972 Jaffe, Ruth (1968). Dissociative phenomena in former concentration camp inmates. *International Journal of Psycho-Analysis*, 49(2-3), 310-312.

973 Jaffe, Ruth (1970). The sense of guilt within Holocaust survivors. *Jewish Social Studies*, 32(4), 307-314.

974 Jagielski, Stanisław (1968). Psychiczne galwanizowanie "muzułmana" [Psychic jolting of "Muslims" (peculiar facies of concentration camp inmates in their terminal phase)]. *Przegląd Lekarski*, 24(1), 106-109.

975 Jagielski, Stanisław (1983). Prof. Stanisław Konopka: Trzy rozdziały w moim zyciu [Prof. Stanislaw Konopka: Three chapters from my life]. *Archiwum Historii Medycyny*, 46(4), 475-480.

976 Jagoda, Zenon (1978). La survie au camp de concentration dans l'appréciation d'anciens prisonniers d'Auschwitz-Birkenau [Survival in concentration camp as viewed by former prisoners of Auschwitz-Birkenau]. In: *Medizinische Untersuchungen der Spätfolgen des Krieges und des NS-Regimes bei Jugendlichen und Kindern von ehemaligen KZ-Häftlingen und Verfolgten* [Medical Research of the Late Effects of the War and National Socialism Regime on Youth and Children of Former Concentration Camp Inmates and Persecuted Persons]. Wien: Internationale Föderation der Widerstandskämpfer. [VI Internationaler Medizinischer Kongress der FIR. Prague, 1976].

977 Jagoda, Zenon (1987). Selbsthilfe und "Volksmedizin" im Konzentrationslager [Self-help and "Folk Medicine" in concentration camps]. In: Hamburger Institut für Sozialforschung (Eds.), *Die Auschwitz-Hefte. Texte der polnischen Zeitschrift "Przegląd Lekarski" über historische, psychische und medizinische Aspekte des Lebens und Sterbens in Auschwitz. Band 2*. [The Auschwitz Journal. Text of the Polish Journal "Medical Review" on Historical, Psychic and Medical Aspects of Life and Death in Auschwitz. Volume 2]. Weinheim and Basel: Beltz, pp. 149-187.

978 Jagoda, Zenon; Kłodziński, Stanisław; and Masłowski, Jan (1973). Śmiech w obozie koncentracyjnym [Laughter in a concentration camp]. *Przegląd Lekarski*, 30(1), 84-99.

979 Jagoda, Zenon; Kłodziński, Stanisław; and Masłowski, Jan (1974). Życie kulturalne w obozie Oświęcimskim [Cultural life at the Auschwitz concentration camp]. *Przegląd Lekarski*, 31(1), 19-39.

980 Jagoda, Zenon; Kłodziński, Stanisław; and Masłowski, Jan (1975). Używki w obozie oświęcimskim [Drug addiction at the Auschwitz camp]. *Przegląd Lekarski*, 32(1), 40-67.

981 Jagoda, Zenon; Kłodziński, Stanisław; and Masłowski, Jan (1976). Stereotypy zachowań u byłych więźniów obozu oświęcimskiego [Behavioral stereotypes in former inmates of Nazi concentration camps]. *Przegląd Lekarski*, 33(1), 46-71.

982 Jagoda, Zenon; Kłodziński, Stanisław; and Masłowski, Jan (1977). Przetrwanie obozu w ocenic byłych więźniow Oświecimia-Brzezinki [Survival in the camp evaluated by ex-prisoners from Auschwitz-Birkenau]. *Przegląd Lekarski*, 34(1), 77-108.

983 Jagoda, Zenon; Kłodziński, Stanisław; and Masłowski, Jan (1977). Sny więźiów obozu oświęcimskiego [Dreams of prisoners from concentration camp Auschwitz]. *Przegląd Lekarski*, 34(1), 28-66.

984 Jagoda, Zenon; Kłodziński, Stanisław; and Masłowski, Jan (1978). Przyjaźnie oświęcimskie [Friendships made at the Auschwitz concentration camps]. *Przegląd Lekarski*, 35(1), 32-77.

985 Jagoda, Zenon; Kłodziński, Stanisław; and Masłowski, Jan (1978). Słownik Oświęcimski (C-C). Makieta [The Auschwitz vocabulary. A model]. *Przegląd Lekarski*, 35(1), 78-94.

986 Jagoda, Zenon; Kłodziński, Stanisław; and Masłowski, Jan (1978). Stereotype Verhaltensweisen der ehemaligen Häftlinge des KZ Auschwitz Birkenau [Stereotypical behavior in former prisoners of the concentration camp Auschwitz-Birkenau]. In: *Medizinische Untersuchungen der Spätfolgen des Krieges und des NS-Regimes bei Jugendlichen und Kindern von ehemaligen KZ-Häftlingen und Verfolgten* [Medical Research of the Late Effects of the War and National Socialism Regime on Youth and Children of Former Concentration Camp Inmates and Persecuted Persons]. Wien: Internationale Föderation der Widerstandskämpfer. [VI Internationaler Medizinischer Kongress der FIR. Prague, 1976].

987 Jagoda, Zenon; Kłodziński, Stanisław; and Masłowski, Jan (1980). Agresja i agresywność w obozie oswięcimskim [Aggression and aggressiveness in Auschwitz]. *Przegląd Lekarski*, 37(1), 43-75.

988 Jagoda, Zenon; Kłodziński, Stanisław; and Masłowski, Jan (1981). Stosunek ofiar Oświęcimia-Brzezinki do prześladowców [Attitudes of survivors of the Auschwitz-Birkenau camps to their former persecutors]. *Przegląd Lekarski*, 38(1), 37-62.

989 Jagoda, Zenon; Kłodziński, Stanisław; and Masłowski, Jan (1987). "bauernfuss, goldzupa, himmelautostrada." Zum Krematoriumsesperanto, der Sprache polnischer KZ-Häftlinge ["Bauernfus, goldzupa, himelautostrada": Esperanto of the crematoria, the language of Polish concentration camp prisoners]. In: Hamburger Institut für Sozialforschung (Eds.), *Die Auschwitz-Hefte. Texte der polnischen Zeitschrift "Przegląd Lekarski" über historische, psychische und medizinische Aspekte des Lebens und Sterbens in Auschwitz. Band 2* [The Auschwitz Journal. Text of the Polish Journal "Medical Review" on Historical, Psychic and Medical Aspects of Life and Death in Auschwitz. Volume 2]. Weinheim and Basel: Beltz, pp. 241-260.

990 Jagoda, Zenon; Kłodziński, Stanisław; and Masłowski, Jan (1987). "Die Nächte gehören uns nicht..." Häftlingsträume in Auschwitz und im Leben danach [The nights don't belong to us - concentration camp inmates dreams in Auschwitz and life after]. In: Hamburger Institut

für Sozialforschung (Eds.), *Die Auschwitz-Hefte. Texte der polnischen Zeitschrift "Przegląd Lekarski" über historische, psychische und medizinische Aspekte des Lebens und Sterbens in Auschwitz. Band 2* [The Auschwitz Journal. Text of the Polish Journal "Medical Review" on Historical, Psychic and Medical Aspects of Life and Death in Auschwitz. Volume 2]. Weinheim and Basel: Beltz, pp. 189-239.

991 Jagoda, Zenon; Kłodziński, Stanisław; and Masłowski, Jan (1987). Opfer und Peiniger [Victims and torturers]. In: Hamburger Institut für Sozialforschung (Eds.), *Die Auschwitz-Hefte. Texte der polnischen Zeitschrift "Przegląd Lekarski" über historische, psychische und medizinische Aspekte des Lebens und Sterbens in Auschwitz. Band 1* [The Auschwitz Journal. Text of the Polish Journal "Medical Review" on Historical, Psychic and Medical Aspects of Life and Death in Auschwitz. Volume 1]. Weinheim and Basel: Beltz, pp. 53-88.

992 Jagoda, Zenon; Kłodziński, Stanisław; and Masłowski, Jan (1987). Das Überleben im Lager aus der Sicht ehemaliger Häftlinge von Auschwitz-Birkenau [Camp survival evaluated by ex-prisoners from Auschwitz-Birkenau]. In: Hamburger Institut für Sozialforschung (Eds.), *Die Auschwitz-Hefte. Texte der polnischen Zeitschrift "Przegląd Lekarski" über historische, psychische und medizinische Aspekte des Lebens und Sterbens in Auschwitz. Band 1* [The Auschwitz Journal. Text of the Polish Journal "Medical Review" on Historical, Psychic and Medical Aspects of Life and Death in Auschwitz. Volume 1]. Weinheim and Basel: Beltz, pp. 13-51.

993 Jagoda, Zenon; Kłodziński, Stanisław; and Masłowski, Jan (1987). Verhaltensstereotype ehemaliger Häftlinge des Konzentrationslagers Auschwitz [Stereotypes of behavior of former prisoners of the concentration camp Auschwitz]. In: Hamburger Institut für Sozialforschung (Eds.), *Die Auschwitz-Hefte. Texte der polnischen Zeitschrift "Przegląd Lekarski" über historische, psychische und medizinische Aspekte des Lebens und Sterbens in Auschwitz. Band 2* [The Auschwitz Journal. Text of the Polish Journal "Medical Review" on Historical, Psychic and Medical Aspects of Life and Death in Auschwitz. Volume 2]. Weinheim and Basel: Beltz, pp. 25-59.

994 Jakubik, Andrzej (1981). Obraz własnej osoby a pobyt w hitlerowskich obozach koncentracyjnych. Problemy teoretyczno-metodologiczne [Self-image and confinement in Hitlerite concentration camps: Theoretical and methodological problems]. *Przegląd Lekarski*, 38(1), 15-26.

995 Jakubik, Andrzej (1986). Badania, empiryczne nad obrazem własnym u byłych więźniów hitlerowskich obozów koncentracyjnych

[Empirical studies of self concept in former prisoners of Nazi concentration camps]. *Przegląd Lekarski*, 43(1), 20-28.

996 Jakubik, Andrzej (1988). Leczenie astenii poobozowej [Treatment of post-concentration camp asthenia]. *Przegląd Lekarski*, 45(1), 21-24.

997 Jakubik, Andrzej (1995). Zur Behandlung des KZ-Syndroms [Treatment of concentration camp syndrome]. In: Hamburger Institut für Sozialforschung (Eds.), *Die Auschwitz-Hefte. Ergänzungsband. Texte der polnischen Zeitschrift "Przegląd Lekarski" über historische, psychische und medizinische Aspekte des Lebens und Sterbens in Auschwitz* [The Auschwitz Journal. Supplementary volume. Text of the Polish Journal "Medical Review" on Historical, Psychic and Medical Aspects of Life and Death in Auschwitz]. Weinheim and Basel: Rogner and Bernhard, pp. 19-21.

998 Jakubik, Andrzej, and Ryn, Zdzisław (1973). Pseudomedyczne eksperymenty w obozach hitlerowskich. Bibliografia polska 1945-1971 [Pseudomedical experiments in Nazi concentration camps: Polish bibliography, 1945-1971]. *Przegląd Lekarski*, 30(1), 72-75.

999 Jańkowski, Jerzy; Turska-Karbowska, Grażyna; and Żukowski, Wojciech (1989). Stan zdrowia tzw. dzieci Zamojszczyzny [Health status of so-called children from the Zamość district]. *Przegląd Lekarski*, 46(1), 13-15.

1000 Janota, O. (1946). Conséquences de la deuxieme guerre mondiale en Tchecoslovaquie au point de vue psychiatrique [Consequences of the second world war in Czechoslovakia from a psychiatric point of view]. *Presse Médicale*, 49, 667-668.

1001 Jaroszewski, Zdzisław, and Tarmanowska, Benigna (1981). Dzieci w Instytucie Higieny Psychicznej (w Warszawie, 1943-1944) [Children at the Institute for Mental Hygiene (Warsaw, 1943-1944)]. *Przegląd Lekarski* 38(1), 152-155.

1002 Jaspers, Karl and Augstein, Rudolf (1966). The criminal state and German responsibility. *Commentary*, 41(2), 33-39.

1003 Jędrzejczak, K. (1973). Przewlekłe następstwa psychiczne pobytu w hitlerowskich obozach koncentracyjnych na podstawie badań 214 byłych więzniów [Chronic psychological sequels after incarceration in Hitlerian concentration camps based on the investigation of 214 ex-prisoners]. *Annales Academiae Medicae Stetinensis*, 19, 537-563.

1004 Jekiełek, Wojciech (1966). Akcja pomocy Batalionów Chłopskich dla więź obozu koncentracyjnego Oświęcim-Brzezinka [Supporting action of the "peasant brigade" for the prisoners of the Auschwitz-Birkenau concentration camp]. *Przegląd Lekarski*, 22(1), 120-131.

1005 Jezierska, Maria E. (1967). Zagadnienie małych obozów [Problems of small concentration camps]. *Przegląd Lekarski*, 23(1), 127-216.

1006 Jezierska, Maria E. (1971). It is not permitted to be sick. In: *Auschwitz Anthology. Vol. 2: In Hell They Preserved Human Dignity. Part 2.* Warsaw: International Auschwitz Committee, pp. 193-216.

1007 Jezierska, Maria E. (1978). Warunki sanitarne ewakuacji pieszej więźniów w latach 1944-1945 (teoria i rzeczywistość) [Sanitary conditions prevailing during the evacuation on foot of prisoners in 1944-1945 (Theory and facts)]. *Przegląd Lekarski*, 35(1), 147-154.

1008 Jezierska, Maria E. (1980). Szpital obozu Buchenwald (na podstawie archiwaliów z okresu 3 IV-20 VII 1945 r) [The hospital in the Buchenwald concentration camp (according to the archives for the period of April 3, 1945 to July 20, 1945)]. *Przegląd Lekarski*, 37(1), 76-85.

1009 Jezierska, Maria E. (1986). Z fizjologicznych problemów bytowania w obozie [Physiological problems of everyday life in the concentration camp]. *Przegląd Lekarski*, 43(1), 161-166.

1010 Jockush, Ulrich, and Scholz, Lothar (Eds.) (1992). *Administered Killings at the Time of National Socialism: Involvement, Suppression, Responsibility of Psychiatry and Judicial System.* Regensburg: Roderer, 1992. 146 pp.

1011 Jockush, Ulrich, and Scholz, Lothar (Eds.) (1992). *Verwaltetes Morden im Nationalsozialismus: Verstrickung, Verdrängung, Verantwortung von Psychiatrie und Justiz* [Administered Killings at the Time of National Socialism: Involvement, Suppression, Responsibility of Psychiatry and Judicial System]. Regensburg: Roderer, 1992. 156 pp.

1012 Jofen, Jean (1972). Long-range effects of medical experiments in concentration camps (the effects of administration of estrogens to the mother on the intelligence of offspring). In: *Proceedings of the Fifth World Congress of Jewish Studies, The Hebrew University, Mount Scopus - Givat Ram, Jerusalem, 3-11 August 1969. Vol. 2.* Jerusalem: World Union of Jewish Studies, pp. 55-71.

1013 Jores, A. (1960). In dauernder Angst. Hypertonie, Angina pectoris und vorzeitiger Tod nach apoplektischem Insult [In continuing anxiety: Hypertonia, angina pectoris and premature death after apoplexy attack]. In: March, Hans (Ed.), *Verfolgung und Angst in ihren leib-seelischen Auswirkungen. Dokumente* [Persecution and Anxiety in Their Psychosomatic Forms of Expression. Documentation]. Stuttgart: Klett, pp. 41-45.

1014 Jores, A. (1960). "Der Voodoo-Tod." Angst als Todesursache [The voodoo death: Anxiety as cause of death]. In: March, Hans (Ed.), *Verfolgung und Angst in ihren leib-seelischen Auswirkungen. Dokumente* [Persecution and Anxiety in Their Psychosomatic Forms of Expression. Documentation]. Stuttgart: Klett, pp. 49-51.

1015 Jucovy, Milton E. (1983). The effects of the Holocaust on the second generation: Psychoanalytic studies. *American Journal of Social Psychiatry*, 3(1), 15-20.

1016 Jucovy, Milton E. (1985). Telling the Holocaust story: A link between the generations. *Psychoanalytic Inquiry*, 5(1), 31-49.

1017 Jucovy, Milton E. (1986). The Holocaust. In: Rothstein, Arnold (Ed.), *The Reconstruction of Trauma: Its Significance in Clinical Work*. Madison, CT: International Universities Press, pp. 153-169.

1018 Jucovy, Milton E. (1989). Some controversial issues in Holocaust studies: Psychoanalytic reflections. In: Blum, Harold P.; Weinshel, Edward M.; and Rodman, Robert (Eds.), *The Psychoanalytic Core: Essays in Honor of Leo Rangell, M.D.* Madison, CT: International Universities Press, pp. 453-482.

1019 Jucovy, Milton E. (1989). Therapeutic work with survivors and their children: Recurrent themes and problems. In: Marcus, Paul, and Rosenberg, Alan (Eds.), *Healing Their Wounds: Psychotherapy with Holocaust Survivors and Their Families*. New York: Praeger, pp. 51-66.

1020 Jucovy, Milton E. (1992). Psychoanalytic contributions to Holocaust studies. *International Journal of Psycho-Analysis*, 73(2), 267-282.

1021 Kacyzyński, Antoni (1969). Gościec u więźniów obozów koncentracyjnych w obrazie ówczesnym i aktualnym [Rheumatism in prisoners of concentration camps based on past and present data]. *Przegląd Lekarski*, 25(1), 28-30.

1022 Kacyzyński, Antoni (1975). Der Gelenkrheumatismus bei ehemaligen Häftlingen Hitlerscher Konzentrationslager [Rheumatic arthritis in former prisoners of Hitler-concentration camps]. *Mitteilungen der FIR*, 8, 22-24.

1023 Kahana, Boaz (1992). Late-life adaptation in the aftermath of extreme stress. In: Wykle, May L.; Kahana, Eva F.; and Kowal, Jerome (Eds.), *Stress and Health Among the Elderly*. New York: Springer, pp. 151-171.

1024 Kahana, Boaz; Harel, Zev; and Kahana, Eva F. (1988). Predictors of psychological well-being among survivors of the Holocaust. In: Wilson, John P.; Harel, Zev; and Kahana, Boaz (Eds.), *Human Adaptation to Extreme Stress: From the Holocaust to Vietnam*. New York: Plenum, pp. 171-192.

1025 Kahana, Boaz; Harel, Zev; and Kahana, Eva F. (1989). Clinical and gerontological issues facing survivors of the Nazi Holocaust. In: Marcus, Paul, and Rosenberg, Alan (Eds.), *Healing Their Wounds: Psychotherapy with Holocaust Survivors and Their Families*. New York: Praeger, pp. 197-211.

1026 Kahana, Boaz; Kahana, Eva F.; Harel, Zev; and Segal, Mary (1985). The victim as helper: Prosocial behavior during the Holocaust. *Humboldt Journal of Social Relations*, 13(1-2), 357-373.

1027 Kahana, Eva F.; Kahana, Boaz; Harel, Zev; and Rosner, Tena (1988). Coping with extreme trauma. In: Wilson, John P.; Harel, Zev; and Kahana, Boaz (Eds.), *Human Adaptation to Extreme Stress: From the Holocaust to Vietnam*. New York: Plenum, pp. 55-76.

1028 Kahana, Ralph J. (1981). Reconciliation between the generations: A last chance. *Journal of Geriatric Psychiatry and Neurology*, 14(2), 225-239.

1029 Kahn, Charlotte (1994). The crossroad between research and therapy. In: Kestenberg, Judith S,, and Fogelman, Eva (Eds.), *Children during the Nazi Reign: Psychological Perspective on the Interview Process*. Westport, CT: Prager, pp. 91-108.

1030 Kahn, M.L. (1978). Les problèmes de la seconde generation [The problems of the second generation]. In: *Medizinische Untersuchungen der Spätfolgen des Krieges und des NS-Regimes bei Jugendlichen und Kindern von ehemaligen KZ-Häftlingen und Verfolgten* [Medical Research of the Late Effects of the War and National Socialism Regime on Youth and Children of Former Concentration Camp

Inmates and Persecuted Persons]. Wien: Internationale Föderation der Widerstandskämpfer. [VI Internationaler Medizinischer Kongress der FIR. Prague, 1976].

1031 Kaiser, H. Jurgen (1994). Kompetenz im Lebenslauf alterer Zeitzeugen: Anmerkungen zu methodischen Problemen der Erfassung von Kompetenzerleben [Competence in the life course of older survivors: Comments on methodological problems in assessment of subjective competence]. *Zeitschrift für Gerontologie*, 27(2), 122-128.

1032 Kalechofsky, R. (1991). The social and medical antecedents to the medical experiments in the Nazi concentration camps. In: Berger, Alan L. (Ed.), *Bearing Witness to the Holocaust: 1939-1989*. Lewiston, NY: Edwin Mellen Press, pp. 43-54.

1033 Kalma, J.J. (1946). *Redt de Joden! Wat Gebeurt er met de Joodse Pleegkinderen?* [Save the Jews! What Happens with the Jewish Foster Children?]. Amsterdam: De Arbeiderspers.

1034 Kalman-Pollak, Shulamith (1992). *Signonot hitmodedut im hazichronot hatraumatim b'kerev nitzolim sh'hayoo b'gil hahitbagrut b'shoah* [The coping styles used to deal with traumatic memories of Holocaust survivors who were adolescents during the war]. Unpublished master's thesis, Department of Psychology, Tel Aviv University, Tel Aviv, Israel. 140 pp.

1035 Kamien, Frances (1992). *Inheriting the Holocaust*. Unpublished master's thesis, New York University, 96 pp. *Masters Abstracts International*, 30(2), p. 216. (University Microfilms no. AAC 1346176).

1036 Kamieński, Bogdan (1976). Wspomnienia z Sonderaktion Krakau [Reminiscing about the sonderaktion Krakau]. *Przegląd Lekarski*, 33(1), 171-179.

1037 Kaminer, Hanna, and Lavie, Peretz (1991). Sleep and dreaming in Holocaust survivors: Dramatic decrease in dream recall in well-adjusted survivors. *Journal of Nervous and Mental Disease*, 179(11), 664-669.

1038 Kaminer, Hanna, and Lavie, Peretz (1993). Sleep and dreams in well-adjusted and less adjusted Holocaust survivors. In: Stroebe, Margaret S.; Stroebe, Wolfgang; and Hansson, Robert O. (Eds.), *Handbook of Bereavement: Theory, Research and Intervention*. New York: Cambridge University Press, pp. 331-345.

1039 Kania, S. (1990). Zadośćuczynienie za zbrodnie Trzeciej Rzesy [Compensation for the crimes of the Third Reich]. *Przegląd Lekarski*, 47(1), 27-33.

1040 Kanter, Isaac (1970). Extermination camp syndrome: The delayed type of double-bind: A transcultural study. *International Journal of Social Psychiatry*, 16(4), 275-282.

1041 Kanter, Isaac (1976). Social psychiatry and the Holocaust. *Journal of Psychology and Judaism*, 1(1), 55-66.

1042 Karolini, Tadeusz (1976). Początki rewiru w Gusen [The beginning of the sick bay in the camp Gusen]. *Przegląd Lekarski*, 33(1), 179-183.

1043 Karr, Stephen D. (1973). *Second generation effects of the Nazi Holocaust*. Unpublished doctoral dissertation, California School of Professional Psychology, Berkely, 188 pp. *Dissertation Abstracts International*, 35(6-B), p. 2935. (University Microfilms no. AAC 7330244).

1044 Karson, Esther (1989). *Borderline phenomena in children of Holocaust survivors*. Unpublished doctoral dissertation, California School of Professional Psychology, Los Angeles, 235 pp. *Dissertations Abstracts International*, 51(6-B), p. 3135. (University Microfilms no. AAC 9021427).

1045 Kasahara, Y. (1977). Concentration camp syndrome. *Nippon Rinsho. Japanese Journal of Clinical Medicine*, 35(1), 698-699.

1046 Kaslow, Florence W. (1990). Treating Holocaust survivors. *Contemporary Family Therapy*, 12(5), 393-405.

1047 Kaslow, Florence W. (1995). Descendents of Holocaust victims and perpetrators: Legacies and dialogue. *Contemporary Family Therapy*, 17(3), 275-290.

1048 Kater, Michael H. (1987). The burden of the past: problems of a modern historiography of physicians and medicine in Nazi Germany. *German Studies Review*, 10, 31-57.

1049 Kater, Michael H. (1989). *Doctors Under Hitler*. Chapel Hill, NC: University of North Carolina Press. 426 pp.

1050 Kater, Michael H. (1994). An historical and contemporary view of Jewish doctors in Germany. In: Michalczyk, John J. (Ed.), *Medicine,*

Ethics, and the Third Reich: Historical and Contemporary Issues. Kansas City, MO: Sheed & Ward, pp. 161-166.

1051 Katz, Cipora (1964). Tuberkulose und Deportation [Tuberculosis and deportation]. In: *Ätio-Pathogenese und Therapie der Erschöpfung und vorzeitigen Vergreisung* [The Aetiology, Pathogenesis and Therapy of Exhaustion and Premature Aging]. Wien: Verlag der FIR, pp. 334-336. [IV Internationaler Medizinischer Kongress. Bucharest, 22-27 Juni 1964].

1052 Katz, Cipora, and Keleman, Franklin A. (1981). The children of the Holocaust survivors: Issues of separation. *Journal of Jewish Communal Service*, 58(3), 257-263.

1053 Katz, Jay (1994). Concentration camp experiments: Their relevance for contemporary research with human beings. In: Michalczyk, John J. (Ed.), *Medicine, Ethics, and the Third Reich: Historical and Contemporary Issues*. Kansas City, MO: Sheed & Ward, pp. 73-86.

1054 Kav-Venaki, Sophie; Nadler, Arie; and Gershoni, Hadas (1983). Sharing past traumas: A comparison of communication behaviors in two groups of Holocaust survivors. *International Journal of Social Psychiatry*, 29(1), 49-59.

1055 Kav-Venaki, Sophie; Nadler, Arie; and Gershoni, Hadas (1985). Sharing the Holocaust experience: Communication behaviors and their consequences in families of ex-partisans and ex-prisoners of concentration camps. *Family Process*, 24(2), 273-280.

1056 Kay, Avi (1995). *Genocide and generativity: The effects of the Holocaust experience on generativity (survivorship)*. Unpublished doctoral dissertation, Northwestern University, Evanston, Illinois, 286 pp. *Dissertation Abstracts International*, 56(7-B), p. 4034. (University Microfilms no. AAC 9537455).

1057 Keilson, Hans (1949). Zur Psychologie der jüdischen Kriegswaisen [On the psychology of Jewish war orphans] In: Pfister-Ammende, Maria (Ed.), *Die Psychohygiene, Grundlagen und Ziele* [Psychohygiene, Bases and Purposes]. Bern: Huber, pp. 1-6.

1058 Keilson, Hans (1961). Vooroordeel en haat, een psychologische bijdrage tot het probleem van het anti-semitisme [Prejudice and hate, a psychological contribution to the problem of anti-semitism]. *Maandblad voor de Geestelijke Volksgezondheid*, 3, 83-98.

1059 **Keilson, Hans (1983). Afscheid, herinnering en rouw [Parting,** memory and mourning]. In: *Scheiding en Rouw* [Separation and Mourning]. Utrecht: Stichting ICODO, pp. 16-22.

1060 Keilson, Hans (1985). Oorlogsgevolgen in een medisch kader [War consequences in a medical framework]. In: *Problematiek van Oorlogsgetrofflene* [Problems of War Victims]. Utrecht: Stichting ICODO, pp. 21-28.

1061 Keilson, Hans (1995). Die fragmentierte Psychotherapie eines aus Bergen-Belsen zurück-gekehrten Jungen [The fragmented psychotherapy of a boy survivor from Bergen-Belsen]. *Psyche: Zeitschrift für Psychoanalyse und ihre Anwendungen*, 49(1), 69-84.

1062 Keilson, Hans, and Sarphatie, Herman (1992). *Sequential Traumatization in Children: A Clinical and Statistical Follow-Up Study on the Fate of the Jewish War Orphans in the Netherlands*. Jerusalem: Magnes. 463 pp.

1063 Keinan, Giora; Mikulincer, Mario; and Rybnicki, Abraham (1988). Perception of self and parents by second-generation Holocaust survivors. *Behavioral Medicine*, 14(1), 6-12.

1064 Keller, Robin S. (1988). Children of Jewish Holocaust survivors: Relationship of family communication to family cohesion, adaptability and satisfaction. *Family Therapy*, 15(3), 223-237.

1065 Kempisty, Czesław (1967). Stan zdrowia byłych więźniów ze środowiska wrocławskiego [State of health of former concentration camp inmates from the Wroclaw area]. *Przegląd Lekarski*, 24(1), 96-98.

1066 Kempisty, Czesław (1970). Wyniki badań lekarskich byłych więźniów obozu dla dzieci Łodzi [The results of medical investigations of children-prisoners in Lodz]. *Przegląd Lekarski*, 27(1), 24-27.

1067 Kempisty, Czesław (1971). The Wroclaw environment. In: *Auschwitz Anthology. Vol. 3: It Did Not End in Forty-Five. Part 1*. Warsaw: International Auschwitz Committee, pp. 200-209.

1068 Kempisty, Czesław (1973). Wyniki socjo-medycznych badań potomstwa byłych więźiów hitlerowskich [The results of sociomedical investigations of children of ex-prisoners of the Hitlerian camps]. *Przegląd Lekarski*, 30(1), 12-20.

1069 Kempisty, Czesław (1975). Ergebnisse der 2 sozialmedizinischer Untersuchung der Kinder von Eltern, die in Hitler-Konzentrationslagern interniert waren [Results of the second social-medical examination of children whose parents were prisoners in Hitler's concentration camps]. *Mitteilungen der FIR*, 8, 25-26.

1070 Kempisty, Czesław (1975). Ergebnisse der sozialmedizinischer Untersuchung von Personen, die als Kinder in Nazi Konzentrationslagern waren [Results of social medical examinations of persons who were in Nazi concentration camps as children]. *Mitteilungen der FIR*, 8, 27-29.

1071 Kempisty, Czesław (1978). Ergebnisse der sozialmedizinischer Häftlinge untersuchung der Kinder of KZ Häftlinge [Results of sociomedical examinations of offspring of concentration camp survivors]. In: *Medizinische Untersuchungen der Spätfolgen des Krieges und des NS-Regimes bei Jugendlichen und Kindern von ehemaligen KZ-Häftlingen und Verfolgten* [Medical Research of the Late Effects of the War and National Socialism Regime on Youth and Children of Former Concentration Camp Inmates and Persecuted Persons]. Wien: Internationale Föderation der Widerstandskämpfer. [VI Internationaler Medizinischer Kongress der FIR. Prague, 1976].

1072 Kempisty, Czesław (1979). Wyniki drugiego etapu socjo-medycznych badań potomstwa byłych więźiów obozów hitlerowskich [Results of second phase of sociomedical examinations of offspring of the former inmates of Nazi concentration camps]. *Przegląd Lekarski*, 36(1), 18-25.

1073 Kempisty, Czesław (1983). Causes of war, disability and mortality in former inmates of concentration camps. *Cahiers d'Informations Médicales, Sociales et Juridiques*, 19, 122-123.

1074 Kempisty, Czesław; Kruszczynski, K.; Pilichowski, C.; and Szwarc, Halina (1978). Biologische und oekonomische Folgen der Deportation und Gefangenhaltung der Polen in den Nazi-Konzentrationslagern [Biological and economical sequelae of deportation and imprisonment of Poles in the Nazi concentration camps]. In: *Medizinische Untersuchungen der Spätfolgen des Krieges und des NS-Regimes bei Jugendlichen und Kindern von ehemaligen KZ-Häftlingen und Verfolgten* [Medical Research of the Late Effects of the War and National Socialism Regime on Youth and Children of Former Concentration Camp Inmates and Persecuted Persons]. Wien: Internationale Föderation der Widerstandskämpfer. [VI Internationaler Medizinischer Kongress der FIR. Prague, 1976].

1075 Kempisty, Czesław, and Leszczyńska, Zdisława (1974). Z badań nad płodnością byłych więźniarek obozów hitlerowskich [Investigations of the fertility of female ex-prisoners of Hitlerian camps]. *Przegląd Lekarski*, 31(1), 58-65.

1076 Kempisty, Czesław, and Leszczyńska, Zdisława (1975). Wyniki socjo-medycznych badań byłych deportowanych do pracy przymusowej w Trzeciej Rzeszy [Results of sociomedical studies of persons deported to the Third Reich as slave laborers]. *Przegląd Lekarski*, 32(1), 70-78.

1077 Kempisty, Czesław, and Piotrowska, E. (1977). Problemy gerontologii spolecnej procesie zmian aktywnosci byłych więźniów przechodzących na emeryturę [Socio-gerontological problems following change of activity in ex-prisoners who are about to retire]. *Przegląd Lekarski*, 34(1), 17-25.

1078 Kempisty, Czesław, and Szemraj-Lochyńska, Alicja (1987). Arteriosklerose bei ehemaligen KZ-Häftlingen und ihre Auswirkungen auf den Alterungsprozess und die Mortalität [Arteriosclerosis in former concentration camp inmates and its influence on aging and mortality]. In: Hamburger Institut für Sozialforschung (Eds.), *Die Auschwitz-Hefte. Texte der polnischen Zeitschrift "Przegląd Lekarski" über historische, psychische und medizinische Aspekte des Lebens und Sterbens in Auschwitz. Band 2* [The Auschwitz Journal. Text of the Polish Journal "Medical Review" on Historical, Psychic and Medical Aspects of Life and Death in Auschwitz. Volume 2]. Weinheim and Basel: Beltz, pp. 75-80.

1079 Kenigsberg, Rositta E., and Lieblich, Cathy M. (Eds.) (1992). *The First National Conference on Identification, Treatment and Care of the Aging Holocaust Survivor, March 29-31, 1992: Selected Proceedings*. Miami, FL: Holocaust Documentation and Education Center and Southeast Florida Center on Aging, Florida International University. 99 pp.

1080 Kępiński, Antoni (1970). TZW. "KZ Syndrom." Proba syntezy [The so-called concentration camp syndrome: An attempt at a synthesis]. *Przegląd Lekarski*, 27(1), 18-23.

1081 Kępiński, Antoni (1971). Anus mundi. In: *Auschwitz Anthology. Vol. 1: Inhuman Medicine. Part 2*. Warsaw: International Auschwitz Committee, pp. 1-12.

1082 Kępiński, Antoni (1972). Auschwitz reflections: The railway loading platform. In: *Auschwitz Anthology. Vol. 3: It Did Not End in Forty-Five. Part 2*. Warsaw: International Auschwitz Committee, pp. 81-129.

1083 Kępiński, Antoni (1972). Z niemieckich badań nad następstwami przebywania w obozach hitlerowskich [German studies of sequelae of imprisonment in Nazi concentration camps]. *Przegląd Lekarski*, 29(1), 243-246.

1084 Kępiński, Antoni (1972). A nightmare. In: *Auschwitz Anthology. Vol. 3: It Did Not End in Forty-Five. Part 2*. Warsaw: International Auschwitz Committee, pp. 241-260.

1085 Kępiński, Antoni (1973). Le syndrome concentrationnaire. Essai d'une synthese [The concentration camp syndrome. An attempt at synthesis]. *Cahiers d'Informations Médicales, Sociales et Juridiques*, 1, 3-12.

1086 Kępiński, Antoni (1987). Das sogenamnte KZ-Syndrom: Versuch einer synthese [The so-called concentration camp syndrome: Attempt at a synthesis]. In: Hamburger Institut für Sozialforschung (Eds.), *Die Auschwitz-Hefte. Texte der polnischen Zeitschrift "Przegląd Lekarski" über historische, psychische und medizinische Aspekte des Lebens und Sterbens in Auschwitz. Band 2* [The Auschwitz Journal. Text of the Polish Journal "Medical Review" on Historical, Psychic and Medical Aspects of Life and Death in Auschwitz. Volume 2]. Weinheim and Basel: Beltz, pp. 7-13.

1087 Kępiński, Antoni, and Kłodziński, Stanisław (1973). O dodatniej aktywności psychicznej więźniów [Mental activity of inmates at concentration camps]. *Przegląd Lekarski*, 30(1), 81-84.

1088 Kępiński, Antoni, and Kłodziński, Stanisław (1976). Über die positiven psychischen Reaktionen der Häftlinge [On the positive psychic reactions of inmates]. *Mitteilungen der FIR*, 10, 1-7.

1089 Kępiński, Antoni, and Masłowski, Jan (1966). Okupacyjna tematyka lekarska w polskich publikacjach z lat 1964-1965 [Medical themes from the Nazi occupation times in Polish publications 1964-1965]. *Przegląd Lekarski*, 22(1), 241-247.

1090 Kestenberg, Judith S. (1972). Psychoanalytic contributions to the problem of children of survivors from Nazi persecution. *Israel Annals of Psychiatry and Related Disciplines*, 10(4), 311-325.

1091 Kestenberg, Judith S. (1973). Introductory remarks. In: Anthony, E. James, and Koupernik, Cyrille (Eds.), *The Child in His Family. Vol. 2: The Impact of Disease and Death*. New York: John Wiley & Sons, pp. 359-361.

1092 Kestenberg, Judith S. (1974). Kinder von Überlebenden der Nazi Verfolgengen. Psychoanalytische Beitrage [Children of survivors of Nazi persecutees. Psychoanalytic contribution]. *Psyche: Zeitschrift für Psychoanalyse und ihre Anwendungen*, 28, 249-265.

1093 Kestenberg, Judith S. (1980). Psychoanalyses of children of survivors from the Holocaust: Case presentations and assessment. *Journal of the American Psychoanalytic Association*, 28(4), 775-804.

1094 Kestenberg, Judith S. (1981). The psychological consequences of punitive institutions. *Israel Journal of Psychiatry and Related Sciences*, 18(1), 15-30.

1095 Kestenberg, Judith S. (1982). Die diskriminierende Praxis in der Wiedergutmachung [Discriminating practice in reparations]. *Arbeitshefte Kinderpsychoanal*, 2, 183-214.

1096 Kestenberg, Judith S. (1982). The experience of survivor-parents. In: Bergmann, Martin S., and Jucovy, Milton E. (Eds.), *Generations of the Holocaust*. New York: Basic Books, pp. 46-61.

1097 Kestenberg, Judith S. (1982). Survivor-parents and their children. In: Bergmann, Martin S., and Jucovy, Milton E. (Eds.), *Generations of the Holocaust*. New York: Basic Books, pp. 83-101.

1098 Kestenberg, Judith S. (1982). A metapsychological assessment based on an analysis of a survivor's child. In: Bergmann, Martin S., and Jucovy, Milton E. (Eds.), *Generations of the Holocaust*. New York: Basic Books, pp. 137-158

1099 Kestenberg, Judith S. (1983). History's role in the psychoanalyses of survivors and their children. *American Journal of Social Psychiatry*, 3(1), 24-28.

1100 Kestenberg, Judith S. (1985). Child survivors of the Holocaust - 40 years later: Reflections and commentary. *Journal of the American Academy of Child Psychiatry*, 24(4), 408-412.

1101 Kestenberg, Judith S. (1987). The development of the ego-ideal, its structure in Nazi youth and in persecuted Jewish children. *Issues in Ego Psychology*, 10(2), 22-34.

1102 Kestenberg, Judith S. (1987). Imagining and remembering. *Israel Journal of Psychiatry and Related Sciences*, 24(4), 229-241.

1103 Kestenberg, Judith S. (1988). Introduction to "Child survivors of the Holocaust." *Psychoanalytic Review*, 75(4), 495-497.

1104 Kestenberg, Judith S. (1988). Memories from early childhood. *Psychoanalytic Review*, 75(4), 561-571.

1105 Kestenberg, Judith S. (1989). Coping with losses and survival. In: Dietrich, David R., and Shabad, Peter C. (Eds.), *The Problem of Loss and Mourning: Psychoanalytic Perspectives*. Madison, CT: International Universities Press, pp. 381-403.

1106 Kestenberg, Judith S. (1989). Neue Gedanken zur Transposition. Klinische, therapeutische und entwicklungsbedingte Betrachtungen [New thoughts on transposition: Clinical, therapeutic, and developmental considerations]. *Jahrbuch der Psychoanalyse*, 24, 163-189.

1107 Kestenberg, Judith S. (1989). Transposition revisited: Clinical, therapeutic, and developmental considerations. In: Marcus, Paul, and Rosenberg, Alan (Eds.), *Healing Their Wounds: Psychotherapy with Holocaust Survivors and Their Families*. New York: Praeger, pp. 67-82.

1108 Kestenberg, Judith S. (1991). Kinder unter dem Joch des Nationalsozialismus: Aus der internationalen Forschung der planmassigen Verfolgung von Kindern; gegründet 1981 durch Child Development Research und affiliiert mit dem Psychologie Department der Universität Tel Aviv [Children under the Nazi yoke: From International Research of Systematic Child Persecution, founded in 1981 by Child Development Research and affiliated with the Psychology Department of Tel Aviv University]. *Jahrbuch der Psychoanalyse*, 28, 179-209.

1109 Kestenberg, Judith S. (1992). Children of survivors and child survivors. *Echoes of the Holocaust*, 1, 27-50. [Bulletin of the Jerusalem Center for Research into the Late Effects of the Holocaust. Talbieh Mental Health Center, Jerusalem, Israel].

1110 Kestenberg, Judith S. (1992). Children under the Nazi yoke. *British Journal of Psychotherapy*, 8(4), 374-390.

1111 Kestenberg, Judith S. (1993). Children who survived the war and children of survivors. *ICODO Info*, 10, 5-27.

1112 Kestenberg, Judith S. (1993). Spätfolgen bei verfolgten Kindern [After effects in later life child victims of persecution]. *Psyche: Zeitschrift für Psychoanalyse und ihre Anwendungen*, 47(8), 730-742.

1113 Kestenberg, Judith S. (1993). What a psychoanalyst learned from the Holocaust and genocide. *International Journal of Psycho-Analysis*, 74(6), 1117-1129.

1114 Kestenberg, Judith S. (1994). The diary from the ghetto in Krakow. *Echoes of the Holocaust*, 3, 21-39. [Bulletin of the Jerusalem Center for Research into the Late Effects of the Holocaust. Talbieh Mental Health Center, Jerusalem, Israel].

1115 Kestenberg, Judith S. (1994). Overview of the effect of psychological research interviews on child survivors. In: Kestenberg, Judith S., and Fogelman, Eva (Eds.), *Children during the Nazi Reign: Psychological Perspective on the Interview Process*. Westport, CT: Praeger, pp. 3-33.

1116 Kestenberg, Judith S. (1995). The response of the child to the rescuer. *Echoes of the Holocaust*, 4, 1-8. [Bulletin of the Jerusalem Center for Research into the Late Effects of the Holocaust. Talbieh Mental Health Center, Jerusalem, Israel].

1117 Kestenberg, Judith S., and Brenner, Ira (1986). Children who survived the Holocaust: The role of rules and routines in the development of the superego. *International Journal of Psycho-Analysis*, 67(3), 309-316.

1118 Kestenberg, Judith S., and Brenner, Ira (1988). Le narcissisme comme moyen de survie [Narcissism as a survival strategy]. *Revue Française de Psychanalyse*, 52(6), 1393-1408.

1119 Kestenberg, Judith S., and Fogelman, Eva (Eds.) (1994). *Children during the Nazi Reign: Psychological Perspective on the Interview Process*. Westport, CT: Praeger. 221 pp.

1120 Kestenberg, Judith S., and Gampel, Yolanda (1983). Growing up in the Holocaust culture. *Israel Journal of Psychiatry and Related Sciences*, 20(1-2), 129-146.

1121 Kestenberg, Judith S., and Kestenberg, Milton (1980). Psychoanalyses of children of survivors from the Nazi persecution: The continuing struggle of survivor parents. *Victimology*, 5(2-4), 368-373.

1122 Kestenberg, Judith S., and Kestenberg, Milton (1993). Organized persecution of children. *Echoes of the Holocaust*, 2, 13-23. [Bulletin of the Jerusalem Center for Research into the Late Effects of the Holocaust. Talbieh Mental Health Center, Jerusalem, Israel].

1123 Kestenberg, Judith S.; Kestenberg, Milton; and Amighi, Janet-Kestenberg (1988). The Nazi's quest for death and the Jewish quest for life. In: Braham, Randolph L. (Ed.), *The Psychological Perspectives of the Holocaust and of its Aftermath*. Boulder, CO: Social Science Monographs; and New York: Csengeri Institute for Holocaust Studies of the Graduate School and University Center of the City University of New York, pp. 13-43.

1124 Kestenberg, Milton (1992). The healing power of creativity. *Echoes of the Holocaust*, 1, 51-59. [Bulletin of the Jerusalem Center for Research into the Late Effects of the Holocaust. Talbieh Mental Health Center, Jerusalem, Israel].

1125 Kestenberg, Milton (1994). The effect of interviews on child survivors: Child survivors revisited. In: Kestenberg, Judith S., and Fogelman, Eva (Eds.), *Children during the Nazi Reign: Psychological Perspective on the Interview Process*. Westport, CT: Praeger, pp. 57-71.

1126 Kestenberg, Milton, and Kestenberg, Judith S. (1988). The sense of belonging and altruism in children who survived the Holocaust. *Psychoanalytic Review*, 75(4), 533-560.

1127 Kiedrzyńska, Wanda (1976). Książka porodów w Ravensbrück [A logbook of deliveries at the Ravensbruck camp]. *Przegląd Lekarski*, 33(1), 95-104.

1128 Kieler, Jørgen (1952). Conditions of deportation. In: Helweg-Larsen, Per; Hoffmeyer, Henrik; Kieler, Jørgen; Hess Thaysen, Eigil; Hess Thaysen, Jørn; Thygesen, Paul; and Hertel Wulff, Munke, *Famine Disease in German Concentration Camps, Complications and Sequelae: With Special Reference to Tuberculosis, Mental Disorders and Social Consequences*. Copenhagen: Ejnar Munksgaard, pp. 29-70. [Also published as *Acta Psychiatrica et Neurologica Scandinavica*, Supplementum 83.]

1129 Kieler, Jørgen (1955). Die zelluläre Wirkung des Eiweissmangels durch In-vitro Studien beleuchtet [The cellular reaction of protein deficiency: In vitro studies]. In: Michel, Max (Ed.), *Gesundheitsschäden durch Verfolgung und Gefangenschaft und ihre Spätfolgen: Zusammenstellung der Referate und Ergebnisse der Internationalen Sozialmedizinischen Konferenz über die Pathologie der Ehemaligen Deportierten und Internierten, 5-7 Juni 1954 in Kopenhagen* [Health Damages Caused by Persecution and Internment and the Late Effects: Compilation of the Papers and Results of the International Conference of Social Medicine on the Pathology of

Former Deported and Interned Persons, 5-7 June 1954 in Copenhagen]. Frankfurt am Main: Röderberg, pp. 135-147.

1130 Kieler, Jørgen (1980). Immediate reactions to capture and deportation. *Danish Medical Bulletin*, 27(5), 217-220.

1131 Kieler, Jørgen; Hess Thaysen, Eigil; and Hess Thaysen, Jørn (1952). Treatment of famine disease. In: Helweg-Larsen, Per; Hoffmeyer, Henrik; Kieler, Jørgen; Hess Thaysen, Eigil; Hess Thaysen, Jørn; Thygesen, Paul; and Hertel Wulff, Munke, *Famine Disease in German Concentration Camps, Complications and Sequelae: With Special Reference to Tuberculosis, Mental Disorders and Social Consequences*. Copenhagen: Ejnar Munksgaard, pp. 178-198. [Also published as *Acta Psychiatrica et Neurologica Scandinavica*, Supplementum 83.]

1132 Kieler, Jørgen; Hess Thaysen, Eigil; and Hess Thaysen, Jørn (1955). Behandlung der Hungerkrankheit [Treatment of hunger disease]. In: Michel, Max (Ed.), *Gesundheitsschäden durch Verfolgung und Gefangenschaft und ihre Spätfolgen: Zusammenstellung der Referate und Ergebnisse der Internationalen Sozialmedizinischen Konferenz über die Pathologie der Ehemaligen Deportierten und Internierten, 5-7 Juni 1954 in Kopenhagen* [Health Damages Caused by Persecution and Internment and the Late Effects: Compilation of the Papers and Results of the International Conference of Social Medicine on the Pathology of Former Deported and Interned Persons, 5-7 June 1954 in Copenhagen]. Frankfurt am Main: Röderberg, pp. 324-331.

1133 Kieler, Jørgen; Hess Thaysen, Eigil; Hess Thaysen, Jørn; and Thygesen, Paul (1952). Diseases of repatriation: Recovery from starvation. In: Helweg-Larsen, Per; Hoffmeyer, Henrik; Kieler, Jørgen; Hess Thaysen, Eigil; Hess Thaysen, Jørn; Thygesen, Paul; and Hertel Wulff, Munke, *Famine Disease in German Concentration Camps, Complications and Sequelae: With Special Reference to Tuberculosis, Mental Disorders and Social Consequences*. Copenhagen: Ejnar Munksgaard, pp. 308-329. [Also published as *Acta Psychiatrica et Neurologica Scandinavica*, Supplementum 83.]

1134 Kieler, Jørgen, and Thygesen, Paul (1952). Famine disease: Cardiovascular signs and symptoms. In: Helweg-Larsen, Per; Hoffmeyer, Henrik; Kieler, Jørgen; Hess Thaysen, Eigil; Hess Thaysen, Jørn; Thygesen, Paul; and Hertel Wulff, Munke, *Famine Disease in German Concentration Camps, Complications and Sequelae: With Special Reference to Tuberculosis, Mental Disorders and Social Consequences*. Copenhagen: Ejnar Munksgaard, pp. 161-

169. [Also published as *Acta Psychiatrica et Neurologica Scandinavica*, Supplementum 83.]

1135 Kieler, Jørgen, and Thygesen, Paul (1952). Famine disease: Disorders of the blood. In: Helweg-Larsen, Per; Hoffmeyer, Henrik; Kieler, Jørgen; Hess Thaysen, Eigil; Hess Thaysen, Jørn; Thygesen, Paul; and Hertel Wulff, Munke, *Famine Disease in German Concentration Camps, Complications and Sequelae: With Special Reference to Tuberculosis, Mental Disorders and Social Consequences*. Copenhagen: Ejnar Munksgaard, pp. 170-173. [Also published as *Acta Psychiatrica et Neurologica Scandinavica*, Supplementum 83.]

1136 Kieler, Jørgen, and Thygesen, Paul (1952). Famine disease: Musculature. In: Helweg-Larsen, Per; Hoffmeyer, Henrik; Kieler, Jørgen; Hess Thaysen, Eigil; Hess Thaysen, Jørn; Thygesen, Paul; and Hertel Wulff, Munke, *Famine Disease in German Concentration Camps, Complications and Sequelae: With Special Reference to Tuberculosis, Mental Disorders and Social Consequences*. Copenhagen: Ejnar Munksgaard, pp. 174-177. [Also published as *Acta Psychiatrica et Neurologica Scandinavica*, Supplementum 83.]

1137 Kieler, Jørgen, and Thygesen, Paul (1952). Famine disease: Metabolism. In: Helweg-Larsen, Per; Hoffmeyer, Henrik; Kieler, Jørgen; Hess Thaysen, Eigil; Hess Thaysen, Jørn; Thygesen, Paul; and Hertel Wulff, Munke, *Famine Disease in German Concentration Camps, Complications and Sequelae: With Special Reference to Tuberculosis, Mental Disorders and Social Consequences*. Copenhagen: Ejnar Munksgaard, pp. 178-198. [Also published as *Acta Psychiatrica et Neurologica Scandinavica*, Supplementum 83.]

1138 Kieler, Jørgen, and Thygesen, Paul (1952). Famine disease: Endocrine glands. In: Helweg-Larsen, Per; Hoffmeyer, Henrik; Kieler, Jørgen; Hess Thaysen, Eigil; Hess Thaysen, Jørn; Thygesen, Paul; and Hertel Wulff, Munke, *Famine Disease in German Concentration Camps, Complications and Sequelae: With Special Reference to Tuberculosis, Mental Disorders and Social Consequences*. Copenhagen: Ejnar Munksgaard, pp. 199-206. [Also published as *Acta Psychiatrica et Neurologica Scandinavica*, Supplementum 83.]

1139 Kiełkowski, Roman (1971). Obóz pracy przymusowej i koncentracyjny w Płaszowie [The Plaszow concentration and compulsory labor camp]. *Przegląd Lekarski*, 27(1), 23-26.

1140 Kieta, Mieczysław (1980). Instytut higieny SS i Policji w Oświęcimiu [The SS and Police Institute of Hygiene in Auschwitz]. *Przegląd Lekarski*, 37(1), 172-176.

1141 Kieta, Mieczysław (1987). Das Hygiene-Institut der Waffen-SS und Polizei in Auschwitz [The SS and Police Institute of Hygiene in Auschwitz]. In: Hamburger Institut für Sozialforschung (Eds.), *Die Auschwitz-Hefte. Texte der polnischen Zeitschrift "Przegląd Lekarski" über historische, psychische und medizinische Aspekte des Lebens und Sterbens in Auschwitz. Band 1* [The Auschwitz Journal. Text of the Polish Journal "Medical Review" on Historical, Psychic and Medical Aspects of Life and Death in Auschwitz. Volume 1]. Weinheim and Basel: Beltz, pp. 213-217.

1142 Kijak, Moises (1989). Further discussions of reactions of psychoanalysts to the Nazi persecution, and lessons to be learnt. *International Review of Psycho-Analysis*, 16(2), 213-222.

1143 Kijak, Moises, and Funtowicz, Silvio (1982). The syndrome of the survivor of extreme situations: Definitions, difficulties, hypotheses. *International Review of Psycho-Analysis*, 9(1), 25-33.

1144 Kinsler, Florabel (1981). Second generation effects of the Holocaust: The effectiveness of group therapy in the resolution of the transmission of parental trauma. *Journal of Psychology and Judaism*, 6(1), 53-67.

1145 Kinsler, Florabel (1986). *An Eriksonian and evaluative investigation of the effects of video testimonials upon Jewish survivors of the Holocaust*. Unpublished doctoral dissertation, International College, Los Angeles, California.

1146 Kinsler, Florabel (1988). The loneliness of the Holocaust survivor. *Journal of Psychology and Judaism*, 12(3), 156-177.

1147 Kinsler, Florabel (1995). The emotional and physiological issues of aging in North American Holocaust survivors. In: Lemberger, John (Ed.), *A Global Perspective on Working with Holocaust Survivors and the Second Generation*. Jerusalem: JDC-Brookdale Institute of Gerontology and Human Development, AMCHA, and JDC-Israel, pp. 25-49.

1148 Kinsler, Florabel (1995). Group services for Holocaust survivors and their families. In: Lemberger, John (Ed.), *A Global Perspective on Working with Holocaust Survivors and the Second Generation*. Jerusalem: JDC-Brookdale Institute of Gerontology and Human Development, AMCHA, and JDC-Israel, pp. 59-79.

1149 Kinston, Warren, and Rosser, Rachel (1974). Disaster: Effects on mental and physical state. *Journal of Psychosomatic Research*, 18(6), 437-456.

1150 Kirschenbaum, Martin; Obermeyer, Vera R.; and Lukoff, Christel (1988). Conclusion to special issue on "Children of the Holocaust." *Family Therapy*, 15(3), 285.

1151 Kiwala, Julian (1971). At the end of 1942 and the beginning of 1943. In: *Auschwitz Anthology. Vol. 2: In Hell They Preserved Human Dignity. Part 2*. Warsaw: International Auschwitz Committee, pp. 161-180.

1152 Klebanow, D. (1948). Hunger und psychische Erregung als Ovar-und Keimschädigung [Hunger and psychic excitation as the cause of ovarian and gonadal disturbances]. *Geburtshilfe und Frauenheilkunde*, 8, 812-820.

1153 Kleber, Rolf (1994). Late gevolgen van de Tweede Wereldoorlog [Late consequences from World War II]. *Psycholoog*, 29(4), 125-131.

1154 Klee, E. (1990). "Turning the tap on was no big deal" - The gassing doctors during the Nazi period and afterwards. In: Benz, Wolfgang, and Distel, Barbara (Eds.), *Dachau Review 2. History of Nazi Concentration Camps: Studies, Reports, Documents. Vol. 2*. Brussels: Comité International de Dachau, pp. 46-66.

1155 Klein, F. (1984). Janusz Korczak - Arzt und Erzieher - Ein Symbol gelebter Menschlichkeit für die heutige medizinische und heilpadagogische Praxis [Janusz Korczak - physician and educator - a symbol of humanity in action for today's medical and pedagogical practice]. *Das Offentliche Gesundheitswesen*, 46(5), 224-248.

1156 Klein, Hillel (1967). Psychiatric disturbances of Holocaust survivors. *Israel Annals of Psychiatry and Related Disciplines*, 5(1), 95-96.

1157 Klein, Hillel (1968). Problems in the psychotherapeutic treatment of Israeli survivors of the Holocaust. In: Krystal, Henry (Ed.), *Massive Psychic Trauma*. New York: International Universities Press, pp. 233-248.

1158 Klein, Hillel (1971). Families of survivors in the Kibbutz: Psychological studies. In: Krystal, Henry, and Niederland, William G. (Eds.), *Psychic Traumatization: Aftereffects in Individuals and Communities*. Boston, MA: Little, Brown, pp. 67-92.

1159 Klein, Hillel (1972). Holocaust survivors in Kibbutzim: Readaptation and reintegration. *Israel Annals of Psychiatry and Related Disciplines*, 10(1), 78-91.

1160 Klein, Hillel (1973). Children of the Holocaust: Mourning and bereavement. In: Anthony, E. James, and Koupernik, Cyrille (Eds.), *The Child in His Family. Vol. 2: The Impact of Disease and Death*. New York: John Wiley & Sons, pp. 393-409.

1161 Klein, Hillel (1974). Child victims of the Holocaust. *Journal of Clinical Child Psychology*, 11, 63-72.

1162 Klein, Hillel (1974). Delayed effects and after-effects of severe traumatization. *Israel Annals of Psychiatry and Related Disciplines*, 12(4), 293-303.

1163 Klein, Hillel (1978). Survivors of the Holocaust. *Mental Health and Society*, 5(1-2), 35-45.

1164 Klein, Hillel (1979). Some theoretical and clinical aspects of the Holocaust on survivors and families. In: *Israel-Netherlands Symposium on the Impact of Persecution. Jerusalem, 16-24 October 1977*. Rijswijk: The Netherlands: Ministry of Cultural Affairs, Recreation and Social Welfare, pp. 15-18.

1165 Klein, Hillel (1984). The survivor's search for meaning and identity. In: Gutman, Israel, and Saf, Avital (Eds.), *The Nazi Concentration Camps: Structure and Aims, the Image of the Prisoner, the Jews in the Camps. Proceedings of the Fourth Yad Vashem International Conference, Jerusalem, January 1980*. Jerusalem: Yad Vashem, pp. 543-554.

1166 Klein, Hillel (1985). Los procesos de identification y la renegacion durante el nazismo [Identification processes and denial in the shadow of Nazism]. *Revista de Psicoanalisis*, 42(4), 749-66.

1167 Klein, Hillel (1987). Chaim b'tzel iyum b'hashmada - 40 shana achrei hashoah: Aspektim tipuliyim [Life under existential threat - 40 years after the Holocaust: Therapeutic aspects]. *Sihot: Israel Journal of Psychotherapy*, 1(2), 94-98.

1168 Klein, Hillel (1990). General survey [Psychology of survivors]. In: Gutman, Israel (Ed.), *Encyclopedia of the Holocaust. Vol. 4*. New York: Macmillan, pp. 1426-1428.

1169 Klein, Hillel, and Kogan, Ilany (1986). Identification processes and denial in the shadow of Nazism. *International Journal of Psycho-Analysis*, 67(1), 45-52.

1170 Klein, Hillel, and Kogan, Ilany (1987). Tahalichei hizdahut v'hakchasha b'tzel hanatzizm [Denial and identification processes in survivors of the Holocaust]. *Sihot: Israel Journal of Psychotherapy*, 1(2), 108-111.

1171 Klein, Hillel, and Kogan, Ilany (1989). Some observations on denial and avoidance in Jewish Holocaust and post-Holocaust experience. In: Edelstein, Eliezer L.; Nathanson, Donald L., and Stone, Andrew M. (Eds.), *Denial: A Clarification of Concepts and Research*. New York: Plenum, pp. 299-308.

1172 Klein, Hillel, and Last, Uriel (1974). Cognitive and emotional aspects of the attitudes of American and Israeli youth toward the victims of the Holocaust. *Israel Annals of Psychiatry and Related Disciplines*, 12(2), 111-131.

1173 Klein, Hillel, and Last, Uriel (1978). Attitudes toward persecutor representations in children of traumatized and nontraumatized parents: Cross-cultural comparison. In: Feinstein, Sherman C., and Giovacchini, Peter L. (Eds.), *Adolescent Psychiatry: Developmental and Clinical Studies. Vol. 6*. Chicago, IL: University of Chicago Press, pp. 224-238.

1174 Klein, Hillel, and Reinharz, Shulamit (1972). Adaptation in the kibbutz of Holocaust survivors and their families. In: Miller, Louis (Ed.), *Mental Health in Rapid Social Change*. Jerusalem: Academic Press, pp. 302-319.

1175 Klein, Hillel; Zellermayer, Julius; and Shanan, Joel (1963). Former concentration camp inmates on a psychiatric ward. *Archives of General Psychiatry*, 8, 334-342.

1176 Klein, Judith (1991). "An unseren Schläfen perlt die Angst." Traumberichte in literarischen Werken über das Grauen der Ghettos und Lager ["Anxiety glistens on our brows": Dream narratives in literary works about the horrors of ghettos and concentration camps]. *Psyche: Zeitschrift für Psychoanalyse und ihre Anwendungen*, 45(6), 506-521.

1177 Klein, Marc E. (1987). *Transmission of trauma: The defensive styles of children of Holocaust survivors*. Unpublished doctoral dissertation, California School of Professional Psychology, Berkeley/Alameda, 115 pp. *Dissertation Abstracts International*, 48(12-B), p. 3682. (University Microfilms no. AAC 8802441).

1178 Klein, O. (1948). *Vliv kocentracniho tabora na ethicky charackter zidovske mladeze* [Effects of a concentration camp on the ethical character of young Jewish people]. Unpublished doctoral dissertation, Prague.

1179 Klein-Parker, Fran (1988). Dominant attitudes of adult children of Holocaust survivors toward their parents. In: Wilson, John P.; Harel, Zev; and Kahana, Boaz (Eds.). *Human Adaptation to Extreme Stress: From the Holocaust to Vietnam*. New York: Plenum, pp. 193-218.

1180 Kleinplatz, Morrie M. (1980). *The effects of cultural and individual supports on personality variables among children of Holocaust survivors in Israel and North America*. Unpublished doctoral dissertation, University of Windsor, Ontario, Canada. *Dissertation Abstracts International*, 41(3), p. 1114. (University Microfilms no. AAC 0533560).

1181 Klimkova-Deutschova, E. (1961). Chronicka progresivni astenie jako soucast vlivu valecnych utrap na nervovou soustavu [The chronic progressive asthenia as part of the war stress on the nervous sytem]. *Prakticky Lekar*, 41, 145-152.

1182 Klimkova-Deutschova, E. (1961). Neurologische Beiträge zur Diagnostik und Therapie der Folgezüstande des Krieges [Neurological contributions to the diagnosis and therapy of states resulting from the war]. In: *Die Behandlung der Asthenie und der vorzeitigen Vergreisung bei ehemaligen Widerstandskampfern und KZ-Häftlingen* [Treatment of Asthenia and Premature Aging in Former Resistance Fighters and Concentration Camp Inmates]. Wien: Verlag der FIR, pp. 51-62. [III Internationaler Medizinischer Konferenz. Liege, 17-19 März 1961].

1183 Klimkova-Deutschova, E. (1964). Neurologische Aspekte der Kriegsfolgen und ihre Dynamik [Neurological aspects of war sequels and their dynamics]. In: *Ätio-Pathogenese und Therapie der Erschöpfung und vorzeitigen Vergreisung* [The Aetiology, Pathogenesis and Therapy of Exhaustion and Premature Aging]. Wien: Verlag der FIR, pp. 541-554. [IV Internationaler Medizinischer Konferenz. Bucharest, 22-27 Juni 1964].

1184 Klimkova-Deutschova, E. (1971). Beitrag zu den Erkrankungen des Stützsystems [Contributions to the morbidity of the musculo-skelatal system]. In: Herberg, Hans-Joachim (Ed.), *Spätschäden nach*

Extrembelastungen [Late Damage After Extreme Stress]. Herford: Nicolai, pp. 134-135. [II Internationalen Medizinisch-Juristischen Konferenz. Dusseldorf, 1969].

1185 Klimkova-Deutschova, E. (1971). Neurologische und psychische Folgezüstande des Krieges und der Verfolgung bei Kindern und Jugendlichen [Neurological and psychic states in children and juveniles, resulting from the war and persecution]. In: Herberg, Hans-Joachim (Ed.), *Spätschäden nach Extrembelastungen* [Late Damage After Extreme Stress]. Herford: Nicolai, pp. 252-262. [II Internationalen Medizinische-Juristischen Konferenz. Dusseldorf, 1969].

1186 Klimkova-Deutschova, E. (1973). Neurologische Aspekte von Veränderungen der Knochenstruktur und intrakranialen Kalzifikationen nach Hunger [Neurological aspects of changes in the structure of the bones and intracranial calcification after hunger]. In: *Ermüdung und vorzeitiges Altern: Folge von Extrembelastungen* [Exhaustion and Premature Aging: Result of Extreme Stress]. Leipzig: Barth, pp. 39-47. [V Internationaler Medizinischer Kongress der FIR. Paris, 21-24 September 1970].

1187 Klimkova-Deutschova, E. (1978). Folgen des Krieges bei weiteren Generationen [War consequences in later generations]. In: *Medizinische Untersuchungen der Spätfolgen des Krieges und des NS-Regimes bei Jugendlichen und Kindern von ehemaligen KZ-Häftlingen und Verfolgten* [Medical Research of the Late Effects of the War and National Socialism Regime on Youth and Children of Former Concentration Camp Inmates and Persecuted Persons]. Wien: Internationale Föderation der Widerstandskämpfer. [VI Internationaler Medizinischer Kongress der FIR. Prague, 1976].

1188 Klimkova-Deutschova, E. (1978). Die Situation der Kinder in der Welt [The situation of the children in the world]. *Mitteilungen der FIR*, 14, 7-10.

1189 Kłodziński, Stanisław (1964). Untersuchungen über Lungentuberkulose bei ehemaligen Häftlingen des KZ-Lagers Auschwitz [Examinations of lung tuberculosis in former internees of the concentration camp Auschwitz]. In: *Ätio-Pathogenese und Therapie der Erschöpfung und vorzeitigen Vergreisung* [The Aetiology, Pathogenesis and Therapy of Exhaustion and Premature Aging]. Wien: Verlag der FIR, pp. 288-290. [IV Internationaler Medizinischer Kongress. Bucharest, 22-27 Juni 1964].

1190 Kłodziński, Stanisław (1965). Cel i metodyka badań lekarskich byłych więźniów hitlerowskich obozów koncentracyjnych [Goals and methods of medical examination of ex-prisoners from Hitlerian concentration camps]. *Przegląd Lekarski*, 21(1), 34-36.

1191 Kłodziński, Stanisław (1965). Dur wysypkowy w obozie Oświęcim [Typhus exanthematicus in the camp of Auschwitz]. *Przegląd Lekarski*, 21(1), 46-48.

1192 Kłodziński, Stanisław (1965). Zbrodnicze doświadczenia farmakologiczne na więzniach obozu koncentracyjnego w oświęcimiu [Criminal pharmacological experiments on prisoners of the Auschwitz concentration camp]. *Przegląd Lekarski*, 21(1), 40-46.

1193 Kłodziński, Stanisław (1969). Zbrodnicze doświadczenia z zakresu gruźlicy w Neuengamme. Działalność Kurta Heissmeyera [Criminal experiments on tuberculosis in Hitler's concentration camp Neuengamme: Activities of Kurt Heissmeyer]. *Przegląd Lekarski*, 36(10), 86-91.

1194 Kłodziński, Stanisław (1970). Dr. Stefan Pizlo, wiezien Oswiecimia nr 333 [Dr. Stefan Pizlo, Prisoner No. 333 of the Auschwitz concentration camp]. *Przegląd Lekarski*, 26(1), 258-260.

1195 Kłodziński, Stanisław (1971). Criminal experiments with tuberculosis carried out in Nazi concentration camps. In: *Auschwitz Anthology. Vol. 1: Inhuman Medicine. Part 2*. Warsaw: International Auschwitz Committee, pp. 163-184.

1196 Kłodziński, Stanisław (1971). Criminal pharmacological experiments on inmates of the concentration camp in Auschwitz. In: *Auschwitz Anthology. Vol. 1: Inhuman Medicine. Part 2*. Warsaw: International Auschwitz Committee, pp. 13-45.

1197 Kłodziński, Stanisław (1971). SS-men in the Auschwitz "Health Service." In: *Auschwitz Anthology. Vol. 1: Inhuman Medicine. Part 2*. Warsaw: International Auschwitz Committee, pp. 185-204.

1198 Kłodziński, Stanisław (1971). "Sterilization" and castration with the help of x-rays in the Auschwitz concentration camp. In: *Auschwitz Anthology. Vol. 1: Inhuman Medicine. Part 2*. Warsaw: International Auschwitz Committee, pp. 46-79.

1199 Kłodziński, Stanisław (1971). Phenol in the Auschwitz-Birkenau Concentration Camp. In: *Auschwitz Anthology. Vol. 1: Inhuman Medicine Part 2*. Warsaw: International Auschwitz Committee, pp. 99-119.

1200 Kłodziński, Stanisław (1971). The contribution of the Polish health service to save the life of the prisoners in the Auschwitz concentration camp. In: *Auschwitz Anthology. Vol. 2: In Hell They Preserved Human Dignity. Part 2.* Warsaw: International Auschwitz Committee, pp. 58-96.

1201 Kłodziński, Stanisław (1971). The purpose and methodology of medical examinations of former prisoners of Nazi concentration camps. In: *Auschwitz Anthology. Vol. 3: It Did Not End in Forty-Five. Part 1.* Warsaw: International Auschwitz Committee, pp. 67-75.

1202 Kłodziński, Stanisław (1972). Swoisty stan chorobowy po przebyciu obozów hitlerowskich [Specific diseases after internment in Hitler's camps]. *Przegląd Lekarski*, 29(1), 15-21.

1203 Kłodziński, Stanisław (1973). Verbrecherische Tuberkulose-experimente im Konzentrationslager Neuengamme: Die Tätigkeit von Kurt Heissmeyer [Criminal experiments with tuberculosis in the concentration camp Neuengamme: The activity of Kurt Heissmeyer]. In: *Ermüdung und vorzeitiges Altern: Folge von Extrembelastungen* [Exhaustion and Premature Aging: Result of Extreme Stress]. Leipzig: Barth, pp. 347-348. [V Internationaler Medizinischer Kongress der FIR. Paris, 21-24 September 1970].

1204 Kłodziński, Stanisław (1976). Apteka w obozie kobiecym w Brzezince [Pharmacy at the women's concentration camp of Birkenau]. *Przegląd Lekarski*, 33(1), 90-95.

1205 Kłodziński, Stanisław (1977). Sabotaż w buchenwaldzkim Instytucie Higieny SS Dr. Marian Ciepielowski [Sabotage at the SS Institute of Hygiene at the Buchenwald camp. Dr. Marian Ciepielowski]. *Przegląd Lekarski*, 34(1), 141-145.

1206 Kłodziński, Stanisław (1978). Dr. Mieczyslaw Jaworski. *Przegląd Lekarski*, 35(1), 221-223.

1207 Kłodziński, Stanisław (1981). O orzecznictwie psychiatrycznym wobec prześladowanych przez hitleryzm [Victims of Nazi persecutions in the light of expert judicial opinion]. *Przegląd Lekarski*, 38(1), 221-224.

1208 Kłodziński, Stanisław (1981). Uwagi o sytuacji zdrowotnej robotników przymusowych w Niemczech hitlerowskich [Health status of forced laborers in Hitlerite Germany]. *Przegląd Lekarski*, 38 (1), 62-72.

1209 Kłodziński, Stanisław (1984). Kilka uwag o KZ-syndromie [A few remarks about the K-Z syndrome]. *Przegląd Lekarski*, 41(1), 17-21.

1210 Kłodziński, Stanisław (1984). Patologia pracy w Oświęcimiu-Brzezince [The pathology of work in Auschwitz-Birkenau]. *Przegląd Lekarski*, 41(1), 37-54.

1211 Kłodziński, Stanisław (1984). Zbigniew Sobieszczanski, M.D. *Przegląd Lekarski*, 41(1), 131-136.

1212 Kłodziński, Stanisław (1987). Die erste Vergasung von Häftlingen und Kriegsgefangenen im Konzentrationslager Auschwitz [The first gassing of inmates and prisoners-of-war in concentration camp Auschwitz]. In: Hamburger Institut für Sozialforschung (Eds.), *Die Auschwitz-Hefte. Texte der polnischen Zeitschrift "Przegląd Lekarski" über historische, psychische und medizinische Aspekte des Lebens und Sterbens in Auschwitz. Band 1* [The Auschwitz Journal. Text of the Polish Journal "Medical Review" on Historical, Psychic and Medical Aspects of Life and Death in Auschwitz. Volume 1]. Weinheim and Basel: Beltz, pp. 261-275.

1213 Kłodziński, Stanisław (1987). Phenol. In: Hamburger Institut für Sozialforschung (Eds.), *Die Auschwitz-Hefte. Texte der polnischen Zeitschrift "Przegląd Lekarski" über historische, psychische und medizinische Aspekte des Lebens und Sterbens in Auschwitz. Band 1* [The Auschwitz Journal. Text of the Polish Journal "Medical Review" on Historical, Psychic and Medical Aspects of Life and Death in Auschwitz. Volume 1]. Weinheim and Basel: Beltz, pp. 277-280.

1214 Kłodziński, Stanisław (1987). Der spezifische Krankheitszustand nach KZ-Haft [The specific sickness situation following imprisonment]. In: Hamburger Institut für Sozialforschung (Eds.), *Die Auschwitz-Hefte. Texte der polnischen Zeitschrift "Przegląd Lekarski" über historische, psychische und medizinische Aspekte des Lebens und Sterbens in Auschwitz. Band 2* [The Auschwitz Journal. Text of the Polish Journal "Medical Review" on Historical, Psychic and Medical Aspects of Life and Death in Auschwitz. Volume 2]. Weinheim and Basel: Beltz, pp. 61-67.

1215 Kłodziński, Stanisław (1988). Lekarzen Hitlerowscy, Aquillin Ullrich i Heinrich Bunke, w procesie o tzw eutanazje [The Nazi physicians, Aquillin Ullrich amd Heinrich Bunke in the legal suit concerning euthanasia]. *Przegląd Lekarski*, 45(1), 78-84.

1216 Kłodziński, Stanisław (1989). Postawy ideowe więźniów w Oświecimiu [Ideologic attitudes of prisoners at the Auschwitz concentration camp]. *Przegląd Lekarski*, 46(1), 22-57.

1217 Kłodziński, Stanisław (1990). Doctor of pharmacy Jan Sikorski. *Przegląd Lekarski*, 47(1), 193-197.

1218 Kłodziński, Stanisław (1990). Merytoryczne i psychologiczne znaczenie oświęcimskich listów obozowych [Essential and psychological significance of the letters from the Auschwitz concentration camp]. *Przegląd Lekarski*, 47(1), 33-50.

1219 Kłodziński, Stanisław (1990). Socjologiczne i psychologiczne aspekty handlu w KL Auschwitz-Birkenau [Sociological and psychological aspects of commercial exchange transactions in the Auschwitz-Birkenau concentration camp]. *Przegląd Lekarski*, 47(1), 50-77.

1220 Kłodziński, Stanisław (1995). Häftlingsbriefe aus dem Konzentrationslager Auschwitz. Ihre historische und psychologische Bedeutung [Letters of inmates of the concentration camp Auschwitz: Their historical and psychological meaning]. In: Hamburger Institut für Sozialforschung (Eds.), *Die Auschwitz-Hefte. Ergänzungsband. Texte der polnischen Zeitschrift "Przegląd Lekarski" über historische, psychische und medizinische Aspekte des Lebens und Sterbens in Auschwitz* [The Auschwitz Journal. Supplementary Volume. Text of the Polish Journal "Medical Review" on Historical, Psychic and Medical Aspects of Life and Death in Auschwitz]. Weinheim and Basel: Rogner and Bernhard, pp. 22-26.

1221 Kłodziński, Stanisław, and Kutyba, Janusz (1966). Wstępne wyniki badań stanu zdrowia 100 bylych więźniow Hitlerowskich obozów koncentracyjnych [Preliminary results of a health investigation of 100 ex-prisoners of Hitlerian camps]. *Przegląd Lekarski*, 36(1), 1070-1072.

1222 Kłodziński, Stanisław, and Kutyba, Janusz (1971). Cracow mid-town-old-town district. In: *Auschwitz Anthology. Vol. 3: It Did Not End in Forty-Five. Part 1*. Warsaw: International Auschwitz Committee, pp. 180-190.

1223 Kłodziński, Stanisław, and Masłowski, Jan (1987). Vernichtung durch Arbeit. Zur Pathologie der Arbeit in Konzentrationslager [Destruction by work: Concerning the pathology of work in concentration camp]. In: Hamburger Institut für Sozialforschung (Eds.), *Die Auschwitz-Hefte. Texte der polnischen Zeitschrift "Przegląd Lekarski" über historische, psychische und medizinische Aspekte des Lebens und Sterbens in Auschwitz. Band 2* [The Auschwitz Journal. Text of the Polish Journal "Medical Review" on Historical, Psychic and Medical Aspects of Life and Death in Auschwitz. Volume 2]. Weinheim and Basel: Beltz, pp. 135-148.

1224 Kluge, Erich (1958). Über die Folgen schwere Häftzeiten [On the sequelae of severe imprisonment]. *Nervenarzt*, 29, 462-465.

1225 Kluge, Erich (1961). Über den Defektcharakter von Dauerfolgen schwerer Häftzeiten [Organic defects as chronic sequelae of severe imprisonment]. *Medizinische Sachverstandige*, 57, 185-187.

1226 Kluge, Erich (1963). Über Defektzustände nach schweren Haftzeiten, insbesondere nach KZ-Haft [On impairment after severe incarceration, mainly in concentration camps]. In: Paul, Helmut, and Herberg, Hans-Joachim (Eds.), *Psychische Spätschäden nach Politischer Verfolgung* [Psychological Late Damages Following Political Persecution]. Basel: Karger, pp. 85-94.

1227 Kluge, Erich (1965). Über Ergebnisse bei der Begutachtung Verfolgte [Results of evaluations of persecutees]. *Nervenarzt*, 36, 321.

1228 Kluge, Erich (1971). Über das Problem der Psychotherapie bei chronischen Verfolgungsschäden [The problem of psychotherapy in chronic damage due to persecution]. In: Herberg, Hans-Joachim (Ed.), *Spätschäden nach Extrembelastungen* [Late Damage After Extreme Stress]. Herford: Nicolai, pp. 187-189. [II Internationalen Medizinisch-Juristischen Konferenz. Dusseldorf, 1969].

1229 Kluge, Erich (1972). Das Problem der chronischen Schädigung durch Extrembelastung in der heutigen Psychiatrie [The problem of chronic damage through massive stress in contemporary psychiatry]. *Fortschritte der Neurologie, Psychiatrie*, 40, 1-30.

1230 Kluge, Erich (1973). Über Dauerfolgen schwerer Häftzeiten unter besonderer Berücksichtigung hirnorganischer Störungen [Permanent sequels of severe internment, with special emphasis on organic brain damage]. In: *Ermüdung und vorzeitiges Altern: Folge von Extrembelastungen* [Exhaustion and Premature Aging: Result of Extreme Stress]. Leipzig: Barth, pp. 189-191. [V Internationaler Medizinischer Kongress der FIR. Paris, 21-24 September 1970].

1231 Kluvers, Elouise, and Kluvers, Ingrid (1960). Social aspects of camp pathology. In: *Experts Meeting on the Later Effects of Imprisonment and Deportation, Oslo*. Paris: World Veterans Federation, 131-135.

1232 Kluvers, Elouise, and Kluvers, Ingrid (1979). *Jouw Oorlog, Mij een Zorg* [Your War - I Don't Care]. Baarn: In Den Toren. 155 pp.

1233 Kluyskens, Pierre (1960). Legal aspects of camp pathology. In: *Experts Meeting on the Later Effects of Imprisonment and Deportation, Oslo*. Paris: World Veterans Federation, pp. 137-142.

1234 Kluyskens, Pierre (1961). Legal aspects of the problem: Comparative report. In: *International Conference on the Later Effects of Imprisonment and Deportation Organized by the World Veterans Federation. The Hague, November 20-25, 1961*. The Hague: World Veterans Federation, pp. 167-177.

1235 Koenig, Werner (1964). Chronic or persisting identity diffusion. *American Journal of Psychiatry*, 120(11), 1081-1084.

1236 Koenig, Werner (1966). Über Behandlungsergebnisse der chronisch-reaktiven Depression und anderer psychischer Verfolgungsschäden [Results of the treatment of chronic reactive depression and other psychiatric disturbances due to persecution]. In: Lopez Ibor, Juan J. (Ed.), *Proceedings. Fourth World Congress of Psychiatry, Madrid, 5-11 September 1966*. Amsterdam: Excerpta Medica Foundation, pp. 1816-1818.

1237 Koevary, Hanna Levinsky (1975). A search for home: The road to Israel. In: Steinitz, Lucy Y., and Szonyi, David M. (Eds.), *Living After the Holocaust: Reflections by the Post-War Generation in America*. New York: Bloch, pp. 137-146.

1238 Kogan, Ilany (1988). The second skin. *International Review of Psycho-Analysis*, 15(2), 251-260.

1239 Kogan, Ilany (1989). The search for self. *International Journal of Psycho-Analysis*, 70(4), 661-671.

1240 Kogan, Ilany (1989). Working through the vicissitudes of trauma in the psychoanalysis of Holocaust survivors' offspring. *Sigmund Freud House Bulletin*, 13(2), 25-33.

1241 Kogan, Ilany (1990). Vermitteltes und reales Trauma in der Psychoanalyse von Kindern von Holocaust-überlebenden [Transmitted and real trauma in the psychoanalysis of the children of Holocaust survivors]. *Psyche: Zeitschrift für Psychoanalyse und ihre Anwendungen*, 44(6), 533-544.

1242 Kogan, Ilany (1992). From acting out to words and meaning. *International Journal of Psycho-Analysis*, 73(3), 455-465.

1243 Kogan, Ilany (1993). Curative factors in the psychoanalyses of Holocaust survivors' offspring before and during the Gulf War. *International Journal of Psycho-Analysis*, 74(4), 803-814.

1244 Kogan, Ilany (1995). *The Cry of Mute Children: A Psychoanalytic Perspective of the Second Generation of the Holocaust*. New York: Free Association Books. 178 pp.

1245 Kogan, Ilany (1995). Love and heritage of the past. *International Journal of Psycho-Analysis*, 76(4), 805-823.

1246 Kogon, Eugen (1973). *The Theory and Practice of Hell: The German Concentration Camps and the System Behind Them*. New York: Octogon. 307 pp.

1247 Kolle, K. (1958). Die Opfer der nationalsozialistischen verfolgung in psychiatrischer sight [The victims of the National Socialist persecution in the light of psychiatry]. *Nervenarzt*, 29, 148-158.

1248 Kolle, K. (1958). Psychosen als Schädigungsfolgen [Psychoses as sequelae to damage]. *Fortschritte der Neurologie, Psychiatrie*, 26, 101-120.

1249 Kolodner, Anna (1987). *The socialization of children of concentration camp survivors*. Unpublished doctoral dissertation, Boston University, Boston, Massachusetts, 339 pp. *Dissertation Abstracts International*, 47(12-A), p. 4521. (University Microfilms no. 8707066).

1250 Komenda, Janina (1987). Frauen im Revier von Birkenau [Women's quarters in Birkenau]. In: Hamburger Institut für Sozialforschung (Eds.), *Die Auschwitz-Hefte. Texte der polnischen Zeitschrift "Przegląd Lekarski" über historische, psychische und medizinische Aspekte des Lebens und Sterbens in Auschwitz. Band 1* [The Auschwitz Journal. Text of the Polish Journal "Medical Review" on Historical, Psychic and Medical Aspects of Life and Death in Auschwitz. Volume 1]. Weinheim and Basel: Beltz, pp. 185-197.

1251 Konieczy, Alfred (1986). Z księgi zmarłych szpitala obozowego w Kolcach [Death registry in the concentration camp hospital in Kolce]. *Przegląd Lekarski*, 43(1), 101-105.

1252 Kor, Eva (1994). The personal, public, and political dimensions of being a Mengele guinea pig. In: Michalczyk, John J. (Ed.), *Medicine, Ethics, and the Third Reich: Historical and Contemporary Issues*. Kansas City, MO: Sheed & Ward, pp. 101-105.

1253 Koranyi, Erwin (1969). Psychodynamic theories of the "survivor syndrome." *Canadian Psychiatric Association Journal*, 14(2), 165-174.

1254 Koranyi, Erwin (1969). A theoretical view of the survivor syndrome. *Diseases of the Nervous System*, 30, 115-118.

1255 Korczyńska, Adela (1980). Przyczynek do zagadnienia pomocy więźiom Oświęcimia-Brzezinka [Contribution to the problem of help to the prisoners of the Auschwitz-Birkenau concentration camp]. *Przegląd Lekarski*, 37(1), 113-118.

1256 Kornhuber, H. (1961). Psychologie und Psychiatrie der Kriegsgefangenschaft [The psychology and psychiatry of prisoners of war]. In: Gruhle, Hans W. (Ed.), *Psychiatrie der Gegenwart: Forschung und Praxis. Band 3: Soziale und angewandte Psychiatrie* [Psychiatry in the Present: Research and Practice. Vol. 3: Social and Applied Psychiatry]. Berlin: Springer.

1257 Kościuszkowa, Janina (1971). Children in the Auschwitz concentration camp. In: *Auschwitz Anthology. Vol. 2: In Hell They Preserved Human Dignity. Part 2.* Warsaw: International Auschwitz Committee, pp. 217-224.

1258 Kosiński, Jerzy (1988). Rewiry w Gablonz-Reinowitz i w Reichenau, filiach Gross-Rosen [Hospitals at Gablonz-Reinowits and Reichenau, branches of the Gross-Rosen concentration camp]. *Przegląd Lekarski*, 45(1), 52-56.

1259 Kover, Elihu (1995). Community-based services for elderly Holocaust survivors. In: Lemberger, John (Ed.), *A Global Perspective on Working with Holocaust Survivors and the Second Generation.* Jerusalem: JDC-Brookdale Institute of Gerontology and Human Development, AMCHA, and JDC-Israel, pp. 51-58.

1260 Kover, Elihu (1995). Self-help community services. In: Lemberger, John (Ed.), *A Global Perspective on Working with Holocaust Survivors and the Second Generation.* Jerusalem: JDC-Brookdale Institute of Gerontology and Human Development, AMCHA, and JDC-Israel, pp. 151-155.

1261 Kowalski, Stanisław (1968). Wstępne wyniki badań byłych więźniów hitlerowskich obozów kocentracyjnych [Preliminary results of an investigation of ex-prisoners from Hitlerian concentration camps]. *Przegląd Lekarski*, 25(1), 54-55.

1262 Kowalski, Stanisław (1971). The Warsaw centre. In: *Auschwitz Anthology. Vol. 3: It Did Not End in Forty-Five. Part 1.* Warsaw: International Auschwitz Committee, pp. 152-162.

1263 Kral, Vojtech A. (1947). An epidemic of encephalitis in the concentration camp Terezin (Theresienstadt) during the winter 1943-1944. *Journal of Nervous and Mental Disease*, 105, 403-413.

1264 Kral, Vojtech A. (1948). O epidemii encefalitidy v Terezinskem ghetu [On the epidemic of encephalitis in the ghetto of Terezin]. *Casopis Lekaru Ceskych*, 87, 1-15.

1265 Kral, Vojtech A. (1949). Beobachtungen bei einer grossen Enzephalitisepidemie [Observations on a large epidemic of encephalitis]. *Schweizer Archiv für Neurologie und Psychiatrie*, 64, 281-328.

1266 Kral, Vojtech A. (1951). Psychiatric observations under severe chronic stress. *American Journal of Psychiatry*, 108, 185-192.

1267 Kral, Vojtech A.; Pazder, Larry H.; and Wigdor, B.T. (1967). Long-term effects of a prolonged stress experience. *Canadian Psychiatric Association Journal*, 12(2), 175-181.

1268 Kraus, Ota B., and Kulka, Erich (1966). *Death Factory: A Document on Auschwitz*. Oxford and New York: Pergamon. 284 pp.

1269 Kraus, Rolf D. (1989). Truth but not art? German autobiographical writings of the survivors of concentration camps, ghettos and prisons. In: *Remembering for the Future: Working Papers and Addenda. Vol. 3: The Impact of the Holocaust and Genocide on Jews and Christians*. Oxford: Pergamon, pp. 2958-2972.

1270 Krell, Robert (1979). Holocaust families: The survivors and their children. *Comprehensive Psychiatry*, 20(6), 560-568.

1271 Krell, Robert (1982). Family therapy with children of concentration camp survivors. *American Journal of Psychotherapy*, 36(4), 513-522.

1272 Krell, Robert (1983). Aspects of psychologic trauma in Holocaust survivors and their children. In: Grobman, Alex, and Landes, Daniel (Eds.), *Genocide: Critical Issues of the Holocaust: A Companion to the Film "Genocide."* Chappaqua, NY: Rossell, pp. 371-380.

1273 Krell, Robert (1984). Holocaust survivors and their children: Comments on psychiatric consequences and psychiatric terminology. *Comprehensive Psychiatry*, 25(5), 521-528.

1274 Krell, Robert (1985). Holocaust survivors and their children: Comments on psychiatric consequences and psychiatric terminology.

In: Chess, Stella, and Thomas, Alexander (Eds.), *Annual Progress in Child Psychiatry and Child Development*. New York: Brunner/Mazel, pp. 631-641.

1275 Krell, Robert (Ed.) (1985). Child survivors of the Holocaust: 40 years later. *Journal of the American Academy of Child Psychiatry*, 24(4), 378-412.

1276 Krell, Robert (1985). Introduction to "Child survivors of the Holocaust: 40 years later." *Journal of the American Academy of Child Psychiatry*, 24(4), 378-380.

1277 Krell, Robert (1985). Therapeutic value of documenting child survivors. *Journal of the American Academy of Child Psychiatry*, 24(4), 397-400.

1278 Krell, Robert (1985). Therapeutic value of documenting child survivors. In: Chess, Stella, and Thomas, Alexander (Eds.), *Annual Progress in Child Psychiatry and Child Development*. New York: Brunner/Mazel, pp. 281-288.

1279 Krell, Robert (1986). Post-traumatic stress disorders: Victims of different wars. *ICODO Info*, 3(1), 5-10.

1280 Krell, Robert (1989). Alternative therapeutic approaches to Holocaust survivors. In: Marcus, Paul, and Rosenberg, Alan (Eds.), *Healing Their Wounds: Psychotherapy with Holocaust Survivors and Their Families*. New York: Praeger, pp. 215-226.

1281 Krell, Robert (1990). Holocaust survivors: A clinical perspective. *Psychiatric Journal of the University of Ottawa*, 15(1), 18-21.

1282 Krell, Robert (1992). Aging Holocaust survivors: Memory, nostalgia, and treatment issues: A keynote address. In: Kenigsberg, Rositta E., and Lieblich, Cathy M. (Eds.), *The First National Conference on Identification, Treatment and Care of the Aging Holocaust Survivor, March 29-31, 1992: Selected Proceedings*. Miami, FL: Holocaust Documentation and Education Center and Southeast Florida Center on Aging, Florida International University, pp. 22-31.

1283 Krell, Robert (1992). The aging child survivor and the problems of memory/nostalgia. In: Kenigsberg, Rositta E., and Lieblich, Cathy M. (Eds.), *The First National Conference on Identification, Treatment and Care of the Aging Holocaust Survivor, March 29-31, 1992: Selected Proceedings*. Miami, FL: Holocaust Documentation and Education Center and Southeast Florida Center on Aging, Florida International University, pp. 37-41.

1284 Krell, Robert (1993). Child survivors of the Holocaust: Strategies of adaptation. *Canadian Journal of Psychiatry*, 38(6), 384-389.

1285 Krell, Robert (1994). The psychiatric treatment of Holocaust survivors. In: Charny, Israel W. (Ed.), *The Widening Circle of Genocide. Genocide: A Critical Bibliographic Review: Vol. 3*. New Brunswick, NJ: Transaction, pp. 245-271.

1286 Krell, Robert (1995). Children who survived the Holocaust: Reflections of a child survivor/psychiatrist. *Echoes of the Holocaust*, 4, 14-21. [Bulletin of the Jerusalem Center for Research into the Late Effects of the Holocaust. Talbieh Mental Health Center, Jerusalem, Israel].

1287 Krell, Robert, and Rabkin, Leslie (1979). The effects of sibling death on the surviving child: A family perspective. *Family Process*, 18(4), 471-477.

1288 Kren, George (1979). Psychohistory and the Holocaust. *Journal of Psychohistory*, 6(3), 409-417.

1289 Kren, George (1989). The Holocaust survivor and psychoanalysis. In: Marcus, Paul, and Rosenberg, Alan (Eds.), *Healing Their Wounds: Psychotherapy with Holocaust Survivors and Their Families*. New York: Praeger, pp. 3-21.

1290 **Kren, George, and Rappoport, Leon (1994). *The Holocaust and the Crisis of Human Behavior.* New York: Holmes & Meier. 176 pp.**

1291 Kret, Józef (1971). The doctors found a way out. In: *Auschwitz Anthology. Vol. 2: In Hell They Preserved Human Dignity. Part 1*. Warsaw: International Auschwitz Committee, pp. 76-106.

1292 Krętowski, Józef; Killmar, Marian; Znosko, Konstanty; Karbowski, Jan; and Kościk-Grenda, Maria (1981). Pomoc społeczna i lekarska kombatantom w Białymstoku [Social and medical aid provided to combatants in the Bialystok area]. *Przegląd Lekarski*, 38(1), 30-33.

1293 Kretschmer, Manfred (1992). Grafeneck - 50 Jahre danach [Grafeneck - 50 years after]. In: Jockush, Ulrich, and Scholz, Lothar (Eds.), *Verwaltetes Morden im Nationalsozialismus: Verstrickung, Verdrängung, Verantwortung von Psychiatrie und Justiz* [Administered Killings at the Time of National Socialism: Involvement, Suppression, Responsibility of Psychiatry and Judicial System]. Regensburg: Roderer, pp. 111-113.

1294 Kretschmer, Manfred (1992). Grafeneck - 50 years after. In: Jockush, Ulrich, and Scholz, Lothar (Eds.), *Administered Killings at the Time of National Socialism: Involvement, Suppression, Responsibility of Psychiatry and Judicial System*. Regensburg: Roderer, pp. 102-104.

1295 Kreuzer, W. (1972). *Über Beziehungen zwischen körperlichen Noxen und psychischen Dauerschäden nach schweren Häftzeiten* [On the relationship between physical noxious stimuli and psychic permanent damage after severe imprisonment]. Unpublished doctoral dissertation, Johannes Gutenberg University of Mainz, Germany.

1296 Kreuzer, W. (1975). Internationale Untersuchungen über psychische Spätschäden [International examination of late psychic damage]. *Mitteilungen der FIR*, 9, 21-32.

1297 Kreuzer, W. (1975). Über Beziehungen zwischen körperlichen Noxen und psychischen Dauerschäden nach schweren Häftzeiten [The relationship between physical and psychic permanent damage after severe incarceration]. *Nervenarzt*, 46, 291-296.

1298 Kropveld, J. (1983). *Het KZ-syndroom* [The concentration camp syndrome]. Unpublished doctoral dissertation, University of Amersterdam, Netherlands.

1299 Krupka-Matuszczyk, Irena (1986), Jeńcy z Lambinowic w szpitalu psychiatrycznym w Lublincu [Prisoners of war from Lamsdorf in the Lublin Psychiatric Hospital]. *Przegląd Lekarski*, 43(1), 83.

1300 Krystal, Henry (1964). The late sequelae of massive psychic trauma. In: *Theme of the First Studies of Concentration Camp Survivors. The Second Wayne State University Workshop on the Late Sequelae of Massive Psychic Traumatization*. Detroit, MI: Wayne State University.

1301 Krystal, Henry (Ed.) (1968). *Massive Psychic Trauma*. New York: International Universities Press. 369 pp.

1302 Krystal, Henry (1968). Patterns of psychological damage. In: Krystal, Henry (Ed.), *Massive Psychic Trauma*. New York: International Universities Press, pp. 1-7.

1303 Krystal, Henry (1968). Psychic sequelae of massive psychic trauma. In: Lopez Ibor, Juan J. (Ed.), *Proceedings. Fourth World Congress of Psychiatry, Madrid 5-11 September 1966. Vol. 2*. New York: Excerpta Medica Foundation.

1304 Krystal, Henry (1970). Trauma: Considerations of its intensity and chronicity. In: Krystal, Henry, and Niederland, William G. (Eds.), *Psychic Traumatization: Aftereffects in Individuals and Communities*. Boston, MA: Little, Brown, pp. 11-28.

1305 Krystal, Henry (1971). Review of the findings and implications of this symposium. In: Krystal, Henry, and Niederland, William G. (Eds.), *Psychic Traumatization: Aftereffects in Individuals and Communities*. Boston, MA: Little, Brown, pp. 217-229.

1306 Krystal, Henry (1978). Trauma and affects. In: Eissler, Ruth S.; Freud, Anna; Kris, Marianne; and Neubauer, Peter B. (Eds.), *Psychoanalytic Study of the Child. Vol. 33*. New Haven, CT: Yale University Press, pp. 81-116.

1307 Krystal, Henry (1981). Integration and self-healing in post-traumatic states. *Journal of Geriatric Psychiatry and Neurology*, 14(2), 165-189.

1308 Krystal, Henry (1984). Integration and self-healing in post-traumatic states. In: Luel, Steven A., and Marcus, Paul (Eds.), *Psychoanalytic Reflections on the Holocaust: Selected Essays*. New York, Ktav, pp. 113-134.

1309 Krystal, Henry (1985). Trauma and the stimulus barrier. *Psychoanalytic Inquiry*, 5(1), 131-161.

1310 Krystal, Henry (1991). Integration and self-healing in post-traumatic states: A ten year retrospective. *American Imago*, 48(1), 93-118.

1311 Krystal, Henry (1993). Beyond the DSM III--R: Therapeutic considerations in post-traumatic stress disorder. In: Wilson, John P., and Raphael, Beverley (Eds.), *International Handbook of Traumatic Stress Syndromes*. New York: Plenum, pp. 841-854.

1312 Krystal, Henry (1995). Trauma and aging: A thirty-year follow-up. In: Caruth, Cathy (Ed.), *Trauma: Explorations in Memory*. Baltimore, MD: Johns Hopkins University Press, pp. 76-99.

1313 Krystal, Henry, and Niederland, William G. (1968). Clinical observations on the "survivor syndrome." *International Journal of Psycho-Analysis*, 49(2-3), 313-315.

1314 Krystal, Henry, and Niederland, William G. (1968). Clinical observations on the survivor syndrome. In: Krystal, Henry (Ed.), *Massive Psychic Trauma*. New York: International Universities Press, pp. 327-348.

1315 Krystal, Henry, and Niederland, William G. (Eds.) (1971). *Psychic Traumatization: Aftereffects in Individuals and Communities*. Boston, MA: Little, Brown. 236 pp.

1316 Krystal, Henry, and Petty, Thomas A. (1963). The dynamics of the adjustment to migration. *Psychiatric Quarterly*, 37, 118.

1317 Krystal, Henry, and Petty, Thomas A. (1968). The psychological complications of convalescence. In: Krystal, Henry (Ed.), *Massive Psychic Trauma*. New York: International Universities Press, pp. 277-296.

1318 Krzywicki, Janusz (1965). Stan uzębienia u byłych więźniów obozów hitlerowskich [The dental status of ex-prisoners of Hitlerian camps]. *Przegląd Lekarski*, 21(1), 36-37.

1319 Krzywicki, Janusz (1978). Gebissuntersuchungen bei Personen die als Kinder und Jugendliche in Haft waren [Examinations of the dental status in persons who as children or adolescents were in concentration camp imprisonment]. In: *Medizinische Untersuchungen der Spätfolgen des Krieges und des NS-Regimes bei Jugendlichen und Kindern von ehemaligen KZ-Häftlingen und Verfolgten* [Medical Research of the Late Effects of the War and National Socialism Regime on Youth and Children of Former Concentration Camp Inmates and Persecuted Persons]. Wien: Internationale Föderation der Widerstandskämpfer, pp. 83-84. [VI Internationaler Medizinischer Kongress der FIR. Prague, 1976].

1320 Kubica, Antoni (1989). Dr. Josef Mengele i ślady jego zbrodni [Dr. Josef Mengele and the traces of his crimes]. *Przegląd Lekarski*, 46(1), 96-106.

1321 Kuch, Klaus, and Cox, Brian J. (1992). Symptoms of PTSD in 124 survivors of the Holocaust. *American Journal of Psychiatry*, 149(3), 337-340.

1322 Kudejko, J. (1972). Gruźlica toczniowa po szczepieniu doświadczalnym w obozie u byłej więźniarki Majdanka [Tuberculosis luposa following an experimental vaccination at the concentration camp of Majdanek]. *Przegląd Dermatologiczny*, 59(1), 43-45.

1323 Kuffel, Edwin (1970). Ostatnie dni w obozie Ebensee [Last days at the Ebensee concentration camp]. *Przegląd Lekarski*, 26(1), 236-238.

1324 Kuhn, E.V.; Brodan, V.; Honzak, R.; Rysanek, K.; and Vojtechnosky, M. (1978). Metabolische Auswirkung des

Schlafentzugs [Metabolic effects of sleep deprivation]. In: *Medizinische Untersuchungen der Spätfolgen des Krieges und des NS-Regimes bei Jugendlichen und Kindern von ehemaligen KZ-Häftlingen und Verfolgten* [Medical Research of the Late Effects of the War and National Socialism Regime on Youth and Children of Former Concentration Camp Inmates and Persecuted Persons]. Wien: Internationale Föderation der Widerstandskämpfer. [VI Internationaler Medizinischer Kongress der FIR. Prague, 1976].

1325 Kuilman, M. (1985). Symptomatologie van oorlogs traumata [Symptomology of war trauma]. In: *Problematiek van Oorlogsgetrofflene* [Problems of War Victims]. Utrecht: Stichting ICODO, pp. 29-39.

1326 Kuilman, M. (1987). Dillemas bij de psychiatrische diagnostiek van oorlogsgetroffenen [Dilemmas in the psychiatric diagnosis of war victims]. In: *Medical Causality and Late Consequences of War*. Utrecht: Stichting ICODO, pp. 9-16.

1327 Kulcsar, I. Shlomo (1968). The psychopathology of Adolf Eichmann. In: Lopez Ibor, Juan J. (Ed.), *Proceedings. Fourth World Congress of Psychiatry, Madrid 5-11 September 1966*. New York, Excerpta Medica Foundation, pp. 1687-1689.

1328 Kulcsar, I. Shlomo (1978). De Sade and Eichman. In: Charny, Israel W. (Ed.), *Strategies Against Violence: Design for Nonviolent Change*. Boulder, CO: Westview, pp. 19-33.

1329 Kulcsar, I. Shlomo; Kulcsar, Shoshanna; and Szondi, Lipot (1966). Adolf Eichmann and the Third Reich. In: Slovenko, Ralph (Ed.), *Crime, Law and Corrections*. Springfield, IL: Thomas, pp. 16-52.

1330 Kulisiewicz, Alexander (1974). Z zagadnień psychopatologii muzyki i pieśni w obozach hitlerowskich [Psychopathology of music and songs in Nazi concentration camps]. *Przegląd Lekarski*, 31(1), 39-45.

1331 Kulisiewicz, Alexander (1975). Dalsze przyczynki do zagadnień psychopatogii muzyki i pieśni w obozach hitlerowskich [Further contributions to the problems of psychopathology of music and songs in Nazi camps]. *Przegląd Lekarski*, 32(1), 33-40.

1332 Kulisiewicz, Alexander (1977). Muzyka i pieśń jako współczynnik samoobrony psychicznej więźniów w obozach hitlerowskich [Music and songs as a factor of self-defence among inmates of Nazi concentration camps]. *Przegląd Lekarski*, 34(1), 66-77.

1333 Kulisiewicz, Alexander (1979). Dalsze przyczynki do zagadnień muzyki i pieśni w zakresie samoobrony psychicznej więźnów w obozach hitlerowskich [Further contributions of music and songs as an instrument of self-defence in Nazi concentration camps]. *Przegląd Lekarski*, 36(1), 38-50.

1334 Kundrats, Anne-Geale H. (1982). *Attribution of meaning to life in extremis*. Unpublished doctoral dissertation, University of Toronto, Ontario, Canada. *Dissertation Abstracts International*, 44(1-B), p. 290. (University Microfilms no. AAC 0551443).

1335 Kuperstein, Elana E. (1981). Adolescents of parent survivors of concentration camps: A review of the literature. *Journal of Psychology and Judaism*, 6(1), 7-22.

1336 Kurimay, Tamas (1990). Illegality 1988. *Contemporary Family Therapy*, 12(5), 381-391.

1337 Kurth, W. (1973). Zur Frage der chronischen Dauerbelastung bei Verfolgten mit der Folge der Frühalterung [The question of chronic stress in persecutees with the consequences of premature aging]. In: *Ermüdung und vorzeitiges Altern: Folge von Extrembelastungen* [Exhaustion and Premature Aging: Result of Extreme Stress]. Leipzig: Barth, pp. 198-200. [V Internationaler Medizinischer Kongress der FIR. Paris, 21-24 September 1970].

1338 Kurth, W. (1978). Späte Schäden bei in Kindheit oder Jugend verfolgter [Delayed damage in survivors who were persecuted during childhood or youth]. In: *Medizinische Untersuchungen der Spätfolgen des Krieges und des NS-Regimes bei Jugendlichen und Kindern von ehemaligen KZ-Häftlingen und Verfolgten* [Medical Research of the Late Effects of the War and National Socialism Regime on Youth and Children of Former Concentration Camp Inmates and Persecuted Persons]. Wien: Internationale Föderation der Widerstandskämpfer, pp. 13-20. [VI Internationaler Medizinischer Kongress der FIR. Prague, 1976].

1339 Kurtz, Helen-Chaya (1989). Las victimas del holocausto en Israel: Una vision general de sus problemas de adaptacion y de los problemas de sus familias [The Holocaust victim in Israel: A general view of their adjustment problems and of the problems of their family]. *Psicopatologia*, 9(1), 27-30.

1340 Kusnetzoff, Juan C. (1985). "Que tiene el Holocausto que ver conmigo?" Una contribucion al estudia de percepticidio ["What does the Holocaust have to do with me?" A contribution to the study of percepticide]. *Revista de Psicoanalisis*, 42(2), 321-333.

1341 Kutscher, Karin (1995). Psychische Folgen extremer menschlicher Verunsicherung am Beispiel des Holocaust [Psychic consequences of extreme human insecurity using the Holocaust as an example]. *Zeitschrift für Individualpsychologie*, 20(2), 92-106.

1342 Kuzak, Zygmunt (1979). Nachtwächter [Nightwatcher]. *Przegląd Lekarski*, 36(1), 159-162.

1343 Kuzak, Zygmunt (1981). Z duchowych przeżyć więźnia [Spiritual experiences of a prisoner]. *Przegląd Lekarski*, 38(1), 159-162.

1344 Kyle, N., and Hoppe, Klaus (1969). *Religiosity and ethnocentric idealism in survivors of severe persecution*. [Paper presented at the International Psychological Congress, London, 1969].

1345 Lach-Kamininńska, Janina (1969). W więzieniu i w obozach hitlerowskich (1943-1945) [In Nazi prisons and concentration camps (1943-1945)]. *Przegląd Lekarski*, 25(1), 167-172.

1346 Ladee, George A. (1985). Kontakt tussen arts en oorlogsgetroffenen in het kader van een keuring [Contact between physician and war victim in the framework of a medical examination]. In: *Problematiek van Oorlogsgetrofflene* [Problems of War Victims]. Utrecht: Stichting ICODO, pp. 40-44.

1347 Lagerwey, Mary D. (1994). *Gold encrusted chaos: An analysis of Auschwitz memoirs*. Unpublished doctoral dissertation, Western Michigan University, Kalamazoo, Michigan, 120 pp. *Dissertation Abstracts International*, 55(6-A), p. 1699. (University Microfilms no. AAC 9429014).

1348 Lagnado, Lucette Matalon, and Dekel, Sheila Cohn (1991). *Children of the Flames: Dr. Josef Mengele and the Untold Story of the Twins at Auschwitz*. New York and London: Penguin. 320 pp.

1349 Landau, A. (1961). Schlafkur bei chronischer Asthenie und vorzeitiger Vergreisung bei ehemaligen KZ-Häftlingen und Internierten [Sleeping cure in chronic asthenia and premature senility in ex-concentration camp inmates and prisoners]. In: *Die Behandlung der Asthenie und der vorzeitigen Vergreisung bei ehemaligen Widerstandskämpfern und KZ-Häftlingen*. [Treatment of Asthenia and Premature Aging in Former Resistance Fighters and Concentration Camp Inmates]. Wien: Verlag der FIR, pp. 63-67. [III Internationale Medizinische Konferenz. Liege, 17-19 März 1961].

1350 Landau, Orith (1995). *Family patterns of second generation Holocaust survivors*. Unpublished doctoral dissertation, Yeshiva University, New York, 144 pp. *Dissertation Abstracts International*, 56(10-A), p. 4147. (University Microfilms no. AAC 9604901).

1351 Landgarten, Helen B. (1981). Group art therapy with children of Holocaust survivors. *Clinical Art Therapy*, 208-245.

1352 Lange, A. (1982). Re-attributie in de directieve gezinstherapie met een oorlogsslachtoffer [Restructuring in directive family therapy with a war victim]. *Tijdschrift Direktieve Therapie*, 4, 288-303.

1353 Lange, A. (1984). Directieve psychotherapie bij oorlogsgetroffenen [Directive psychotherapy with war victims]. In: Dane, Jan (Ed.), *Keerzijde van de bevrijding: Opstellen over de maatschappelijke, psycho-sociale en medische aspekten van de problematiek van oorlogsgetroffenen* [The Other Side of Liberation: Essays on the Social, Psychosocial and Medical Aspects of the Problems of War Victims]. Deventer: Van Loghum Slaterus, pp. 118-144.

1354 Lange, Moshe (1995). Silence therapy with Holocaust survivors and their families. *Australian and New Zealand Journal of Family Therapy*, 16(1), 1-10.

1355 Langer, Lawrence L. (1991). *Holocaust Testimonies: The Ruins of Memory*. New Haven, CT: Yale University Press. 216 pp.

1356 Langeveld, Martin J. (1977). Favorable assimilation of profound psychic shock. *Acta Paedopsychiatrica*, 43(1), 7-14.

1357 Langfeldt, G. (1946). Psychiatric observations and experiences during German occupation of Norway. *Acta Psychiatry*, 21, 459-471.

1358 Lansen, Johan (1991). Gruppentherapie mit der Zweiten Generation von Holocaust-Überlebenden [Group therapy with second generation of Holocaust survivors]. In: Stoffels, Hans (Ed.), *Schicksale der Verfolgten: Psychische und somatische Auswirkungen von Terrorherrschaft* [The Fate of Persecuted Persons: Psychic and Somatic Effects of Terror Reign]. Berlin: Springer.

1359 Lansen, Johan (1993). The second generation: Dutch examinations and professional care. *Echoes of the Holocaust*, 2, 46-59. [Bulletin of the Jerusalem Center for Research into the Late Effects of the Holocaust. Talbieh Mental Health Center, Jerusalem, Israel].

1360 Lansen, Johan (1995). Delayed and long-term effects of persecution suffered in childhood and youth. *Echoes of the Holocaust*, 4, 30-35. [Bulletin of the Jerusalem Center for Research into the Late Effects of the Holocaust. Talbieh Mental Health Center, Jerusalem, Israel].

1361 Lansen, Johan, and Cels, J.P. (1992). Psycho-educative group psychotherapy for Jewish child survivors of the Holocaust and non-Jewish survivors of Japanese concentration camps. *Israel Journal of Psychiatry and Related Sciences*, 29(1), 22-32.

1362 Lantz, Jim (1992). Using Frankl's concepts with PTSD clients. *Journal of Traumatic Stress*, 5(3), 485-490.

1363 Larsen, Helweg; Hoffmeyer, Henrik; Kieler, Jørgen; Hess Thaysen, Eigil; Hess Thaysen, Jørn; Thygesen, Paul; and Hertel Wulff, Munke (1955). Die sozialen Folgeerscheinungen der Deportation [The social implications of deportation]. In: Michel, Max (Ed.), *Gesundheitsschäden durch Verfolgung und Gefangenschaft und ihre Spätfolgen: Zusammenstellung der Referate und Ergebnisse der Internationalen Sozialmedizinischen Konferenz über die Pathologie der Ehemaligen Deportierten und Internierten, 5-7 Juni 1954 in Kopenhagen* [Health Damages Caused by Persecution and Internment and the Late Effects: Compilation of the Papers and Results of the International Conference of Social Medicine on the Pathology of Former Deported and Interned Persons, 5-7 June 1954 in Copenhagen]. Frankfurt am Main: Röderberg, pp. 256-267.

1364 Laska, Vera (1994). The stations of the cross. In: Michalczyk, John J. (Ed.), *Medicine, Ethics, and the Third Reich: Historical and Contemporary Issues*. Kansas City, MO: Sheed & Ward, pp. 129-142.

1365 Last, Uriel (1989). The transgenerational impact of Holocaust trauma: Current state of the evidence. *International Journal of Mental Health*, 17(4), 72-89.

1366 Last, Uriel, and Klein, Hillel (1974). Cognitive and emotional aspects of the attitudes of American and Israeli youth towards the victims of the Holocaust. *Israel Annals of Psychiatry and Related Disciplines*, 12(2), 111-131.

1367 Last, Uriel, and Klein, Hillel (1981). Impact de l'Holocauste: Transmission aux enfants du cevu des parents [Impact of the Holocaust transmission of parental experience to the children]. *Evolution Psychiatrigue*, 46(2), 373-388.

1368 Last, Uriel, and Klein, Hillel (1984). Impact of parental Holocaust traumatization on offsprings' reports of parental child-rearing practices. *Journal of Youth and Adolescence*, 13(4), 267-283.

1369 Latell, Sue R. (1990). *The effects of World War II trauma and cultural self-hate on German children whose parents lived through Nazi Germany*. Unpublished master's thesis, Simon Fraser University, Burnaby, British Columbia, Canada. *Masters Abstracts International*, 31(1), p. 42. (University Microfilms no. AAC MM69579).

1370 Latkowski, B.D.E.; Najwer, P.; and Zalewski, P. (1978). Étude et éstimation oto-laryngologique des anciens prisonniers des camps de concentration soumis aux experiences pseudo-médicales [Oto-laryngological investigations in ex-concentration camp prisoners submitted to pseudo-medical experiments]. In: *Medizinische Untersuchungen der Spätfolgen des Krieges und des NS-Regimes bei Jugendlichen und Kindern von ehemaligen KZ-Häftlingen und Verfolgten* [Medical Research of the Late Effects of the War and National Socialism Regime on Youth and Children of Former Concentration Camp Inmates and Persecuted Persons]. Wien: Internationale Föderation der Widerstandskämpfer. [VI Internationaler Medizinischer Kongress der FIR. Prague, 1976].

1371 Laub, Dori (1991). Truth and testimony: The process and the struggle. *American Imago*, 48(1), 75-91.

1372 Laub, Dori (1992). Bearing witness, or the vicissitudes of listening. In: Felman, Shoshana, and Laub, Dori (Eds.), *Testimony: Crises of Witnessing in Literature, Psychoanalysis and History*. New York and London: Routledge, pp. 57-74.

1373 Laub, Dori (1992). An event without a witness: Truth, testimony and survival. In: Felman, Shoshana, and Laub, Dori (Eds.), *Testimony: Crises of Witnessing in Literature, Psychoanalysis and History*. New York and London: Routledge, pp. 74-92.

1374 Laub, Dori (1995). Die zweite Holocaust: Das Leben ist bedrohlich [The second Holocaust: When life threatens]. *Psyche: Zeitschrift für Psychoanalyse und ihre Anwendungen*, 49(1), 18-40.

1375 Laub, Dori, and Auerhahn, Nanette C. (1984). Reverberations of genocide: Its expressions in the conscious and unconscious of post-Holocaust generations. In: Luel, Steven A., and Marcus, Paul (Eds.), *Psychoanalytic Reflections on the Holocaust: Selected Essays*. New York, Ktav, pp. 151-167.

1376 Laub, Dori, and Auerhahn, Nanette C. (1989). Failed empathy: A central theme in the survivor's Holocaust experience. *Psychoanalytic Psychology*, 6(4), 377-400.

1377 Laub, Dori, and Auerhahn, Nanette C. (1993). Knowing and not knowing massive psychic trauma: Forms of traumatic memory. *International Journal of Psychoanalysis*, 74(2), 287-302.

1378 Laub, Dori, and Podell, Daniel (1995). Art and trauma. *International Journal of Psycho-Analysis*, 76(5), 991-1005.

1379 Laufer, Moses (1973). The analysis of a child of survivors. In: Anthony, E. James, and Koupernik, Cyrille (Eds.), *The Child in His Family. Vol. 2: The Impact of Disease and Death*. New York: John Wiley & Sons, pp. 263-273.

1380 Lavie, Peretz, and Kaminer, Hanna (1991). Dreams that poison sleep: Dreaming in Holocaust survivors. *Dreaming. Journal of the Association for the Study of Dreams*, 1(1), 11-21.

1381 Lax, Sandra (1983). *An historical review of the literature on children of Holocaust survivors and some implications for social work.* Unpublished master's thesis, School of Social Work, Carleton University, Ottawa, Ontario, Canada.

1382 Laznička, M. (1973). Ergebnisse einer 23jährigen Beobachtung des Gesundheitszustands von Teilnehmern an der Tschechoslowakischen Widerstandsbewegung im 2. Weltkrieg in einem Landkreis [Results of a 23 year health observation on members of the Czechoslovak resistance movement in World War II in a rural area]. In: *Ermüdung und vorzeitiges Altern: Folge von Extrembelastungen* [Exhaustion and Premature Aging: Result of Extreme Stress]. Leipzig: Barth, pp. 349-360. [V Internationaler Medizinischer Kongress der FIR. Paris, 21-24 September 1970].

1383 Laznička, M. (1973). Pozdní následky valky na zdravi príslušniků druhého odboje v dynamickém vyvoji 25 let [Late sequelae of war on the health of freedom fighters: Dynamic evolution during 25 years]. *Casopis Lekaru Ceskych*, 112, 129-133.

1384 Laznička, M. (1978). Spätfolgen des Krieges an der Gesundheit von Teilnehmern am zweiten Tschechoslowakischen Widerstandskampf in der dynamischen Enfaltung von dreissig Jahren [Late sequelae of war on the health of participants of the second Czechoslovak resistance fight. A dynamic follow up of 30 years]. In: *Medizinische Untersuchungen der Spätfolgen des Krieges und des NS-Regimes bei*

Jugendlichen und Kindern von ehemaligen KZ-Häftlingen und Verfolgten [Medical Research of the Late Effects of the War and National Socialism Regime on Youth and Children of Former Concentration Camp Inmates and Persecuted Persons]. Wien: Internationale Föderation der Widerstandskämpfer. [VI Internationaler Medizinischer Kongress der FIR. Prague, 1976].

1385 Laznička, M. (1979). Zdravotni stav ucastniku druhého ceskowlovenskeho odboje v prubehu triatriceti let v jednom okresu [State of health in members of Czechoslovakia's 2nd world war resistance movement as followed up in one district over a period of 33 years]. *Casopis Lekaru Ceskych*, 118(49), 1518-1522.

1386 Lederer, Wolfgang (1965). Entwurzelungsdepression ohne Depression, Fettleibigkeit und andere psychosomatische Depressions-Aquivalente [Depression of uprooting without depression, obesity and other psychosomatic equivalents of depression]. *Nervenarzt*, 36, 118-122.

1387 Lederer, Wolfgang (1965). Persecution and compensation: Theoretical and practical implications of the "persecution syndrome." *Archives of General Psychiatry*, 12, 464-474.

1388 Lee, Barbara S. (1988). Holocaust survivors and internal strengths. *Journal of Humanistic Psychology*, 28(1), 67-96.

1389 Legros, J.J.; Franchimont, P.; and Claessens, J.J. (1978). Profil neuroendocrine de l'ancien prisonnier de guerre (P.G.) hospitalisé [The neuroendocrinological profile of hospitalized ex-prisoners of war]. In: *Medizinische Untersuchungen der Spätfolgen des Krieges und des NS-Regimes bei Jugendlichen und Kindern von ehemaligen KZ-Häftlingen und Verfolgten* [Medical Research of the Late Effects of the War and National Socialism Regime on Youth and Children of Former Concentration Camp Inmates and Persecuted Persons]. Wien: Internationale Föderation der Widerstandskämpfer. [VI Internationaler Medizinischer Kongress der FIR. Prague, 1976].

1390 Lehman, M. (1966). Survivor of inhumane Nazi treatment discusses aftermath at seminar here. *NIH Record*, 18(16).

1391 Lehnert, Gerhard (1970). *Spätfolgen nach extremen Lebensverhältnissen. Untersuchungen zu Fragen der Voralterung und einer Beeintrachtigung des andrenokortikalen Regelkreises* [Late Sequelae After Extreme Life Situations: Investigations on the Premature Senility and the Influence on the Adrenocortical System]. Stuttgart: Georg Thieme. 57 pp.

1392 Leiser, Erwin (1982). *Leben nach dem Überleben: Dem Holocaust entrinnen - Begegnen und Schicksale* [Life After Survival: Distancing the Holocaust Experiences and Consequences]. Konigstein im Taunus: Athenaum. 184 pp.

1393 Lekkerkerker, E.C. (1946). Oorlogspleegkinderen [War foster children]. *Maandblad voor de Geestelijke Volksgezondheid*, 10, 227-236.

1394 Lekova, L. (1978). Die Verbreitung des Diabetes unter den Widerstandskämpfern Plovdiv [The distribution of diabetes among resistance fighters in the county of Plovdiv]. In: *Medizinische Untersuchungen der Spätfolgen des Krieges und des NS-Regimes bei Jugendlichen und Kindern von ehemaligen KZ-Häftlingen und Verfolgten* [Medical Research of the Late Effects of the War and National Socialism Regime on Youth and Children of Former Concentration Camp Inmates and Persecuted Persons]. Wien: Internationale Föderation der Widerstandskämpfer. [VI Internationaler Medizinischer Kongress der FIR. Prague, 1976].

1395 Leliefeld, H. (1978). Immateriele hulpverlening aan oorlogsgetroffen [Non-material assistance to war victims]. *Maandblad voor de Geestelijke Volksgezondheid*, 12, 883-887.

1396 Leliefeld, H. (1980). *Overlevenden van het concentratiekamp Dachau 1945-1980, een orienterend onderzoek naar ziekte, sterfte, doodsoorzaken en gebruik van wettelijke regelingen* [Survivors of the Concentration Camp Dachau 1945-1980: An Orienting Research for Disease, Mortality, Causes of Death and the Use of Compensation Laws]. Leiden: Uitgave Nederlands Instituut voor Praeventieve Gezondheidszorg TNO. [NIPG/TNO Projekt 540, Deelrapport I].

1397 Leliefeld, H. (1981). The impact of persecution: Review. In: *Israel-Netherlands Symposium on the Impact of Persecution. Dalfsen, Amsterdam, 14-18 April 1980*. Rijswijk: The Netherlands: Ministry of Cultural Affairs, Recreation and Social Welfare, pp. 15-18.

1398 Leliefeld, H. (1982). *Nederlandse gevangenen van het concentratiekamp Dachau 1941-1979, onderzoek naar mortaliteit en doodsoorzaken* [Dutch Prisoners of the Concentration Camp Dachau, 1941-1979: Research on Mortality and the Causes of Death]. Leiden: Uitgave Nederlands Instituut voor Praeventieve Gezondheidszorg TNO. [Deelrapport II].

1399 Lemberger, John (Ed.) (1995). *A Global Perspective on Working with Holocaust Survivors and the Second Generation.* Jerusalem: JDC-

Brookdale Institute of Gerontology and Human Development, AMCHA, and JDC-Israel. 459 pp.

1400 Lemberger, John (1995). Israel's aging Holocaust survivors. In: Lemberger, John (Ed.), *A Global Perspective on Working with Holocaust Survivors and the Second Generation*. Jerusalem: JDC-Brookdale Institute of Gerontology and Human Development, AMCHA, and JDC-Israel, pp. 103-110.

1401 Lemberger, John (1995). The view from Israel. In: Lemberger, John (Ed.), *A Global Perspective on Working with Holocaust Survivors and the Second Generation*. Jerusalem: JDC-Brookdale Institute of Gerontology and Human Development, AMCHA, and JDC-Israel, pp. 157-162.

1402 Lempp, Robert (1971). Die Bedeutung organischer und psychischer Insulte in Krieg und Verfolgung während der Kindheit und Jugend [The importance of organic and psychic traumatization of children and adolescents during the war and persecution]. In: Herberg, Hans-Joachim (Ed.), *Spätschäden nach Extrembelastungen* [Late Damage After Extreme Stress]. Herford: Nicolai, pp. 241-251. [II Internationalen Medizinisch-Juristischen Konferenz. Dusseldorf, 1969].

1403 Lempp, Robert (1979). *Extrembelastungen in Kindes- und Jugendalter (Über Psychosoziale Spätfolgen nach Nationalsozialistischer Verfolgung in Kindes- und Jugendalter anhand von Aktengutachten)* [Extreme Stress in Children and Youth: On Psychosocial Late Effects Following National Socialism Persecution in Childhood and Youth By Means of Examination of Records]. Bern: Huber.

1404 Lempp, Robert (1995). Delayed and long-term effects of persecution suffered in childhood and youth. *Echoes of the Holocaust*, 4, 30-35. [Bulletin of the Jerusalem Center for Research into the Late Effects of the Holocaust. Talbieh Mental Health Center, Jerusalem, Israel].

1405 Lenski, Mordecai (1959). Problems of disease in the Warsaw Ghetto. In: Esh, Shaul (Ed.), *Yad Vashem Studies on the European Jewish Catastrophe and Resistance. Vol. 3*. Jerusalem, Yad Vesham, pp. 283-293.

1406 Leon, Gloria Rakita (1990). Post-traumatic stress disorder in a concentration camp survivor. In: *Case Histories of Psychopathology. 4th edition*. Boston, MA: Allyn & Bacon, pp. 109-124.

1407 Leon, Gloria Rakita; Butcher, James; Kleinman, Max; Goldberg, Alan; and Almagor, Moshe (1981). Survivors of the Holocaust and their children: Current status and adjustment. *Journal of Personality and Social Psychology*, 41(3), 503-516.

1408 Lerner, Barron H., and Rothman, David J. (1995). Medicine and the Holocaust: Learning more of the lessons. *Annals of Internal Medicine*, 122(10), 793-794.

1409 Lerner, Mitchell (1989). *Themes in the life world of children of survivors of the Holocaust*. Unpublished doctoral dissertation, York University, North York, Ontario, Canada. *Dissertation Abstracts International*, 50(9-A), p. 3063. (University Microfilms no. AAC 566839).

1410 Leśniak, Elżbieta; Leśniak, Roman; and Ryn, Zdzisław (1983). Nurt oświęcimski w twórczości Antoniego Kępinskiego [The Auschwitz theme in the works of Antoni Kępinski]. *Przegląd Lekarski*, 40(12), 849-854.

1411 Leśniak, Roman (1965). Poobozowe zmiany osobowości byłych więźniów obozu koncentracyjnego Oświęci-Brzezinka [Personality changes after imprisonment in the concentration camp of Auschwitz-Birkenau]. *Przegląd Lekarski*, 21(1), 13-20.

1412 Leśniak, Roman, and Leśniak, Elżbieta (1976). Ucieczki z obozów koncentracyjnch-Analiza psychiatryczno-psychologiczna [Escapes from concentration camps: A psychiatric-psychological analysis]. *Przegląd Lekarski*, 33(1), 17-24.

1413 Leśniak, Roman, and Masłowski, Jan (1974). Psychiatryczna problematyka oboźna problematyka obozów hitlerowskich w pracach Antoniego Kępińskiego [Psychiatric problems in Nazi concentration camps in the works of Antoni Kepinski]. *Przegląd Lekarski*, 31(1), 13-18.

1414 Leśniak, Roman; Orwid, Maria; Szymusik, Adam; and Teutsch, Aleksander (1964). Psychiatrische Studien an ehemaligen Häftlingen des Konzentrationslagers Auschwitz [Psychiatric studies of ex-concentration camp prisoners]. In: *Ätio-Pathogenese und Therapie der Erschöpfung und vorzeitigen Vergreisung* [The Aetiology, Pathogenesis and Therapy of Exhaustion and Premature Aging]. Wien: Verlag der FIR, pp. 351-357. [IV Internationaler Medizinischer Kongress. Bucharest, 22-27 Juni 1964].

1415 Leśniak, Roman; Orwid, Maria; Szymusik, Adam; Teutsch, Aleksander; Gątarski, Julian; Dominik, Małgorzata; and Mitarski, Jan (1971). Przegląd Krakowskich studiow psychiatrycznch byłych więźniów koncentracyjnych [Review of the Cracow psychiatric studies of former prisoners of concentration camps]. *Anali Klinicke Bolnice "Dr. M. Stojanovic,"* 10, 207-209.

1416 Leśniak, Roman; Orwid, Maria; Szymusik, Adam; Teutsch, Aleksander; Gątarski, Julian; and Dominik, Małgorzata (1973). Resumé der Krakower psychiatrischer Untersuchungen ehemaliger Konzentrationslagerhäftlinge [Review of the Cracow psychiatric investigations of ex-concentration camp prisoners]. In: *Ermüdung und vorzeitiges Altern: Folge von Extrembelastungen* [Exhaustion and Premature Aging: Result of Extreme Stress]. Leipzig: Barth, pp. 201-203. [V Internationaler Medizinischer Kongress der FIR. Paris, 21-24 September 1970].

1417 Lester, David (1986). Suicide: The concentration camp and the survivors. *Israel Journal of Psychiatry and Related Sciences*, 23(3), 221-223.

1418 Leszcycki, Stanisław (1971). Report of a midwife from Auschwitz. In: *Auschwitz Anthology. Vol. 2: In Hell They Preserved Human Dignity. Part 2.* Warsaw: International Auschwitz Committee, pp. 181-192.

1419 Letourmy, R. (1961). Die Procaintherapie bei der vorzeitigen Vergreisung der ehemaligen Deportierten und bei seniler Asthenie [Procaine treatment of premature senility in ex-deportees and of senile asthenics]. In: *Die Behandlung der Asthenie und der vorzeitigen Vergreisung bei ehmaligen Widerstandskämpfern und KZ-Häftlingen* [Treatment of Asthenia and Premature Aging in Former Resistance Fighters and Concentration Camp Inmates]. Wien: Verlag der FIR, pp. 203-220. [III Internationaler Medizinische Konferenz. Liege, 17-19 März 1961].

1420 Levav, Itzhak, and Abramson, J.H. (1984). Emotional distress among concentration camp survivors: A community study in Jerusalem. *Psychological Medicine*, 14(1), 215-218.

1421 Leventhal, Gloria, and Ontell, Marsha K. (1989). A descriptive demographic and personality study of second generation Jewish Holocaust survivors. *Psychological Reports*, 64(3, pt 2), 1067-1073.

1422 Levi, Joan-Seif (1994). The combined effects of interviews and group participation by the interviewer. In: Kestenberg, Judith S., and

Fogelman, Eva (Eds.), *Children during the Nazi Reign: Psychological Perspective on the Interview Process*. Westport, CT: Praeger, pp. 109-117.

1423 Levine, Howard (1982). Toward a psychoanalytic understanding of children of survivors of the Holocaust. *Psychoanalytic Quarterly*, 51(1), 70-92.

1424 Levinger, L. (1962). Psychiatrische Untersuchungen in Israel an 800 Fällen mit Gesundheitsschäden-forderungen wegen Nazi Verfolgung [Psychiatric investigations in Israel of 800 persons claiming health damages because of persecution by the Nazis]. *Nervenarzt*, 33, 75-80.

1425 Lewin, Carroll M. (1993). Negotiated selves in the Holocaust. *Ethos*, 21(3), 295-318.

1426 Lichtenberg, Pesach, and Marcus, Esther-Lee (1994). Paranoid psychosis in a Holocaust survivor. In: Brink, Terry L. (Ed.), *Holocaust Survivors' Mental Health*. New York: Harworth, pp. 41-46. [Published as a special issue of *Clinical Gerontologist*, 14(3).]

1427 Lichtman, Helen G. (1983). *Children of survivors of the Nazi Holocaust: A personality study*. Unpublished doctoral dissertation, Yeshiva University, New York, 220 pp. *Dissertation Abstracts International*, 44(11-B), p. 3532. (University Microfilms no. AAC 8405004).

1428 Lichtman, Helen G. (1984). Parental communication of Holocaust experiences and personality characteristics among second generation survivors. *Journal of Clinical Psychology*, 40(4), 914-924.

1429 Lichtmann, Ana (1990). Los psicoanalistas y el fenomeno naxi: Acerca de la "condicion necesaria" y la "condicion suficiente." [Psychoanalysts and the phenomenon of Nazism: on the "necessary condition" and the "sufficient condition"]. *Revista de Psicoanalisis*, 47(5-6), 945-953.

1430 Liebenau, Kenneth P. (1992). *A comparison of third generation descendants of Holocaust survivor's scores with the norms on self-esteem, locus of control, behavioral and social problems*. Unpublished doctoral dissertation, California School of Professional Psychology, Fresno, 126 pp. *Dissertation Abstracts International*, 53(4-B), p. 2067. (University Microfilms no. AAC 9221117).

1431 Lifton, Robert Jay (1968). The survivors of the Hiroshima disaster and the survivors of Nazi persecution. In: Krystal, Henry (Ed.),

Massive Psychic Trauma. New York: International Universities Press, pp. 168-203.

1432 Lifton, Robert Jay (1970). Jews as survivors. In: *History and Human Survival: Essays on the Young and Old, Survivors and the Dead, Peace and War, and on Contemporary Psychohistory*. New York: Random House, pp. 195-207.

1433 Lifton, Robert Jay (1978). Witnessing survival. *Social Forces*, 15, 40-44.

1434 Lifton, Robert Jay (1979). Survivor experience and traumatic syndrome. In: *The Broken Connection: On Death and the Continuity of Life*. New York: Simon and Schuster, pp. 163-178.

1435 Lifton, Robert Jay (1979). Victimization and mass violence. In: *The Broken Connection: On Death and the Continuity of Life*. New York: Simon and Schuster, pp. 302-334.

1436 Lifton, Robert Jay (1980). The concept of the survivor. In: Dimsdale, Joel E. (Ed.), *Survivors, Victims and Perpetrators: Essays on the Nazi Holocaust*. Washington, D.C.: Hemisphere, pp. 113-126.

1437 Lifton, Robert Jay (1980). On the consciousness of Holocaust. *Psychohistory Review*, 9(1), 3-22.

1438 Lifton, Robert Jay (1982). Medicalized killing in Auschwitz. *Psychiatry*, 45(4), 283-297.

1439 Lifton, Robert Jay (1983). The doctors of Auschwitz: The biomedical vision. *Psychohistory Review*, 11(2-3), 36-46.

1440 Lifton, Robert Jay (1986). *The Nazi Doctors: Medical Killing and the Psychology of Genocide*. New York: Basic Books. 576 pp.

1441 Lifton, Robert Jay (1986). Reflections on genocide. *Psychohistory Review*, 14(3), 39-54.

1442 Lifton, Robert Jay (1988). Life unworthy of life: Nazi racial views. In: Braham, Randolph L. (Ed.), *The Psychological Perspectives of the Holocaust and of its Aftermath*. Boulder, CO: Social Science Monographs; and New York: Csengeri Institute for Holocaust Studies of the Graduate School and University Center of the City University of New York, pp. 1-11.

1443 Lifton, Robert Jay (1993). From Hiroshima to the Nazi doctors: The evolution of psychoformative approaches to understanding traumatic stress syndromes. In: Wilson, John P., and Raphael, Beverley (Eds.), *International Handbook of Traumatic Stress Syndromes*. New York: Plenum, pp. 11-23.

1444 Lifton, Robert Jay, and Hackett, Amy (1990). Psychology of survivors in Israel. In: Gutman, Israel (Ed.), *Encyclopedia of the Holocaust. Vol. 3*. New York: Macmillan, pp. 1127-1132.

1445 Lifton, Robert Jay, and Markusen, Eric (1990). *The Genocidal Mentality*. New York: Basic Books. 346 pp.

1446 Lifton, Robert Jay, and Olsen, Eric (1976). The human meaning of total disaster: The Buffalo Creek experience. *Psychiatry*, 39(1), 1-18.

1447 Lijtenstein, Marcos (1992). Holocausti [Holocaust]. *Revista Uruguaya de Psicoanalisis*, 75, 183-186.

1448 Linden, R. Ruth (1990). *Making stories making selves: The Holocaust, identity and memory*. Unpublished doctoral dissertation, Brandeis University, Waltham, Massachusetts, 409 pp. *Dissertation Abstracts International,* 50(7-A), p. 2255. (University Microfilms no. AAC 8922195).

1449 Lindy, Jacob D.; Grace, Mary C.; and Green, B.L. (1981). Survivors: Outreach to a reluctant population. *American Journal of Orthopsychiatry*, 51(3), 468-478.

1450 Lingens, Ella (1961). Expert examination of psychic damages attributable to political persecution. In: *International Conference on the Later Effects of Imprisonment and Deportation Organized by the World Veterans Federation. The Hague, November 20-25, 1961*. The Hague: World Veterans Federation, pp. 111-112.

1451 Lingens, Ella (1963). KZ-Häftling und Gesellschaft [Concentration camp survivors and the society]. In: Paul, Helmut, and Herberg, Hans-Joachim (Eds.), *Psychische Spätschäden nach Politischer Verfolgung* [Psychological Late Damages Following Political Persecution]. Basel: Karger, pp. 21-36.

1452 Lingens, Ella (1967). Die situation in Österreich [The situation in Austria]. In: Herberg, Hans-Joachim (Ed.), *Die Beurteilung von Gesundheitsschäden nach Gefangenschaft und Verfolgung* [The Assessment of Health Damages Following Internment and

Persecution]. Herford: Nicolai, pp. 21-28. [Internationalen Medizinisch-Juristischen Symposiums in Köln].

1453 Lingens, Ella (1971). Die Begutachtung arteriosklerotischer Herzkreislaufleiden [Evaluation of arteriosclerotic vascular disease]. In: Herberg, Hans-Joachim (Ed.), *Spätschäden nach Extrembelastungen* [Late Damage After Extreme Stress]. Herford: Nicolai, pp. 115-118. [II Internationalen Medizinisch-Juristische Konferenz. Dusseldorf 1969].

1454 Lingens, Ella (1971). Das Problem der "herrschenden Lehrmeinung" im Begutachtungsverfahren aus medizinischer Sicht [The problem of the "accepted view" in the practice of medical expertise]. In: Herberg, Hans-Joachim (Ed.), *Spätschäden nach Extrembelastungen* [Late Damage After Extreme Stress]. Herford: Nicolai, pp. 293-297. [II Internationalen Medizinisch-Juristischen Konferenz. Dusseldorf, 1969].

1455 Lingens, Ella (1986). An exchange of letters between Ernst Federn and Robert Waelder: On the psychology of mass murderers. *Sigmund Freud House Bulletin*, 10(1), 3-34.

1456 Link, Nan; Victor, Bruce S.; and Binder, Renee L. (1985). Psychosis in children of Holocaust survivors: Influence of the Holocaust in the choice of themes in their psychoses. *Journal of Nervous and Mental Disease*, 173(2), 115-117.

1457 Linne, M. (1967). Aus der Entschädigungspraxis zum Begschlussgesetz [Some samples of restitution according to the German restitution laws]. In: Herberg, Hans-Joachim (Ed.), *Die Beurteilung von Gesundheitsschäden nach Gefangenschaft und Verfolgung* [The Assessment of Health Damages Following Internment and Persecution]. Herford: Nicholai, pp. 46-51. [Internationalen Medizinisch-Juristischen Symposiums in Köln].

1458 Lipkowitz, Marvin H. (1973). The child of two survivors. A report of an unsuccessful therapy. *Israel Annals of Psychiatry and Related Disciplines*, 11(2), 141-155.

1459 Lipscombe, F.M. (1945). Medical aspects of Belsen concentration camp. *Lancet*, 2, 313-315.

1460 Lipstadt, Deborah E. (1989). Children of Jewish survivors of the Holocaust: The evolution of a new-found consciousness. In: *Encyclopedia Judaica Year Book 1988/9*. Jerusalem: Keter, pp. 139-150.

1461 Litman, Shalom (1992). The Holocaust survivor and the second generation 45 years after. In: Jockush, Ulrich, and Scholz, Lothar (Eds.), *Administered Killings at the Time of National Socialism: Involvement, Suppression, Responsibility of Psychiatry and Judicial System*. Regensburg: Roderer, pp. 61-81.

1462 Litman, Shalom (1992). Holocaust-Überlebende und "Zweite Generation": 45 Jahre danach [The Holocaust survivor and the second generation 45 years after]. In: Jockush, Ulrich, and Scholz, Lothar (Eds.), *Verwaltetes Morden im Nationalsozialismus: Verstrickung, Verdrängung, Verantwortung von Psychiatrie und Justiz* [Administered Killings at the Time of National Socialism: Involvement, Suppression, Responsibility of Psychiatry and Judicial System]. Regensburg: Roderer, pp. 63-85.

1463 Lobel, Thelma E.; Kav-Venaki, Sophie; and Yahiam, M. (1985). Guilt feelings and locus of control of concentration camp survivors. *International Journal of Social Psychiatry*, 31(3), 170-175.

1464 Łobowski, Witold (1970). Wstępne wyniki badania lekarskiego byłych więźniów koncentracynych [Preliminary results of medical examinations of former inmates of Hitler's concentration camps]. *Przegląd Lekarski*, 26(1), 28-29.

1465 Løchen, Einar A. (1968). Psychometric patterns. In: Strøm, Axel (Ed.), *Norwegian Concentration Camp Survivors*. Oslo: Universitetsforlaget, and New York: Humanities Press, pp. 132-155.

1466 Loewenberg, Peter (1971). The psychohistorical origins of the Nazi youth cohort. *American Historical Review*, 76, 1457-1502.

1467 Lohman, H.M., and Rosenkotter, Lutz (1982). Psychoanalyse in Hitlerdeutschland. Wie war es wirklich? [Psychoanalysis in Hitler Germany: How was it exactly?]. *Psyche: Zeitschrift für Psychoanalyse und ihre Anwendungen*, 36(11), 961-988.

1468 Lombard, Pearl (1985). Oubli des langues et des mathematiques [Forgetting languages and mathematics]. *Revue Française de Psychanalyse*, 49(3), 889-895.

1469 Lomranz, Jacob (1990). Long-term adaptation to traumatic stress in light of adult development and aging perspectives. In: Parris Stephens, Mary Ann; Crowther, Janis H.; Hobfoll, Stevan E.; and Tennenbaum, Daniel L. (Eds.), *Stress and Coping in Later-Life Families*. New York: Hemisphere, pp. 99-121.

1470 Lomranz, Jacob (1995). Endurance and living: Long-term effects of the Holocaust. In: Hobfoll, Stevan E.; and de Vries, Marten W. (Eds.), *Extreme Stress and Communities: Impact and Intervention*. Amsterdam: Kluwer, pp. 325-352.

1471 Lomranz, Jacob; Shmotkin, Dov; Zechovoy, Amnon; and Rosenberg, Eliot (1985). Time orientation in Nazi concentration camp survivors: Forty years after. *American Journal of Orthopsychiatry*, 55(2), 230-236.

1472 Lønnum, Arve (1960). An analytical survey of the literature published on the delayed effects of internment in concentration camps and their possible relation to the nervous system. In: *Experts Meeting on the Later Effects of Imprisonment and Deportation, Oslo*. Paris: World Veterans Federation, pp. 21-53.

1473 Lønnum, Arve (1963). Om KZ syndromet [On the concentration camp syndrome]. *Nordisk Medicin*, 69, 480-484.

1474 Lønnum, Arve (1968). Neurological disorders. In: Strøm, Axel (Ed.), *Norwegian Concentration Camp Survivors*. Oslo, Universitetsforlaget, and New York: Humanities Press, pp. 85-123.

1475 Lønnum, Arve (1971). Wirbelsäulenspätschäden nach multiplen Traumen [Late sequelae in the columna vetebralis after multiple traumatizations]. In: Herberg, Hans-Joachim (Ed.), *Spätschäden nach Extrembelastungen* [Late Damage After Extreme Stress]. Herford: Nicolai, pp. 136-138. [II Internationalen Medizinisch-Juristische Konferenz. Dusseldorf, 1969].

1476 Lønnum, Arve (1971). Neurologische Størungen bei Norwegischen Konzentrationslagerhäftlingen [Neurological disturbances in Norwegian ex-concentration camp prisoners]. In: Herberg, Hans-Joachim (Ed.), *Spätschäden nach Extrembelastungen* [Late Damage After Extreme Stress]. Herford: Nicolai, pp. 153-164. [II Internationalen Medizinisch-Juristischen Konferenz. Dusseldorf, 1969].

1477 Lønnum, Arve, and Oyen, O. (1973). Uber die neuen Kriegspensionerungsgesetze in Norwegen [On the new Norwegian law of war pensions]. In: *Ermüdung vorzeites Altern: Folge von Extrembelastungen* [Exhaustion and Premature Aging: Result of Extreme Stress]. Leipzig: Barth, pp. 361-365. [V Internationalen Medizinischer Kongress der FIR. Paris, 21-24 September 1970].

1478 Lorenzer, Alfred (1966). Zum begriff der "traumatischen Neurose" [The problem of "traumatic neurosis"]. *Psyche: Zeitschrift für Psychoanalyse und ihre Anwendungen*, 20, 481-492.

1479 Lorenzer, Alfred (1968). Some observations on the latency of symptoms in patients suffering from persecution sequelae. *International Journal of Psycho-Analysis*, 49(2-3), 316-318.

1480 Lorska, Dorota (1971). Block 10 in Auschwitz. In: *Auschwitz Anthology. Vol. 1: Inhuman Medicine. Part 2*. Warsaw: International Auschwitz Committee, pp. 80-98.

1481 Lorska, Dorota (1987). Block 10 in Auschwitz. In: Hamburger Institut für Sozialforschung (Eds.), *Die Auschwitz-Hefte. Texte der polnischen Zeitschrift "Przegląd Lekarski" über historische, psychische und medizinische Aspekte des Lebens und Sterbens in Auschwitz. Band 1* [The Auschwitz Journal. Text of the Polish Journal "Medical Review" on Historical, Psychic and Medical Aspects of Life and Death in Auschwitz. Volume 1]. Weinheim and Basel: Beltz, pp. 209-212.

1482 Lovenstein, A. (1989). *The hypnotic communication of trauma in families of the Holocaust*. Unpublished doctoral dissertation, School of Professional Psychology, University of Denver.

1483 Lovinger, Mark (1986). *Expression of hostility in children of Holocaust survivors*. Unpublished doctoral dissertation, Case Western Reserve University, Cleveland, Ohio, 101 pp. *Dissertation Abstracts International*, 47(8-B), p. 3530. (University Microfilms no. AAC 8627851).

1484 Lowin, Robin G. (1983). *Cross-generational transmission of pathology in Jewish families of Holocaust survivors*. Unpublished doctoral dissertation, California School of Professional Psychology, San Diego, 204 pp. *Dissertation Abstracts International*, 44(11-B), p. 3533. (University Microfilms no. AAC 8404702).

1485 Luchterhand, Elmer G. (1953). *Prisoner behavior and social system in Nazi concentration camps*. Unpublished doctoral dissertation, University of Wisconsin, Madison, Wisconsin. *Dissertation Abstracts International*, WI-1953, p. 250. (University Microfilms no. AAC 0191130).

1486 Luchterhand, Elmer G. (1964). Survival in the concentration camp: An individual or group phenomenon? In: Rosenberg, Bernard; Gerver, Israel; and Howton, F. William (Eds.), *Mass Society in*

Crisis: Social Problems and Social Pathology. New York: Macmillan, pp. 223-224.

1487 Luchterhand, Elmer G. (1966). The gondola-car transports. *International Journal of Social Psychiatry*, 13, 1-28.

1488 Luchterhand, Elmer G. (1967). Prisoner behavior and social system in the Nazi concentration camps. *International Journal of Social Psychiatry*, 13, 245-264.

1489 Luchterhand, Elmer G. (1970). Early and late effects of imprisonment in Nazi concentration camps: Conflicting interpretations in survivor research. *Social Psychiatry*, 5, 102-110.

1490 Luchterhand, Elmer G. (1971). Sociological approaches to massive stress in natural and man-made disasters. *International Psychiatry Clinics*, 8, 29-53.

1491 Luchterhand, Elmer G. (1980). Social behavior of concentration camp prisoners: Continuities and discontinuities with pre- and post-camp life. In: Dimsdale, Joel E. (Ed.), *Survivors, Victims and Perpetrators: Essays on the Nazi Holocaust*. Washington, D.C.: Hemisphere, pp. 259-282.

1492 Ludowyk Gyomroi, Edith (1963). The analysis of a young concentration camp victim. In; Eissler, Ruth S.; Hartmann, Heinz; Freud, Anna; and Kris, Marianne (Eds.), *Psychoanalytic Study of the Child. Vol. 18*. New York: International Universities Press, pp. 484-510.

1493 Ludzki, M. (1977). Children of survivors. *Jewish Spectator*, 2(3), 41-43.

1494 Luel, Steven A. (1984). Living with the Holocaust: Thoughts on revitalization. In: Luel, Steven A., and Marcus, Paul (Eds.), *Psychoanalytic Reflections on the Holocaust: Selected Essays*. New York: Ktav, pp. 169-178.

1495 Luel, Steven A., and Marcus, Paul (Eds.) (1984). *Psychoanalytic Reflections on the Holocaust: Selected Essays*. New York: Ktav. 238 pp.

1496 Luel, Steven A., and Marcus, Paul (1984). Psychoanalysis and the Holocaust: An introduction. In: Luel, Steven A., and Marcus, Paul (Eds.), *Psychoanalytic Reflections on the Holocaust: Selected Essays*. New York: Ktav, pp. 1-8.

1497 Lungershausen, E., and Matiar-Vahar, H. (1968). Erlebnisreaktive psychische Dauerschäden nach Kriegsgefangenschaft und Deportation [Experiential-reactive permanent psychic damages following captivity and deportation]. *Nervenarzt*, 39, 123.

1498 Lustigman, Michael (1974). *The fifth business: Survival as a way of life. An investigation of concentration camp survivors*. Unpublished doctoral dissertation, York University, Canada. *Dissertation Abstracts International*, 36(10-A), p. 6976. (University Microfilms no. AAC 0584331).

1499 Lustigman, Michael (1975). The fifth business: The business of surviving in extremity. *Human Context*, 7(3), 426-440.

1500 Luthe, R. (1968). Erlebnisreaktiver Persönlichkeitswandel als Begriff der Begutachtung im Entschädigungsrecht [Personality changes as a concept reactive in expert statements and restitution law]. *Nervenarzt*, 39, 465-467.

1501 Luthe, R. (1970). Die Determinationsstruktur von Persönlichkeitsfehaltung und ihre Beurteilung im Wiedergutmachungsrecht [Structure-shaping of pathological personality and its evaluation according to the restitution law]. *Fortschritte der Neurologie, Psychiatrie*, 38, 165-192.

1502 Lutwack, Patricia A. (1984). *The psychology of survival: Effective coping strategies used in Nazi concentration camps*. Unpublished doctoral dissertation, University of Florida, Gainesville, 204 pp. *Dissertation Abstracts International*, 45(7-B), p. 2314. (University Microfilms no. AAC 8421042).

1503 Macardle, Dorothy (1949). *Children of Europe: A Study of the Children of Liberated Countries - Their Wartime Experiences, Their Reactions, and Their Needs, With a Note on Germany*. London: Gollancz. 349 pp.

1504 Maciejewski, Zdzisław M. (1975). Wyniki badań ginekologicznych byłych więźniarek mieszkających w Koszalinie [Results of gynecologic examinations of former women inmates living in Koszalin]. *Przegląd Lekarski*, 32(1), 67-70.

1505 Magids, Debbie M. (1995). *Personality comparison between offspring of hidden survivors of the Holocaust and offspring of American Jewish parents*. Unpublished doctoral dissertation, Fordham University, Bronx, New York, 89 pp. *Dissertation Abstracts International*, 55(11-B), p. 5077. (University Microfilms no. AAC 9511236).

1506 Majer, Diemut (1992). The judiciary between adaptation and conflict demonstrated by the example of "Euthanasia." In: Jockush, Ulrich, and Scholz, Lothar (Eds.), *Administered Killings at the Time of National Socialism: Involvement, Suppression, Responsibility of Psychiatry and Judicial System*. Regensburg: Roderer, pp. 26-39.

1507 Majer, Diemut **(1992). Justiz zwischen Anpassung und Konflikt am Beispiel der "Euthanasie" [The judiciary between adaptation and** conflict demonstrated by the example of "Euthanasia"]. In: Jockush, Ulrich, and Scholz, Lothar (Eds.), *Verwaltetes Morden im Nationalsozialismus: Verstrickung, Verdrängung, Verantwortung von Psychiatrie und Justiz* [Administered Killings at the Time of National Socialism: Involvement, Suppression, Responsibility of Psychiatry and Judicial System]. Regensburg: Roderer, pp. 26-40.

1508 Major, Ellinor F. (1990). Effects of the Holocaust on the second generation: A study including control groups of Norwegian born Jewish Holocaust survivors and their children. In: Lundeberg, Jan-Erik; Otto, Ulf; and Rybeck, Bo (Eds.), *Wartime Medical Services: Second International Conference. Stockholm, Sweden, 25-29 June 1990: Proceedings*. Stockholm: Forsvarets forskningsanstalt (FOA), pp. 31-156.

1509 Major, Ellinor F. (1996). The impact of the Holocaust on the second generation: Norwegian Jewish Holocaust survivors and their children. *Journal of Traumatic Stress*, 9(3), 441-445.

1510 Makowski, Antoni (1967). Wspomnienia lekarza z obozów koncentracyjnych w Monowicach, Buchenwaldzie i Zwiebergen-Langensteinie [Reminiscences of a physician from the concentration camps in Monowice, Buchenwald and Zwieberg-Langenstein]. *Przegląd Lekarski*, 23(1), 212-222.

1511 Makowski, Antoni (1969). I oddział wewnętrzny szpitala obozu koncentracyjnego Buna-Monowice [First ward of internal medicine in the hospital of the concentration camp in Buna-Monowice]. *Przegląd Lekarski*, 25(1), 71-75.

1512 Makowski, Antoni (1970). Niektóre osiągnięcia organizacyjne szpitala obozowego w Monowicach [Some specific achievements in the organization of the sick bay in Monowice (Auschwitz III)]. *Przegląd Lekarski*, 17(1), 165-168.

1513 Makowski, Antoni (1972). Z zagadnień zdrowotnch obozu Buna-Monowice w świetle zachowanych dokumentów [Health problems at the Buna-Monowice concentration camp in the light of existing documents]. *Przegląd Lekarski*, 29(1), 45-51.

1514 Maller, O. (1964). The late psychopathology of former concentration camp inmates. *Psychiatria et Neurologia*, 148, 140-177.

1515 Mandell, Havi B. (1995). *Homeward from exile: The experience of homecoming for adult survivors of childhood trauma*. Unpublished doctoral dissertation, The Union Institute, Cincinnati, Ohio, 250 pp. *Dissertation Abstracts International*, 56(2-B), p. 1114. (University Microfilms no. AAC 9519602).

1516 Mandula, Rachel (1995). A bribe, living-bread, and a white tablecloth. *Contemporary Family Therapy*, 17(4), 469-482.

1517 Mangiameli, G.C. (1978). Interpretation cybernetique des hallucinations chez les survivants [Cybernetical interpretation of survivor's hallucinations]. In: *Medizinische Untersuchungen der Spätfolgen des Krieges und des NS-Regimes bei Jugendlichen und Kindern von ehemaligen KZ-Häftlingen und Verfolgten* [Medical Research of the Late Effects of the War and National Socialism Regime on Youth and Children of Former Concentration Camp Inmates and Persecuted Persons]. Wien: Internationale Föderation der Widerstandskämpfer. [VI Internationaler Medizinischer Kongress der FIR. Prague, 1976].

1518 Maniakówna, Maria (1970). W oświęcimskim bloku nr 11 [In the Auschwitz concentration camp Block No. 11]. *Przegląd Lekarski*, 26(1), 208-212.

1519 Mant, A.K. (1978). Genocide. *Journal of the Forensic Science Society*, 18(1-2), 13-17.

1520 Maoz, Benjamin (1987). Hatipul b'totzaot meucharot shel histatrut b'zeman hashoah b'Holland [The treatment of late effects of hiding during the Holocaust in the Netherlands]. *Sichot: Israel Journal of Psychotherapy*, 1(2), 112-115.

1521 March, Hans (1959). Zur Frage der Neurosen Begutachtung; ein kasuistischer Beitrag [Expert statements in neuroses: A casuistic contribution]. *Medizinische Wochenschrift*, 10, 428-432.

1522 March, Hans (Ed.) (1960). *Verfolgung und Angst in ihren leib-seelischen Auswirkungen. Dokumente* [Persecution and Anxiety in Their Psychosomatic Forms of Expression. Documentation]. Stuttgart: Klett. 273 pp.

1523 March, Hans (1960). Eine Jüdin unter dem Nazi-Terror. Angst und Parkinsontremor [A Jewish woman under Nazi terror: Anxiety and

Parkinson's tremor]. In: March, Hans (Ed.), *Verfolgung und Angst in ihren leib-seelischen Auswirkungen. Dokumente* [Persecution and Anxiety in Their Psychosomatic Forms of Expression. Documentation]. Stuttgart: Klett, pp. 114-129.

1524 March, Hans (1960). Anlage und Schicksalseinflüsse. Halbseitenlähmung [Tendency and fate: Haemiplegia]. In: March, Hans (Ed.), *Verfolgung und Angst in ihren leib-seelischen Auswirkungen. Dokumente* [Persecution and Anxiety in Their Psychosomatic Forms of Expression. Documentation]. Stuttgart: Klett, pp. 84-93.

1525 March, Hans (1960). Nach China verschlagen. Asthma-bronchiale als Verfolgungsleiden [Banished to China: Bronchial asthma as a result of persecution]. In: March, Hans (Ed.), *Verfolgung und Angst in ihren leib-seelischen Auswirkungen. Dokumente* [Persecution and Anxiety in Their Psychosomatic Forms of Expression. Documentation]. Stuttgart: Klett, pp. 94-113.

1526 March, Hans (1960). Die Bedeutung der Anamnese in der Gutachterpraxis. Traumatische Hirnleistungsschwäche und Epilepsie [The importance of the anamnesis in the expert statements: Traumatic brain damage and epilepsy]. In: March, Hans (Ed.), *Verfolgung und Angst in ihren leib-seelischen Auswirkungen. Dokumente* [Persecution and Anxiety in Their Psychosomatic Forms of Expression. Documentation]. Stuttgart: Klett, pp. 130-147.

1527 March, Hans (1960). Zweierlei Mass: Abnorme Erlebnisreaktion oder vitaler Persönlichkeitsbruch? [Two criteria: Abnormal reaction to experiences or personality breakdown?]. In: March, Hans (Ed.), *Verfolgung und Angst in ihren leib-seelischen Auswirkungen. Dokumente* [Persecution and Anxiety in Their Psychosomatic Forms of Expression. Documentation]. Stuttgart: Klett, pp. 148-157.

1528 March, Hans (1960). Die Schicksale zweier Juden und ein Beispielgutachten: Zum Problem der Neurosen-Begutachtung [The fate of two Jews and an example of an expert statement on the problem of evaluation of neuroses]. In: March, Hans (Ed.), *Verfolgung und Angst in ihren leib-seelischen Auswirkungen. Dokumente* [Persecution and Anxiety in Their Psychosomatic Forms of Expression. Documentation]. Stuttgart: Klett, pp. 158-191.

1529 March, Hans (1960). Ein schlichter Widerstandskämpfer. Paranoide Geistesstörung als Haftfolge [A modest resistance fighter: Paranoid psychosis as a result of imprisonment]. In: March, Hans (Ed.), *Verfolgung und Angst in ihren leib-seelischen Auswirkungen.*

Dokumente [Persecution and Anxiety in Their Psychosomatic Forms of Expression. Documentation]. Stuttgart: Klett, pp. 195-211.

1530 March, Hans (1960). Fünfundzwanzigmal vergewaltigt. Chronisch reaktiver Depressionszustand [Raped fifty times: A chronic-reactive depressive state]. In: March, Hans (Ed.), *Verfolgung und Angst in ihren leib-seelischen Auswirkungen. Dokumente* [Persecution and Anxiety in Their Psychosomatic Forms of Expression. Documentation]. Stuttgart: Klett, pp. 212-234.

1531 March, Hans (1960). Ein Mensch auf der Flucht - ein Bildbericht. Schwerhörigkeit, schwerste neurotische Lebenshemmung [A man on the run: Picture of a state - Hearing difficulties, severe neurotic inhibitions]. In: March, Hans (Ed.), *Verfolgung und Angst in ihren leib-seelischen Auswirkungen. Dokumente* [Persecution and Anxiety in Their Psychosomatic Forms of Expression. Documentation]. Stuttgart: Klett, pp. 235-268.

1532 March, Hans (Ed.) (1968). *Medizin und Menschlichkeit: Bausteine ärztlicher Diagnostik* [Medicine and Humaneness: Building Blocks of Medical Diagnosis]. Herford: Nicolai. 149 pp.

1533 Marcinkowski, T. (1989). Wspomnienie z obozu przejściowego w Pruszkowie [Reminiscences of the stay in the transit camp in Pruszków]. *Przegląd Lekarski*, 46(1), 159-163.

1534 Marcus, Paul (1984). Jewish consciousness after the Holocaust. In: Luel, Steven A., and Marcus, Paul (Eds.), *Psychoanalytic Reflections on the Holocaust: Selected Essays*. New York: Ktav, pp. 179-198.

1535 Marcus, Paul, and Rosenberg, Alan (1988). The Holocaust survivor's faith and religious behavior and some implications for treatment. *Holocaust and Genocide Studies*, 3(4), 413-430.

1536 Marcus, Paul, and Rosenberg, Alan (1988). A philosophical critique of the "survivor syndrome" and some implications for treatment. In: Braham, Randolph L. (Ed.), *The Psychological Perspectives of the Holocaust and of its Aftermath*. Boulder, CO: Social Sciences Monographs; and New York: Csengeri Institute for Holocaust Studies of the Graduate School and University Center of the City University of New York, pp. 53-78.

1537 Marcus, Paul, and Rosenberg, Alan (Eds.) (1989). *Healing Their Wounds: Psychotherapy with Holocaust Survivors and Their Families*. New York: Praeger. 304 pp.

1538 Marcus, Paul, and Rosenberg, Alan (1989). Treatment issues with survivors and their offspring: An interview with Anna Ornstein. In: Marcus, Paul, and Rosenberg, Alan (Eds.), *Healing Their Wounds: Psychotherapy with Holocaust Survivors and Their Families*. New York: Praeger, pp 105-116.

1539 Marcus, Paul, and Rosenberg, Alan (1989). The religious life of Holocaust survivors and its significance for psychotherapy. In: Marcus, Paul, and Rosenberg, Alan (Eds.), *Healing Their Wounds: Psychotherapy with Holocaust Survivors and Their Families*. New York: Praeger, pp. 227-256.

1540 Marcus, Paul, and Rosenberg, Alan (1994). Reevaluating Bruno Bettelheim's work on the Nazi concentration camps: The limits of his psychoanalytic approach. *Psychoanalytic Review*, 81, 537-563.

1541 Marcus, Paul, and Rosenberg, Alan (1995). The value of religion in sustaining the self in extreme situations. *Psychoanalytic Review*, 82(1), 81-105.

1542 Marcus, Paul, and Wineman, Irene (1985). Psychoanalysis encountering the Holocaust. *Psychoanalytic Inquiry*, 5(1), 85-98.

1543 Marcus, S. (1961). Study carried out in England on a group of 300 young refugees. In: *International Conference on the Later Effects of Imprisonment and Deportation Organized by the World Veterans Federation. The Hague, November 20-25, 1961*. The Hague: World Veterans Federation, pp. 158-159.

1544 Marin, Bernd (1980). A post-Holocaust "anti-Semitism without anti-Semites?": Austria is a case in point. *Political Psychology*, 2(2), 57-74.

1545 Markiewicz, Aleksandra (1979). Long term effects of severe oppression: The living victims of World War II. *Michigan Academician*, 12(2), 123-135.

1546 Marks, Jane (1993). *The Hidden Children: The Secret Survivors of the Holocaust*. New York: Fawcett Columbine. 308 pp.

1547 Martino, C., and Sciarra, M.A. (1964). Psycho-pathologische und gerichtsmedizinische Erwägungen über die chronischen Reaktionsdepressionen bei ehemaligen internierten und deportierten [Psychopathology and forensic discussions on the chronic depression reactive in ex-deportees and prisoners]. In: *Ätio-Pathogenese und Therapie der Erschöpfung und vorzeitigen Vergreisung* [The

Aetiology, Pathogenesis and Therapy of Exhaustion and Premature Aging]. Wien: Verlag der FIR, pp. 344-350. [IV Internationaler Medizinischer Kongress. Bucharest, 22-27 Juni 1964].

1548 Masłowski, Jan (1976). Trzydziesta rocznica wyzwolenia Oświęcimia-Brzezinki w Towarzystwie Lekarski Krakowskim [30th anniversary of the liberation of the Auschwitz camp. Commemorative services organized by the Cracow Medical Society]. *Przegląd Lekarski*, 33(1), 200-212.

1549 Masłowski, Jan (1978). Okupacyjna tematyka lekarska w polskich publikacjach z roku 1977 [Medical subjects relating to the Nazi occupation in Polish publications in 1977]. *Przegląd Lekarski*, 35(1), 237-253.

1550 Masłowski, Jan (1980). Okupacyna tematyka lekarska w polskich publikacjach z roku 1979 [Medical subjects relating to the Nazi occupation in Polish publications in 1979]. *Przegląd Lekarski*, 37(1), 213-218.

1551 Masłowski, Jan (1981). Antoni Kępiński w latach 1939-1947 [Antoni Kepinski during the years 1939-1947]. *Przegląd Lekarski*, 38(1), 126-137.

1552 Masłowski, Jan (1981). Okupacyjna tematyka lekarska w polskich publikacjach z roku 1980 [Medical subjects relating to the Nazi occupation in Polish publications published in 1980]. *Przegląd Lekarski*, 38(1), 229-248.

1553 Masłowski, Jan (1984). Okupacyjna tematyka lekarska w polskich publikacjach z roku 1983 [Medical subjects relating to the Nazi occupation in Polish publications published in 1983]. *Przegląd Lekarski*, 41(1), 159-177.

1554 Masłowski, Jan (1984). Patologia pracy w Auschwitz-Birkenau [The pathology of work in Auschwitz-Birkenau]. *Przegląd Lekarski*, 41(1), 37-54

1555 Masłowski, Jan (1985). Z nowszego piśmiennictwa o martyrologii dzieci [Modern literature on the martyrdom of children]. *Przegląd Lekarski*, 42(1), 201-205.

1556 Masłowski, Jan; Paryski, E.R.; Kurgan, A.; and Michalski, E. (1981). Tresc poprzednich zesytow poswieconych zagadnieniom lekarskim okresu okupacji hitlerowskiej [Contents of preceding issues devoted to medical problems of the Nazi occupation]. *Przegląd Lekarski*, 38(1), 249-269.

1557 Matussek, Paul (1961). Die Konzentrationslagerhaft als Belastungssituation [Imprisonment in concentration camps as a stress situation]. *Nervenarzt*, 32, 538-542.

1558 Matussek, Paul (1963). Die Ruckgliederung von Verfolgten. Die Bewältigung ihres Schicksals [Rehabilitation of persecutees. Coping with their fate]. *Therapiewoche*, 1109-1113.

1559 Matussek, Paul (1969). Spätfolgen bei KZ-Häftlingen [Late effects in concentration camp prisoners]. *Bild der Wissenschaft*, 803-809.

1560 Matussek, Paul (1971). *Die Konzentrationslagerhaft und ihre Folgen* [Internment in Concentration Camps and its Consequences]. Berlin: Springer. 272 pp.

1561 Matussek, Paul (1971). Late symptomatology among former concentration camp inmates. In: Arieti, Silvano (Ed.), *The World Biennial of Psychiatry and Psychotherapy*. New York: Basic Books.

1562 Matussek, Paul (1971). Psychoreaktive Störungen bei ehemaligen KZ-Häftlingen [Psychoreactive disturbances in ex-concentration camp prisoners]. In: Herberg, Hans-Joachim (Ed.), *Spätschäden nach Extrembelastungen* [Late Damage After Extreme Stress]. Herford: Nicolai, pp. 182-186. [II Internationalen Medizinish-Juristischen Konferenz. Dusseldorf, 1969].

1563 Matussek, Paul (1975). Psychische Schäden bei Konzentrationslagerhäftlingen [Psychic damages in concentration camp prisoners]. In: *Psychiatrie der Gegenwart* [Psychiatry in the Present]. Berlin: Springer, pp. 387-427.

1564 Matussek, Paul (1975). *Internment in Concentration Camps and Its Consequences*. New York: Springer. 269 pp.

1565 Matussek, Paul (1977). Bedrängnis und Bewältigung im Spiegel des Einzelschicksals. Individuelle Stressreaktion bei ehemaligen KZ Häftlingen [Stress and coping as seen in individual fates: Individual stress reactions in ex-concentration camp prisoners]. *Klinische Wochenschrift*, 55, 869-876.

1566 Matussek, Paul; Grigat, R.; Haibock, H.; and Halbach, G. (1973). Late effects of concentration camp stress. *International Research Communication System*, 39-72.

1567 Matuszewski, H.; Ślizowska, H.; and Batycka, U. (1990). Stan zrdowia byłych więźniów hitlerowskiego obozu dla dzieci w Łodzi

[Health status of former prisoners of the Nazi concentration camp for children in Lodz]. *Przegląd Lekarski*, 47(1), 12-15.

1568 Matuszewski, H.; Ślizowska, H.; and Bajka, J. (1990). Własna ocena stanu zdrowia byłych więźiów hitlerowskich obozów koncentracyjnych [Self assessment of health status by former prisoners of the Nazi concentration camps]. *Przegląd Lekarski*, 47(1), 12-15.

1569 Mazor, Aviva; Gampel, Yolanda; Enright, R.D.; and Orenstein, Ruth (1990). Holocaust survivors: Coping with post-traumatic memories in childhood and 40 years later. *Journal of Traumatic Stress*, 3(1), 1-14.

1570 Mazor, Aviva, and Tal, Ido (1996). Intergenerational transmission: The individuation process and the capacity for intimacy of adult children of Holocaust survivors. *Contemporary Family Therapy*, 18(1), 95-113.

1571 McCord, Janet S. (1995). *A study of the suicides of eight Holocaust survivor/writers*. Unpublished doctoral dissertation, Boston University, Massachusetts, 347 pp. *Dissertation Abstracts International*, 56(6-A), p. 2228. (University Microfilms no. AAC 9536848).

1572 **Meed,** Benjamin (1992). Holocaust survivors and aging: A keynote address. In: Kenigsberg, Rositta E., and Lieblich, Cathy M. (Eds.), *The First National Conference on Identification, Treatment and Care of the Aging Holocaust Survivor, March 29-31, 1992: Selected Proceedings*. Miami, FL: Holocaust Documentation and Education Center and Southeast Florida Center on Aging, Florida International University, pp. 16-21.

1573 Meadow, Diane (1981). The preparatory interview: A client-focused approach with children of Holocaust survivors. *Social Work with Groups*, 4(3-4), 135-144.

1574 Meed, Rita G. (1988). *The impact of kinship group experience on the identity, self-esteem, alienation, and subjective well-being on children of Holocaust survivors*. Unpublished doctoral dissertation, Long Island University, Brookville, New York, 147 pp. *Dissertation Abstracts International*, 49(7-B), p. 2927. (University Microfilms no. AAC 8807500).

1575 Meerloo, Joost A. (1963). Delayed mourning in victims of extermination camps. *Journal of the Hillside Hospital*, 12, 96-98.

1576 Meerloo, Joost A. (1963). Neurologism and denial of psychic trauma in extermination camp survivors. *American Journal of Psychiatry*, 120, 65-66.

1577 Meerloo, Joost A. (1968). Delayed mourning in victims of extermination camps. In: Krystal, Henry (Ed.), *Massive Psychic Trauma*. New York: International Universities Press, pp. 70-72.

1578 Meerloo, Joost A. (1969). Persecution trauma and the reconditioning of emotional life: A brief survey. *American Journal of Psychiatry*, 125(9), 1187-1191.

1579 Meerloo, Joost A. (1975). Hoe het concentratiekamp zijn slachtoffers programmeert [How the concentration camp programs its victims]. *Arts en Wereld*, 8, 14-32.

1580 Meltzer, Donald (1968). Terror, persecution, dread - A dissection of paranoid anxieties. *International Journal of Psycho-Analysis*, 49, 396-401.

1581 Melville, J. (1979). The scars of the survivors. *New Society*, 3, 15-18.

1582 Mende, Walter (1962). Grenzen der seelischen Belastbarkeit [The limits of psychological tolerance]. *Medizinische Klinik*, 57, 1636-1640.

1583 Mende, Walter (1963). Gutachterliche Probleme bei der Beurteilung erlebnisreaktiver Schädigungen [Problems of expert evaluation in cases of traumatization caused by life events]. In: Paul, Helmut, and Herberg, Hans-Joachim (Eds.), *Psychische Spätschäden nach Politischer Verfolgung* [Psychological Late Damages Following Political Persecution]. Basel: Karger, pp. 281-292.

1584 Mende, Walter (1971). Begutachtungsfragen bei erlebnisreaktiven Störungen [Problems of expert evaluation of disturbances due to life events]. In: Herberg, Hans-Joachim (Ed.), *Spätschäden nach Extrembelastungen* [Late Damage After Extreme Stress]. Herford: Nicolai, pp. 190-192. [II Internationaler Medizinisch-Juristischen Konferenz. Dusseldorf, 1969].

1585 Merowitz, Martin (1981). Words before we go: The experience of Holocaust and its effect on communication in the aging survivor. *Journal of Geriatric Psychiatry*, 14(2), 241-244.

1586 Meyer, J. (1961). Die abnormalen Erlebnisreaktionen im Kriege bei Truppe und Zivilbevölkerung [The abnormal experience and reactions in war by soldiers and the civilian population]. In: Gruhle, Hans W. (Ed.), *Psychiatrie der Gegenwart: Forschung und Praxis. Band 3: Soziale und angewandte Psychiatrie* [Psychiatry in the Present: Research and Practice. Vol. 3: Social and Applied Psychiatry]. Berlin: Springer.

1587 Meyer, Joachim-Ernst (1988). The fate of the mentally ill in Germany during the Third Reich. *Psychological Medicine*, 18(3), 575-581.

1588 Meyer-Lindenberg, Johannes (1991). The Holocaust and German Psychiatry. *British Journal of Psychiatry*, 159, 7-12.

1589 Meyerowitz, Hilda (1947). Case work services for adolescent newcomers. *Jewish Social Services Quarterly*, 24, 136-146.

1590 Meyroune, Claude (1961). Die Bedeutung der Aufstellung periodischer Gesundheitsbilanzen für die Bekämpfung des vorzeitigen Alterns [The importance of periodical health evaluations in the battle against premature aging]. In: *Die Behandlung der Asthenie und der vorzeitigen Vergreisung bei ehemaligen Widerstandskämpfern und KZ-Häftlingen* [Treatment of Asthenia and Premature Aging in Former Resistance Fighters and Concentration Camp Inmates]. Wien: Verlag der FIR, pp. 245-254. [III Internationaler Medizinische Konferenz. Liege, 17-19 März 1961].

1591 Mianowska, Aleksandra (1987). Szpitale jenieckie w Krakowie i na Słąskow [Hospitals for prisoners in Cracow and Silesia]. *Przegląd Lekarski*, 44(1), 150-154.

1592 Mianowska, Aleksandra (1990). Żolnierze-żydzi w szpitalach jenieckich w Krakowie [Soldiers-Jews in the hospitals for prisoners of war in Cracow]. *Przegląd Lekarski*, 47(1), 149-160.

1593 Michalczyk, John J. (Ed.) (1994). *Medicine, Ethics and the Third Reich: Historical and Contemporary Issues*. Kansas City, MO: Sheed & Ward. 258 pp.

1594 Michalczyk, John J. (1994). Euthanasia in Nazi propaganda films: Selling murder. In: Michalczyk, John J. (Ed.), *Medicine, Ethics, and the Third Reich: Historical and Contemporary Issues*. Kansas City, MO: Sheed & Ward, pp. 64-70

1595 Micheels, Louis J. (1985). Bearer of the secret. *Psychoanalytic Inquiry*, 5(1), 21-30.

1596 Michel, Max (Ed.), (1955). *Gesundheitsschäden durch Verfolgung und Gefangenschaft und ihre Spätfolgen: Zusammenstellung der Referate und Ergebnisse der Internationalen Sozialmedizinischen Konferenz über die Pathologie der Ehemaligen Deportierten und Internierten, 5-7 Juni 1954 in Kopenhagen* [Health Damages Caused by Persecution and Captivity and the Late Effects: Compilation of the Papers and Results of the International Conference of Social Medicine on the Pathology of Former Deported and Interned Persons, 5-7 June 1954 in Copenhagen]. Frankfurt am Main: Röderberg. 382 pp.

1597 Michel, Max (1955). Spätschäden und Summationsschäden [Late and summation sequelae]. In: Michel, Max (Ed.), *Gesundheitsschäden durch Verfolgung und Gefangenschaft und ihre Spätfolgen: Zusammenstellung der Referate und Ergebnisse der Internationalen Sozialmedizinischen Konferenz über die Pathologie der Ehemaligen Deportierten und Internierten, 5-7 Juni 1954 in Kopenhagen* [Health Damages Caused by Persecution and Captivity and the Late Effects: Compilation of the Papers and Results of the International Conference of Social Medicine on the Pathology of Former Deported and Interned Persons, 5-7 June 1954 in Copenhagen]. Frankfurt am Main: Röderberg, pp. 48-51.

1598 Michel, Max (1955). Einige Probleme der Begutachtung von Verfolgungsschäden deutscher Opfer des Nazi Regimes [Some problems in the evaluation of persecution-caused damages in German victims of the Nazi regime]. In: Michel, Max (Ed.), *Gesundheitsschäden durch Verfolgung und Gefangenschaft und ihre Spätfolgen: Zusammenstellung der Referate und Ergebnisse der Internationalen Sozialmedizinischen Konferenz über die Pathologie der Ehemaligen Deportierten und Internierten, 5-7 Juni 1954 in Kopenhagen* [Health Damages Caused by Persecution and Captivity and the Late Effects: Compilation of the Papers and Results of the International Conference of Social Medicine on the Pathology of Former Deported and Interned Persons, 5-7 June 1954 in Copenhagen]. Frankfurt am Main: Röderberg, pp. 297-316.

1599 Miecznikowski, Andrzej (1987). Uwagi o opiece lekarskiej nad więźniami w okupowanym Lwowie [Health care for prisoners in occupied Lvov]. *Przegląd Lekarski*, 44(1), 148-150.

1600 Milčinski, Jane Z. (1970). Crisis in medical ethics. In: *Auschwitz Anthology. Vol. 1: Inhuman Medicine. Part 1*. Warsaw: International Auschwitz Committee, pp. 123-146.

1601 Milikowski, Herman (Ed.) (1973). *Sociologie als Verzet, Over KZ-Syndroom, Gezinsproblemen, Sociale en Seksuele Relaties en Agressie*

[Sociology of Resistance, About the Concentration Camp Syndrome, Family Problems, Social and Sexual Reactions and Aggression]. Amsterdam: Van Gennep.

1602 Milikowski, Herman (1973). Het KZ-syndroom en de psychiatrische mythen [The concentration camp syndrome and psychiatric myths]. In: Milikowski, Herman (Ed.), *Sociologie als Verzet, Over KZ-Syndroom, Gezinsproblemen, Sociale en Seksuele Relaties en Agressie* [Sociology of Resistance, About the Concentration Camp Syndrome, Family Problems, Social and Sexual Reactions and Aggression]. Amsterdam: Van Gennep, pp. 87-122.

1603 Milikowski, Herman (1973). Daarom wil ik pleiten voor verzetstherapie [Therefore I wish to plead for resistance therapy]. In: Milikowski, Herman (Ed.), *Sociologie als Verzet, Over KZ-Syndroom, Gezinsproblemen, Sociale en Seksuele Relaties en Agressie* [Sociology of Resistance, About the Concentration Camp Syndrome, Family Problems, Social and Sexual Reactions and Aggression]. Amsterdam: Van Gennep, pp. 141-149.

1604 Miller, Louis (1981). Social roots of persecution. In: *Israel-Netherlands Symposium on the Impact of Persecution. Dalfsen, Amsterdam 14-18 April 1980*. Rijswijk, The Netherlands: Ministry of Cultural Affairs, Recreation and Social Welfare, pp. 21-26.

1605 Minkowski, Eugene (1946). L'Anésthesie affective [Affective anesthesia]. *Annales Médico-Psychologiques*, 104, 80-88.

1606 Minkowski, Eugene (1948). Les conséquences psychologiques et psychopathologiques de la guerre et du Nazisme [The psychologic and psychopathologic consequences of war and Nazism]. *Schweizer Archiv für Neurologie und Psychiatrie*, 61, 280.

1607 Mischel, Ellis (1979). Personal reflections on the Holocaust and Holocaust survivors. *American Journal of Psychoanalysis*, 39(4), 369-376.

1608 Mitscherlich, Alexander (1963). Die Vorurteilskrankheit [The sickness of prejudice]. *Psyche: Zeitschrift für Psychoanalyse und ihre Anwendungen*, 16, 241.

1609 Mitscherlich, Alexander, and Mielke, Fred (1949). *Doctors of Infamy: The Story of the Nazi Medical Crimes*. New York: Henry Schuman. 172 pp.

1610 Mitscherlich, Alexander, and Mitscherlich, Margarete (1975). *The Inability to Mourn: Principles of Collective Behavior*. New York: Grove. 322 pp.

1611 Mitscherlich-Nielsen, Margarete (1981). Die Vergangenheit in der Gegenwart [The past within the present] *Psyche: Zeitschrift für Psychoanalyse und ihre Anwendungen*, 35(7), 611-615.

1612 Mitscherlich-Nielsen, Margarete (1989). The inability to mourn today. In: Dietrich, David R., and Shabad, Peter C. (Eds.), *The Problem of Loss and Mourning: Psychoanalytic Perspectives*. Madison, CT: International Universities Press, pp. 405-426.

1613 Mitscherlich-Nielsen, Margarete (1993). Was Konnen wir aus der vergangenheit lernen? [What can we learn from the past?] *Psyche: Zeitschrift für Psychoanalyse und ihre Anwendungen*, 47(8), 743-753.

1614 Mock-Degen, M. (1980). De ethische aspekten van een psychiatrisch onderzoek, kanttekeningen bij het proefschrift over de Joodse oorlogswezen [The ethical aspects of a psychiatric research, margin notes on a proof manuscript concerning Jewish war foster children]. *Maandblad voor de Geestelijke Volksgezondheid*, 35(4), 290-301.

1615 Modai, Ilan (1994). Forgetting childhood: A defense mechanism against psychosis in a Holocaust survivor. In: Brink, Terry L. (Ed.), *Holocaust Survivors' Mental Health*. New York: Haworth, pp. 67-71. [Published as a special issue of *Clinical Gerontologist*, 14(3).]

1616 Mollhaff, G. (1975). About insurance medical evaluation of psychoreactive disturbances. *Rechtsmed*, 46(6), 291-296.

1617 Monnickendam, M. (1981). Formal non material services for the traumatized and the social setting in Israel. In: *Israel-Netherlands Symposium on the Impact of Persecution. Dalfsen, Amsterdam, 14-18 April 1980*. Rijswijk: The Netherlands: Rijswijk, Ministry of Cultural Affairs, Recreation and Social Welfare, pp. 43-46.

1618 Mor, Naomi (1990). Holocaust messages from the past. *Contemporary Family Therapy*, 12(5), 371-379.

1619 Moric-Petrovic, Slavka (1961). Neuropsychiatric after-effects on a group of participants in the people's liberation war of Yugoslavia. In: *International Conference on the Later Effects of Imprisonment and Deportation Organized by the World Veterans Federation. The Hague, November 20-25, 1961*. The Hague: World Veterans Federation, pp. 96-99.

1620 Morosow, V.M. (1958). Late sequelae in former deportees and concentration camp survivors. *Journal of Neuropathology and Psychiatry*, 58(3), 373-380.

1621 Morse, Deleres O. (1981). *Studying the Holocaust and human behavior: Effects on early adolescent self-esteem. Locus of control, acceptance of self and others, and philosophy of human nature.* Unpublished doctoral dissertation, California School of Professional Psychology, Fresno, 200 pp. *Dissertation Abstracts International*, 42(10-B), p. 4209. (University Microfilms no. AAC 8204014)

1622 Moses, Rafael (1983). A fifty year span: Some reflections on Israelis and Germans. *Israel Journal of Psychiatry and Related Sciences*, 20(1-2), 155-167.

1623 Moses, Rafael (1984). An Israeli psychoanalyst looks back in 1983. In: Luel, Steven A., and Marcus, Paul (Eds.), *Psychoanalytic Reflections on the Holocaust: Selected Essays*. New York: Ktav, pp. 53-70.

1624 Moses, Rafael (Ed.) (1993). *Persistent Shadows of the Holocaust: The Meaning to Those Not Directly Affected*. Madison, CT: International Universities Press. 288 pp.

1625 Moses, Rafael, and Cohen, Yechezkel (1993). An Israeli view. In: Moses, Rafael (Ed.), *Persistent Shadows of the Holocaust: The Meaning to Those Not Directly Affected*. Madison, CT: International Universities Press, pp. 119-140.

1626 Moska, Dionizy (1974). Polenlagry na Górnym Śląsku [Concentration camps for Polish nationals in Upper Silesia]. *Przegląd Lekarski*, 31(1), 134-139.

1627 Moskovitz, Sarah (1983). *Love Despite Hate: Child Survivors of the Holocaust and Their Adult Lives*. New York: Schocken. 245 pp.

1628 Moskovitz, Sarah (1985). Longitudinal follow-up of child survivors of the Holocaust. *Journal of the American Academy of Child Psychiatry*, 24(4), 401-407.

1629 Moskovitz, Sarah (1988). Barriers to gratitude. In: *Remembering for the Future: Working Papers and Addenda. Vol. 1: Jews and Christians during and After the Holocaust*. Oxford: Pergamon, pp. 494-505.

1630 Moskovitz, Sarah, and Krell, Robert (1990). Child survivors of the Holocaust: Psychological adaptations to survival. *Israel Journal of Psychiatry and Related Sciences*, 27(2), 81-91.

1631 Moskovitz, Thomas B. (1992). *The intergenerational transmission of self-efficacy among families of Jewish survivors of the Holocaust.* Unpublished doctoral dissertation, Miami Institute of Psychology, *Dissertation Abstracts International*, 53(4-B), p. 2071. (University Microfilms no. AAC 9218175).

1632 Mostysser, Toby (1975). Growing up in America with a Holocaust heritage. *Jewish Digest*, 21, 3-6.

1633 Mostysser, Toby (1975). The weight of the past: Reminiscences of a survivor's child. In: Steinitz, Lucy Y., and Szonyi, David M. (Eds.), *Living After the Holocaust: Reflections by the Post-War Generation in America*. New York: Bloch, pp. 3-21.

1634 Moynier, Guttieres (1964). Studie über die Folgen organischer Störungen infolge des Lebens in der Illegalität [Study on the sequels of organic disturbances caused by life in illegality]. In: *Ätio-Pathogenese und Therapie der Erschöpfung und vorzeitigen Vergreisung* [The Aetiology, Pathogenesis and Therapy of Exhaustion and Premature Aging]. Wien: Verlag der FIR, pp. 88-89. [IV Internationaler Medizinischer Kongress. Bucharest, 22-27 Juni 1964].

1635 Mulder, Dirk (1983). The uselessness of general diagnostic concepts. In: Ayalon, Ofra; Eitinger, Leo; Lansen, Johan; Sunier, Armand; and others, *The Holocaust and its Perseverance: Stress, Coping and Disorder*. Assen, The Netherlands: Van Gorcum, pp. 17-24.

1636 Muller, Uri F., and Yahav, Aviva L. (1989). Object relations, Holocaust survival and family therapy. *British Journal of Medical Psychology*, 62(1), 13-21.

1637 Müller-Hegemann, D. (1961). Die Heilbehandlung der Asthenie bei den ehemaligen Deportierten und Widerstandskämpfern [The treatment of asthenia in former deportees and resistance fighters]. In: *Die Behandlung der Asthenie und der vorzeitigen Vergreisung bei ehemaligen Widerstandskämpfern und KZ-Häftlingen* [Treatment of Asthenia and Premature Aging in Former Resistance Fighters and Concentration Camp Inmates]. Wien: Verlag der FIR, pp. 77-79. [III Internationaler Medizinische Konferenz. Liege, 17-19 März 1961].

1638 Müller-Hegemann, D. (1964). Erfahrungen auf dem Gebiete der Begutachtung und Rehabilitation von Verfolgten des Naziregimes

[Evaluation and rehabilitation of persecutees of the Nazi regime]. In: *Ätio-Pathogenese und Therapie der Erschöpfung und vorzeitigen Vergreisung* [The Aetiology, Pathogenesis and Therapy of Exhaustion and Premature Aging]. Wien: Verlag der FIR, pp. 66-72. [IV Internationaler Medizinischer Kongress. Bucharest, 22-27 Juni 1964].

1639 Müller-Hegemann, D. (1966). Uber Schädigungen und Störungen des Nervensystems bei Verfolgten des Naziregimes (VDN) und deren Begutachtung [Traumatizations of the nervous systems in persecutees of the Nazi regime and their evaluation]. *Deutsche Gesundheitswesen*, 21, 561-568.

1640 Müller-Hegemann, D., and Spitzner, G. (1963). Reihenuntersuchungen bei Verfolgten des Naziregimes-mit besondere Berücksichtigung von Einzelhaftfolgen [Serial investigations of persecutees of the Nazi regime with special regard to the sequelae of isolation]. *Deutsche Gesundheitswesen*, 18, 107-116.

1641 Müller-Hill, Benno (1987). Genetics after Auschwitz. *Holocaust and Genocide Studies*, 2(1), 3-20.

1642 Müller-Hill, Benno (1988). *Murderous Science: Elimination by Scientific Selection of Jews, Gypsies, and Others, Germany 1933-1945*. Oxford: Oxford University Press. 208 pp.

1643 Müller-Hill, Benno (1989). From Daedalus to Mengele: The dark side of human genetics. *Genome*, 31(2), 876-878.

1644 Müller-Hill, Benno (1994). Human genetics in Nazi Germany. In: Michalcyzk, John J. (Ed.), *Medicine, Ethics, and the Third Reich: Historical and Contemporary Issues*. Kansas City, MO: Sheed & Ward, pp. 27-34.

1645 Muller-Paisner, Vera (1995). The influence of traumatic memory in the second generation: Myth or reality? In: Lemberger, John (Ed.), *A Global Perspective on Working with Holocaust Survivors and the Second Generation*. Jerusalem: JDC-Brookdale Institute of Gerontology and Human Development, AMCHA, and JDC-Israel, pp. 319-329.

1646 Mury, L. (1973). Untersuchungen psychischer und psychosomatischer Störungen bei ehemaligen Konzentrationslagerhäftlingen 23 Jahre nach der Befreiung [Investigations of psychic and psychosomatic disturbances in ex-concentration camp prisoners, 23 years after the liberation]. In: *Ermüdung und vorzeitiges Altern: Folge von*

Extrembelastungen [Exhaustion and Premature Aging: Result of Extreme Stress]. Leipzig: Barth, pp. 215-246. [V Internationaler Medizinischer Kongress der FIR. Paris, September 1970].

1647 Musaph, Herman (1973). Post concentratiekampsyndroom [The post-concentration camp syndrome]. *Maandblad voor de Geestelijke Volksgezondheid*, 28, 207-217.

1648 Musaph, Herman (1981). The second generation of war victims: Psychopathological problems. *Israel Journal of Psychiatry and Related Sciences*, 18(1), 3-14.

1649 Musaph, Herman (1990). Anniversary reaction as a symptom of grief in traumatized persons. *Israel Journal of Psychiatry and Related Sciences*, 27(3), 175-179.

1650 Nadav, Daniel (1994). Sterilization, euthanasia, and the Holocaust: The brutal chain. In: Michalcyzk, John J. (Ed.), *Medicine, Ethics, and the Third Reich: Historical and Contemporary Issues*. Kansas City, MO: Sheed & Ward, pp. 42-49.

1651 Nadel, C., and Vollhardt, B. (1979). Coping with illness by a concentration camp survivor. *General Hospital Psychiatry*, 2, 175-181.

1652 Nadler, Arie (1987). Validity of transgenerational effects of the Holocaust: Reply to Silverman. *Journal of Consulting and Clinical Psychology*, 55(1), 127-128.

1653 Nadler, Arie, and Ben-Shushan, Dan (1989). Forty years later: Long-term consequences of massive traumatization as manifested by Holocaust survivors from the city and the kibbutz. *Journal of Consulting and Clinical Psychology*, 57(2), 287-293.

1654 Nadler, Arie; Kav-Venaki, Sophie; and Gleitman, Beny (1985). Transgenerational effects of the Holocaust: Externalization of aggression in second generation of Holocaust survivors. *Journal of Consulting and Clinical Psychology*, 53(3), 365-369.

1655 Nagy, Z.; Cochyanova, B.; and Balaz, V. (1978). Gezielte sozialmedizinische Studie unter Teilnehmern des Widerstandskämpfers und ihre dynamischen Elemente [Specific socio-medical study of resistance fighters and its dynamic elements]. In: *Medizinische Untersuchungen der Spätfolgen des Krieges und des NS-Regimes bei Jugendlichen und Kindern von ehemaligen KZ-Häftlingen und Verfolgten* [Medical Research of the Late Effects of the War and National Socialism

Regime on Youth and Children of Former Concentration Camp Inmates and Persecuted Persons]. Wien: Internationale Föderation der Widerstandskämpfer. [VI Internationaler Medizinischer Kongress der FIR. Prague, 1976].

1656 Nathan, Tikva S. (1969). Disturbed parent role in Holocaust survivors. *Israel Annals of Psychiatry and Related Disciplines*, 7(2), 234.

1657 Nathan, Tikva S. (1981). Dor sheny lenitzoley hashoa bemchkarim psychosocialiim [The second generation of Holocaust survivors in psychosocial research]. In: *Studies of the Holocaust Period. Vol. 2.* Tel Aviv: Hakibbutz Hameuchad Publishing House, pp. 13-26.

1658 Nathan, Tikva S. (1990). Children of survivors. In: Gutman, Israel (Ed.), *Encyclopedia of the Holocaust. Vol. 4.* New York: Macmillan, pp. 1432-1434.

1659 Nathan, Tikva S.; Eitinger, Leo; and Winnik, Heinrich Z. (1963). The psychiatric pathology of survivors of the Nazi Holocaust. *Israel Annals of Psychiatry and Related Disciplines*, 1(1), 113-120.

1660 Nathan, Tikva S.; Eitinger, Leo; and Winnik, Heinrich Z. (1964). A psychiatric study of survivors of the Nazi Holocaust: A study of hospitalized patients. *Israel Annals of Psychiatry and Related Disciplines*, 2(1), 47-80.

1661 Nelkin, M. (1971). Survivors of Nazi concentration camps: Psychopathology and views of psychotherapy. *Canadian Journal of Psychiatric Nursing*, 20(6), 560-568.

1662 Nemes, L. (1985). A magyar pszichoanalitikosok sovsa a fasizmus eveiben [Fate of Hungarian psychoanalysts during the Nazi era]. *Orvosi Hetilap*, 126(44), 2730-2732.

1663 Nemeth, M.C. (1971). Psychosis in a concentration camp survivor: A case presentation. *International Psychiatry Clinics*, 8, 135-146.

1664 Neri, Nadia (1989). Identita femminile e sacrificio in Etty Hillesum [Feminine identity and sacrifice in Etty Hillesum]. *Giornale Storico di Psicologia Dinamica*, 13(25), 135-142.

1665 Netter, A. (1961). On the physiopathology of amenorrhea in concentration camps. In: *International Conference on the Later Effects of Imprisonment and Deportation Organized by the World Veterans Federation. The Hague, November 20-25, 1961*. The Hague: World Veterans Federation, pp. 73-77.

1666 Neumann, Micha (1993). Die Psychologie und Psychopathologie der zweiten Generation der Holocaust-überlebenden [The psychology and psychopathology of the second generation of Holocaust survivors]. *Analytische Psychologie*, 24(2), 103-117.

1667 Neurath, P.M. (1951). *Social life in the German concentration camps Dachau and Buchenwald*. Unpublished doctoral dissertation, Columbia University, New York. *Dissertation Abstracts International*, 12(1), p. 111. (University Microfilms no. AAC 0003372).

1668 Newman, Lisa (1979). Emotional disturbance in children of Holocaust survivors. *Social Casework*, 60(1), 43-50.

1669 Nicholls-Goudsmid, Joyce (1988). *Second generation Holocaust survivors and the development of their ego identities*. Unpublished master's thesis, Simon Fraser University, Burnaby, British Columbia, Canada.

1670 Niederland, William G. (1960). Discussion of Klaus Hoppe: The psychodynamics of concentration camp victims. *Psychoanalytic Forum*, 1, 80.

1671 Niederland, William G. (1961). The problem of the survivor. *Journal of the Hillside Hospital*, 10, 233-247.

1672 Niederland, William G. (1964). Psychiatric disorders among persecution victims: A contribution to the understanding of concentration camp pathology and its aftereffects. *Journal of Nervous and Mental Disease*, 139, 458-474.

1673 Niederland, William G. (1966). Ein Blick in die Tiefen der "unbewältigten Vergangenheit Gegenwart" [A look in depth at overcoming the "past in the present"]. *Psyche: Zeitschrift für Psychoanalyse und ihre Anwendungen*, 20, 466.

1674 Niederland, William G. (1968). The psychiatric evaluation of emotional disorders in survivors of Nazi persecution. In: Krystal, Henry (Ed.), *Massive Psychic Trauma*. New York: International Universities Press, pp. 8-22.

1675 Niederland, William G. (1968). An interpretation of the psychological stresses and defenses in concentration camp life and the late after-effects. In: Krystal, Henry (Ed.), *Massive Psychic Trauma*. New York: International Universities Press, pp. 60-70.

1676 Niederland, William G. (1971). Introducing notes on the concept, definition and range of psychiatric trauma. In: Krystal, Henry, and Niederland, William G. (Eds.), *Psychic Traumatization: Aftereffects in Individuals and Communities*. Boston, MA: Little, Brown, pp. 1-9.

1677 Niederland, William G. (1972). Clinical observations on the survivor syndrome. In: Parker, Rolland S. (Ed.), *The Emotional Stress of War, Violence, and Peace*. Pittsburgh, PA: Stanwix House.

1678 Niederland, William G. (1981). The survivor syndrome: Further observations and dimensions. *Journal of the American Psychoanalytic Association*, 29(2), 413-425.

1679 Niederland, William G. (1988). The clinical after effects of the Holocaust in survivors and their offspring. In: Braham, Randolph L. (Ed.), *The Psychological Perspectives of the Holocaust and of its Aftermath*. Boulder, CO: Social Sciences Monographs; and New York: Csengeri Institute for Holocaust Studies of the Graduate School and University Center of the City University of New York, pp. 45-52.

1680 Niedojadło, Eugeniusz (1971). The camp "hospital" in Buna. In: *Auschwitz Anthology. Vol. 2: In Hell They Preserved Human Dignity. Part 2*. Warsaw: International Auschwitz Committee, pp. 46-57.

1681 Nielson, Henrik (1983). Dodelighed 1943-1979 blandt danske modstandsfolk deporteret til tyske koncentrationslejre [Mortality among members of the Danish resistance movement deported to German concentration camps: 1943-1979]. *Ugeskrift for Laeger*, 145(5), 345-350.

1682 Nielson, Henrik (1983). Invaliditet 1946-1979 blandt danske modstandsfolk efter deportation til tyske Koncentrationlej [Disability during the years 1946-1979 among members of the Danish resistance movement deported to German concentration camps]. *Ugeskrift for Laeger*, 145(5), 350-355.

1683 Nielson, Henrik (1983). Invaliditeten og dens forlob 1946-1979 blandt svaert deportationsbelastede KZ-fanger [Disability and its course during the years 1946-1979 among concentration camp prisoners previously exposed to severe stress]. *Ugeskrift for Laeger*, 145(12), 935-940.

1684 Nielson, Henrik, and Madsen, Mette (1983). Deportationsbelastningens og erhvervsplaceringens betydning for overlevende KZ-fangers [The significance of the strain of deportation and the occupation for the post-war mortality and disability of surviving concentration camp prisoners]. *Ugeskrift for Laeger*, 145 (12), 929-934.

1685 Nielson, Henrik, and Sorensen, H. (1984). KZ syndromet i individualle forlöb [The individual course of the concentration camp syndrome]. *Nordisk Psykiatrisk Tidsskrift*, 305-312.

1686 Niewiarowicz, Roman (1970). Wspomnienia o Kotarbińskim - lekarzu i więźniu w obozie koncentracyjnym [Reminiscences about Kotarbinski, physician and concentration camp prisoner]. *Przegląd Lekarski*, 26(1), 266-270.

1687 Niewiarowicz, Roman (1973). Medycyna in articulo mortis w hitlerowskich więzieniach i obozach koncentracyjnych [Medicine in articulo mortis in Nazi prisons and concentration camps]. *Przegląd Lekarski*, 30(1), 179-188.

1688 Nikolic, Dragutin (1961). Epidemiological table of tuberculosis among internees and the consequences of tuberculosis. In: *International Conference on the Later Effects of Imprisonment and Deportation Organized by the World Veterans Federation. The Hague, November 20-25, 1961*. The Hague: World Veterans Federation, pp. 67-68.

1689 Nikolic, Dragutin (1978). Les conséquences tardives de la tuberculose chez les déportés dans les camps de concentration pendant la deuxième guerre mondiale [Late sequels of tuberculosis among the deportees in the concentration camps during World War II]. In: *Medizinische Untersuchungen der Spätfolgen des Krieges und des NS-Regimes bei Jugendlichen und Kindern von ehemaligen KZ-Häftlingen und Verfolgten* [Medical Research of the Late Effects of the War and National Socialism Regime on Youth and Children of Former Concentration Camp Inmates and Persecuted Persons]. Wien: Internationale Föderation der Widerstandskämpfer. [VI Internationaler Medizinischer Kongress der FIR. Prague, 1976].

1690 Niremberski, M. (1946). Psychological investigation of a group of internees at Belsen-Camp. *Journal of Mental Science*, 92, 60-74.

1691 Nissim, Luciana; de Benedetti, L.; and Perretta, G. (1955). Soziale Neu-Eingliederung in Italien (Nazi- und Faschistenopfer) [Social rehabilitation in Italy (victims of Nazis and fascists)]. In: Michel, Max (Ed.), *Gesundheitsschäden durch Verfolgung und Gefangenschaft und ihre Spätfolgen: Zusammenstellung der Referate und Ergebnisse der Internationalen Sozialmedizinischen Konferenz über die Pathologie der Ehemaligen Deportierten und Internierten, 5-7 Juni*

1954 in Kopenhagen [Health Damages Caused by Persecution and Captivity and the Late Effects: Compilation of the Papers and Results of the International Conference of Social Medicine on the Pathology of Former Deported and Interned Persons, 5-7 June 1954 in Copenhagen]. Frankfurt am Main: Röderberg, pp. 238-239.

1692 Noach, Jehudith (1990). *Stress en traumatisering: physiologische, psychische, psychologische en sociale oorlogsproblematiek* [Stress and traumatization: Physiologic, psychiatric, psychologic and social causes of the concentration camp syndrome and other war problems]. Unpublished doctoral dissertation, Leiden University, Leiden, The Netherlands.

1693 Noordhoekhecht, W.G. (1967). Die Situation in den Niederlanden [The situation in the Netherlands]. In: Herberg, Hans-Joachim (Ed.), *Die Beurteilung von Gesundheitsschäden nach Gefangenschaft und Verfolgung* [The Assessment of Health Damages Following Internment and Persecution]. Herford: Nicholai, pp. 29-33. [Internationaler Medizinisch-Juristischen Symposiums in Köln].

1694 Noordhoekhecht, W.G.; Gilbert-Dreyfuss, H.; Ost, Dr.; Fichez, Louis F.; and Katz, Charles (1955). Einige Verkürzte Auszüge aus der Debatte und den späteren Mitteilungen [Some extracts from the debates and later announcements]. In: Michel, Max (Ed.), *Gesundheitsschäden durch Verfolgung und Gefangenschaft und ihre Spätfolgen: Zusammenstellung der Referate und Ergebnisse der Internationalen Sozialmedizinischen Konferenz über die Pathologie der Ehemaligen Deportierten und Internierten, 5-7 Juni 1954 in Kopenhagen* [Health Damages Caused by Persecution and Captivity and the Late Effects: Compilation of the Papers and Results of the International Conference of Social Medicine on the Pathology of Former Deported and Interned Persons, 5-7 June 1954 in Copenhagen]. Frankfurt am Main: Röderberg, pp. 332-337.

1695 Nourok, Andrew J. (1991). *The relationship between ethnic-communal affiliation and effects of post-traumatic stress disorder in children of Holocaust survivors*. Unpublished master's thesis, California State University, Long Beach, 62 pp. *Masters Abstracts International*, 30(1), p. 57. (University Microfilms no. AAC 1345453).

1696 Nowak, Jan (1973). Verbrechen an Kindern und Jugendlichen während der Nazi Okkupationszeit [Crimes against children and adolescents during the Nazi occupation]. In: *Ermüdung und vorzeitiges Altern: Folge von Extrembelastungen* [Exhaustion and Premature Aging: Result of Extreme Stress]. Leipzig: Barth, pp. 376-

386. [V Internationaler Medizinischer Kongress der FIR. Paris, 21-24 September 1970].

1697 Nowak, Jan (1978). Die Problematik des KZ syndroms und eigene Behandlungsmethoden und Erfolge [Problems of the concentration camp syndrome and personal methods of treatment and results]. In: *Medizinische Untersuchungen der Spätfolgen des Krieges und des NS-Regimes bei Jugendlichen und Kindern von ehemaligen KZ-Häftlingen und Verfolgten* [Medical Research of the Late Effects of the War and National Socialism Regime on Youth and Children of Former Concentration Camp Inmates and Persecuted Persons]. Wien: Internationale Föderation der Widerstandskämpfer. [VI Internationaler Medizinischer Kongress der FIR. Prague, 1976].

1698 Nowakowska, Maria (1971). The "Women's Hospital" in Birkenau. In: *Auschwitz Anthology. Vol. 2: In Hell They Preserved Human Dignity. Part 2.* Warsaw: International Auschwitz Committee, pp. 144-160.

1699 Nowakowska, Maria (1975). "Infirmerie des femmes" à Birkenau [The women's sick bay in Birkenau]. *Cahiers d'Informations Médicales, Sociales et Juridiques*, 6, 1-4.

1700 Nowicki, Jerzy (1975). Po oswobodzeniu z obozu w Sandbostel [After the liberation of the Sandbostel camp]. *Przegląd Lekarski*, 32(1), 182-187.

1701 Obadia, Jean Paul (1986). An indefatigable worker. *Revue Française de Psychanalyse*, 50(2), 789-801.

1702 Obermeyer, Vera R. (1988). Outmarriage and cohesion in Jewish Holocaust survivor families. *Family Therapy*, 15(3), 255-269.

1703 Obermeyer, Vera R., and Lukoff, Christel (Eds.) (1988). Special issue: "Children of the Holocaust." *Family Therapy*, 15(3), 197-285.

1704 Obermeyer, Vera R., and Lukoff, Christel (1988). Introduction to special issue on "Children of the Holocaust." *Family Therapy*, 15(3), 197-198.

1705 Ofman, Jacob (1981). *Separation-individuation in children of Nazi Holocaust survivors and its relationship to perceived parental overvaluation.* Unpublished doctoral dissertation, California School of Professional Psychology, Berkeley, 151 pp. *Dissertation Abstracts International*, 42(8-B), p. 3434. (University Microfilms no. AAC 8201496).

1706 Ofri, Irit; Solomon, Zahava; and Dasberg, Haim (1995). Attitudes of therapists toward Holocaust survivors. *Journal of Traumatic Stress*, 8(2), 229-242.

1707 Okner, Debra F., and Flaherty, Joseph F. (1989). Parental communication and psychological distress in children of Holocaust survivors: A comparison between the United States and Israel. *International Journal of Social Psychiatry*, 35(3), 265-273.

1708 Olbrycht, Jan (1970). The Nazi health office actively participated with the SS administration in Auschwitz. In: *Auschwitz Anthology. Vol. 1: Inhuman Medicine. Part 1*. Warsaw: International Auschwitz Committee, pp. 147-205.

1709 Oliner, Marion M. (1982). Hysterical features among children of survivors. In: Bergmann, Martin S., and Jucovy, Milton E. (Eds.), *Generations of the Holocaust*. New York: Basic Books, pp. 267-286.

1710 Oliner, Pearl M., and Oliner, Samuel P. (1991). Righteous people in the Holocaust. In: Charny, Israel W. (Ed.), *Genocide: A Critical Bibliographic Review. Vol. 2*. London: Mansell, pp. 363-385.

1711 Oliner, Samuel P., and Oliner, Pearl M. (1988). *The Altruistic Personality: Rescuers of Jews in Nazi Europe*. New York: Free Press. 419 pp.

1712 Olszyna, Roman (1970). Wstępny wykaz lekarzy obozu. Gross-Rosen [Preliminary list of physicians at the Gross-Rosen concentration camp]. *Przegląd Lekarski*, 26(1), 169-171.

1713 Op den Velde, Wybrand (1987). De causaliteitsbeoordeling van psychische klachten van oorlogs-getroffenen [Judgment of causality of psychic complaints of war victims]. In: *Medical Causality and Late Consequences of War*. Utrecht: Stichting ICODO, pp. 25-34.

1714 Ornstein, Anna (1981). The effects of the Holocaust on life-cycle experiences: The creation and recreation of families. *Journal of Geriatric Psychiatry*, 14(2), 135-154.

1715 Ornstein, Anna (1985). Survival and recovery. *Psychoanalytic Inquiry*, 5(1), 99-130.

1716 Ornstein, Anna (1986). The Holocaust: Reconstruction and the establishment of psychic continuity. In: Rothstein, Arnold (Ed.), *The Reconstruction of Trauma: Its Significance in Clinical Work*. Madison, CT: International Universities Press, pp. 171-199.

1717 Orwid, Maria (1972). Socio-psychiatric consequences of the stay in the concentration camp Auschwitz-Birkenau. In: *Auschwitz Anthology. Vol. 3: It Did Not End in Forty-Five. Part 2.* Warsaw: International Auschwitz Committee, pp. 174-206.

1718 Orwid, Maria; Domagalska-Kurdziel, Ewa; and Petruszewski, Kazimierz (1994). Psychospołeczne następstwa holocaustu w drugim pokoleniu ofiar holocaustu ocalonych w Polsce [Psychosocial effects of the Holocaust on the second generation of Holocaust survivors]. *Psychiatria Polska*, 28(1), 113-129.

1719 Orwid, Maria; Domagalska-Kurdziel, Ewa; and Petruszewski, Kazimierz (1994). Psychospołeczne następstwa holocaustu u osób ocalonych i żyjących w Polsce [Psychosocial effects of the Holocaust on Jewish survivors living in Poland]. *Psychiatria Polska*, 28(1), 91-111.

1720 Orwid, Maria; Domagalska-Kurdziel, Ewa; and Petruszewski, Kazimierz (1995). Psychosocial effects of the Holocaust on Jewish survivors living in Poland. *Psychiatria Polska*, 29(3, supplement), 29-48.

1721 Orwid, Maria; Domagalska-Kurdziel, Ewa; Petruszewski, Kazimierz; Czaplak, Ewa; Izdebski, Ryszard; and Kaminska, Maria (1995). Psychosocial effects of the Holocaust on survivors and the second generation in Poland: Preliminary report. In: Lemberger, John (Ed.), *A Global Perspective on Working with Holocaust Survivors and the Second Generation.* Jerusalem: JDC-Brookdale Institute of Gerontology and Human Development, AMCHA, and JDC-Israel, pp. 205-242.

1722 Orwid, Maria; Szymusik, Adam; and Teutsch, Aleksander (1972). Purpose and method of psychiatric examinations of former prisoners of the Auschwitz concentration camp. In: *Auschwitz Anthology. Vol. 3: It Did Not End in Forty Five. Part 2.* Warsaw: International Auschwitz Committee, pp. 130-142.

1723 Ostwald, Peter, and Bittner, Egon (1968). Life adjustment after severe persecution. *American Journal of Psychiatry*, 124(10), 1393-1400.

1724 Osvik, K. (1961). Indremedisinske funn hos tidligere konsentrasjonsleirfanger [Internal medical findings in ex-concentration camp prisoners]. *Tidsskrift for den Norske Laegeforening. Journal of the Norwegian Medical Association*, 81, 811-812.

1725 Osvik, K. (1961). Study of a group of former Norwegian deportees. Part 5: Internal medical findings in ex-concentration camp inmates. In: *International Conference on the Later Effects of Imprisonment and Deportation Organized by the World Veterans Federation. The Hague, November 20-25, 1961*. The Hague: World Veterans Federation, pp. 122-123.

1726 Oyen, O. (1967). Die Situation in Norwegen [The situation in Norway]. In: Herberg, Hans-Joachim (Ed.), *Die Beurteilung von Gesundheitsschäden nach Gefangenschaft und Verfolgung* [The Assessment of Health Damages Following Internment and Persecution]. Herford: Nicholai, pp. 44-55. [Internationaler Medizinisch-Juristischen Symposiums in Köln].

1727 Paczuła, Tadeusz (1971). The organization and administration of the camp hospital in the concentration camp Auschwitz I. In: *Auschwitz Anthology. Vol. 2: In Hell They Preserved Human Dignity. Part 1*. Warsaw: International Auschwitz Committee, pp. 38-75.

1728 Paczuła, Tadeusz (1987). Organisation und Verwaltung des ersten Häftlingenkrankenhaus in Auschwitz [Organization and management of the first hospital for concentration camp inmates of Auschwitz]. In: Hamburger Institut für Sozialforschung (Eds.), *Die Auschwitz-Hefte: Texte der polnischen Zeitschrift "Przegląd Lekarski" über historische, psychische und medizinische Aspekte des Lebens und Sterbens in Auschwitz. Band 1* [The Auschwitz Journal. Text of the Polish Journal "Medical Review" on Historical, Psychic and Medical Aspects of Life and Death in Auschwitz. Volume 1]. Weinheim und Basel: Beltz, pp. 159-165.

1729 Paldiel, Mordechai (1981). The altruism of Righteous Gentiles. *Holocaust and Genocide Studies*, 3(2), 187-196.

1730 Panasewicz, Józef, and Łuckiewicz, B. (1973). Folgen des Konzentrationslager-Hungerdystrophiesyndroms unter besonderer Berücksichtigung hämotologischer Störungen [Consequences of the concentration camp hunger dystrophy syndrome with special regard to haematological disease]. In: *Ermüdung und Vorzeitiges Altern: Folge von Extrembelastungen* [Exhaustion and Premature Aging: Result of Extreme Stress]. Leipzig: Barth, pp. 56-70. [V Internationaler Medizinischer Kongress der FIR. Paris, 21-24 September 1970].

1731 Parker, Fran K. (1983). *Dominant attitudes of adult children of Holocaust survivors toward their parents*. Unpublished doctoral dissertation, Saybrook Institute, San Francisco, California, 190 pp.

Dissertation Abstracts International, 44(7-B), p. 2230. (University Microfilms no. AAC 8325704).

1732 Pater, J. (1990). Struktura potrzeb u byłych więźniów hitlerowskich obozów koncentracyjnych [Structure of the needs of former prisoners of the Nazi concentration camps]. *Przegląd Lekarski*, 47(1), 20-26.

1733 Paton, Alex (1981). Mission to Belsen. *British Journal of Medical Psychology*, 19, 1656-1659.

1734 Patti, M. (1964). Les facteurs psychoaffectives dans la détermination du syndrome psychosomatique de la déportation et dans l'instauration de la psychose chronique ainsi dite "de ronce artificielle" [Psychoaffective factors in psychosomatic syndromes caused by deportation and in chronic psychoses, the so-called "artificial thorn"]. *Annali di Medicina Navale*, 69, 501-506.

1735 Pattison, E. Mansell (1984). The Holocaust as sin: Requirements in psychoanalytic theory for human evil and mature morality. In: Luel, Steven A., and Marcus, Paul (Eds.), *Psychoanalytic Reflections on the Holocaust: Selected Essays*. New York: Ktav, pp. 71-91.

1736 Paul, Helmut (1957). Der Mechanismus einer Flucht in die Dystrophie [The mechanism of a "flight into dystrophy"]. *Zeitschrift für Psychotherapie und Medizinische Psychologie*, 6(7), 249-257.

1737 Paul, Helmut (1958). Über den psycho-stress [On psychological stress]. *Psychologie und Praxis*, 1, 1-13.

1738 Paul, Helmut (1959). Charakterveränderungen durch Kriegsgefangenschaft und Dystrophie [Changes of character as a result of war imprisonment and dystrophy]. In: Schench, E.G., and Nathusius, W. von (Eds.), *Extrem Lebensverhältnisse und ihre Folgen. Bericht über den 4. Ärztekongress für Pathologie, Therapie und Begutachtung der Heimkehrerkrankheiten in Düsseldorf, 1959* [Extreme Life Conditions and Their Effects. Report on the 4th Physicians Conference on Pathology, Therapy and Survey of Returnees' Diseases in Dusseldorf, 1959]. Verband der Heimkehrer, pp. 41-54.

1739 Paul, Helmut (1959). Die Psyche des Hungernden und des Dystrophikers [The psyche of the starving and dystrophic individual]. In: Schench, E.G., and Nathusius, W. von (Eds.), *Extrem Lebensverhältnisse und ihre Folgen. Bericht über den 4. Ärztekongress für Pathologie, Therapie und Begutachtung der Heimkehrerkrankheiten in Düsseldorf, 1959* [Extreme Life Conditions and Their Effects. Report on the 4th Physicians Conference on Pathology, Therapy and Survey of Returnee's Diseases in Dusseldorf, 1959]. Verband der Heimkehrer, pp. 5-127.

1740 Paul, Helmut (1960). Bemerkungen zum menschlischen Verhalten unter extremen Lebensverhältnissen [Some remarks on human behavior in extreme life situations]. *Arztliche Praxis*, 12, 1-23.

1741 Paul, Helmut (1961). Personality study of former prisoners of war and former internees. In: *International Conference on the Later Effects of Imprisonment and Deportation Organized by the World Veterans Federation. The Hague, November 20-25, 1961*. The Hague: World Veterans Federation, pp. 101-106.

1742 Paul, Helmut (1961). Problems in the classification of personality disorders following imprisonment. In: *International Conference on the Later Effects of Imprisonment and Deportation Organized by the World Veterans Federation. The Hague, November 20-25, 1961*. The Hague: World Veterans Federation, pp. 107-108.

1743 Paul, Helmut (1963). Internationale Erfahrungen mit psychischen Spätschäden [International experience with psychological sequelae]. In: Paul, Helmut, and Herberg, Hans-Joachim (Eds.), *Psychische Spätschäden nach politischer Verfolgung* [Psychological Late Damages Following Political Persecution]. Basel: Karger, pp. 37-84.

1744 Paul, Helmut (1963). Psychologische Untersuchungsergebnisse 15 Jahre nach der Verfolgung [Results of psychological investigations 15 years after the persecution]. In: Paul, Helmut, and Herberg, Hans-Joachim (Eds.), *Psychische Spätschäden nach politischer Verfolgung* [Psychological Late Damages Following Political Persecution]. Basel: Karger, pp. 207-243.

1745 Paul, Helmut (1967). Methodologische Probleme bei der Untersuchung auf psychische Störungen nach Gefangenschaft und Verfolgung [Methodological problems in the investigation of psychological disturbances after imprisonment and persecution]. In: Herberg, Hans-Joachim (Ed.), *Die Beurteilung von Gesundheitsschäden nach Gefangenschaft und Verfolgung* [The Assessment of Health Damages Following Internment and Persecution]. Herford: Nicholai, pp. 77-83. [Internationalen Medizinisch-Juristischen Symposiums in Köln].

1746 Paul, Helmut (1967). Neuere studien zum Thema [Newer studies of the problem]. In: Paul, Helmut, and Herberg, Hans-Joachim (Eds.), *Psychische Spätschäden nach politischer Verfolgung. 2. erweiterte*

Auflage [Psychological Late Damages Following Political Persecution. 2nd enlarged edition]. Basel: Karger, pp. 78-138.

1747 Paul, Helmut (1967). *Vorzeitiger Verschleiss nach Zwangsarbeit unter extremen Verhältnissen* [Premature Aging After Forced Labor Under Extreme Stress]. Mainz: Krausskopf-Verlag.

1748 Paul, Helmut (1971). Das Stressgeschehen in Verfolgung und Gefangenschaft [The experience of stress in persecution and imprisonment]. In: Herberg, Hans-Joachim (Ed.), *Spätschäden nach Extrembelastungen* [Late Damage After Extreme Stress]. Herford: Nicolai, pp. 21-28. [II Internationalen Medizinisch-Juristischen Konferenz. Dusseldorf, 1969].

1749 Paul, Helmut, and Herberg, Hans-Joachim (Eds.) (1963). *Psychische Spätschäden nach politischer Verfolgung* [Psychological Late Damages Following Political Persecution]. Basel: Karger. 313 pp.

1750 Paul, Helmut, and Herberg, Hans-Joachim (1963). Psychische Spätschäden nach Verfolgungseinflüssen in der Kindheit und Jugend [Psychological sequelae after persecution in childhood and youth]. In: Paul, Helmut, and Herberg, Hans-Joachim (Eds.), *Psychische Spätschäden nach politischer Verfolgung* [Psychological Late Damages Following Political Persecution]. Basel: Karger, pp. 179-206.

1751 Paul, Helmut, and Herberg, Hans-Joachim (Eds.) (1967). *Psychische Spätschäden nach politischer Verfolgung. 2. erweiterte Auflage* [Psychological Late Damages Following Political Persecution. 2nd enlarged edition]. Basel: Karger. 396 pp.

1752 Paul-Mengelberg, Maria (1963). Die Bedeutung der graphologischen Diagnostik im Rahmen der Begutachtung Verfolgter [The meaning of the graphological diagnosis in the evaluation of persecutees]. In: Paul, Helmut, and Herberg, Hans-Joachim (Eds.), *Psychische Spätschäden nach politischer Verfolgung* [Psychological Late Damages Following Political Persecution]. Basel: Karger, pp. 245-255.

1753 Paul-Mengelberg, Maria (1967). Schriftpsychologische Begutachtung von Spätschäden nach Gefangenschaft und Verfolgung [Psychological evaluation of handwriting in cases of late damage after imprisonment and persecution]. In: Herberg, Hans-Joachim (Ed.), *Die Beurteilung von Gesundheitsschäden nach Gefangenschaft Verfolgung* [The Assessment of Health Damages Following Internment and Persecution]. Herford: Nicolai, pp. 84-92. [Internationalen Medizinische-Juristischen Symposiums in Köln].

1754 Paul-Mengelberg, Maria (1971). Schreibmotorische Störungen bei ehemaligen Kriegsgefangenen und Verfolgten [Motor disturbances in writing in former prisoners of war and persecutees]. In: Herberg, Hans-Joachim (Ed.), *Spätschäden nach Extrembelastungen* [Late Damage After Extreme Stress]. Herford: Nicolai, pp. 206-217. [II Internationalen Medizinisch-Juristischen Konferenz. Dusseldorf, 1969].

1755 Pawełczyźska, Anna (1973). Przemiany stuktury społecznej a możliwość przeżycia w Oswięcimie [Social structural changes and prospects for survival at the Auschwitz concentration camp]. *Przegląd Lekarski*, 30(1), 76-81.

1756 Pawłowski, Bolesław (1974). Uwagi o szpitalu obozowym w Wiener Neudorf [The concentration camp hospital at Wiener Neudorf]. *Przegląd Lekarski*, 31(1), 195-200.

1757 Pawłowski, Boleslaw (1976). Nieznane epizody z obozu w Aflenz [Some unknown episodes at the Aflenz concentration camp]. *Przegląd Lekarski*, 33(1), 188-194.

1758 Pawłowski, Bolesław (1979). Przybycie do Mauthausen [Arrival in Mauthausen]. *Przegląd Lekarski*, 36(1), 156-159.

1759 Pedersen, S. (1949). Psychological reactions to extreme social displacement (refugee neuroses). *Psychoanalytic Review*, 36, 344-354.

1760 Pennebaker, James W.; Barger, Steven D.; and Tiebout, John (1989). Disclosure of traumas and health among Holocaust survivors. *Psychosomatic Medicine*, 51(5), 577-589.

1761 Perel, Esther, and Saul, Jack (1989). A family therapy approach to Holocaust survivor families. In: Marcus, Paul, and Rosenberg, Alan (Eds.), *Healing Their Wounds: Psychotherapy with Holocaust Survivors and Their Families*. New York: Praeger, pp. 135-152.

1762 Peretz, D. (1954). Gormim psihosomatiyim b'alveset [Psychosomatic factors in amenorrhea]. *Harefuah*, 46, 189-192.

1763 Peretz, Tamar; Baider, Lea; Ever-Hadani, Pnina; and Kaplan De-Nour, Atara (1994). Psychological distress in female cancer patients with Holocaust experience. *General Hospital Psychiatry*, 16(6), 413-418.

1764 Perl, Gisella (1984). ***I Was a Doctor in Auschwitz.*** Salem, NH: Ayer. 189 pp.

1765 Perl, J.L., and Kahn, M.W. (1983). The effects of compensation on psychiatric disability. *Social Science and Medicine*, 17(7), 439-443.

1766 Peskin, Harvey (1981). Observations on the First International Conference on Children of Holocaust Survivors. *Family Process*, 20(4), 391-394.

1767 Peters, Uwe H. (1989). Die psychischen Folgen der Verfolgung: Das Uberlebenden-Syndrom [The psychological sequelae of persecution: The survivor syndrome]. *Fortschritte der Neurologie, Psychiatrie*, 57(5), 169-191.

1768 Pfäfflin, Friedemann; Rüb, Herbert; and Göpfert, Matthias (1992). Universitätspsychiatrie und Nationalsozialismus [University psychiatric hospitals and National Socialism]. In: Jockush, Ulrich, and Scholz, Lothar (Eds.), *Verwaltetes Morden im Nationalsozialismus: Verstrickung, Verdrängung, Verantwortung von Psychiatrie und Justiz* [Administered Killings at the Time of National Socialism: Involvement, Suppression, Responsibility of Psychiatry and Judicial System]. Regensburg: Roderer, pp. 40-60.

1769 Pfäfflin, Friedemann; Rüb, Herbert; and Göpfert, Matthias (1992). University psychiatric hospitals and National Socialism. In: Jockush, Ulrich, and Scholz, Lothar (Eds.), *Administered Killings at the Time of National Socialism: Involvement, Suppression, Responsibility of Psychiatry and Judicial System*. Regensburg: Roderer, pp. 41-62.

1770 Pfister-Ammende, Maria (1961). Psychologie und Psychiatrie der Internierung und des Flüchtlingsdaseins [Psychology and psychiatry of internment and being a refugee]. In: Gruhle, Hans W. (Ed.), *Psychiatrie der Gegenwart: Forschung und Praxis. Band 3: Soziale und angewandte Psychiatrie* [Psychiatry in the Present: Research and Practice. Vol. 3: Social and Applied Psychiatry]. Berlin: Springer.

1771 Phillips, Russel E. (1978). Impact of Nazi Holocaust on children of survivors. *American Journal of Psychotherapy*, 32(3), 370-378.

1772 Picker, Richard (1993). Psychotherapy and the Nazi past: A search for concrete forms. In: Heimannsberg, Barbara, and Schmidt, Christoph J. (Eds.), *The Collective Silence: German Identity and the Legacy of Shame*. San Francisco, CA: Jossey Bass.

1773 Piekara, Arkadiusz H. (1979). Epizody z tzw. Sonderaktion Krakau [Episodes from the so-called sonderaktion Krakau]. *Przegląd Lekarski*, 36(1), 146-148.

1774 Piekut-Warszawska, Elżbieta (1971). Reminiscences of a nurse. In: *Auschwitz Anthology. Vol. 2: In Hell They Preserved Human Dignity. Part 3*. Warsaw: International Auschwitz Committee, pp. 1-12.

1775 Piekut-Warszawska, Elżbieta (1987). Kinder in Auschwitz: Erinnerungen einer Krankenschwester [Children in Auschwitz: Recollections of a Nurse]. In: Hamburger Institut für Sozialforschung (Eds.), *Die Auschwitz-Hefte: Texte der polnischen Zeitschrift "Przegląd Lekarski" über historische, psychische und medizinische Aspekte des Lebens und Sterbens in Auschwitz. Band 1* [The Auschwitz Journal. Text of the Polish Journal "Medical Review" on Historical, Psychic and Medical Aspects of Life and Death in Auschwitz. Volume 1]. Weinheim und Basel: Beltz, pp. 227-229.

1776 Pilcz, Maria (1975). Understanding the survivor family: An acknowledgement of the positive dimensions of the Holocaust legacy. In: Steinitz, Lucy Y., and Szonyi, David M. (Eds.), *Living After the Holocaust: Reflections by Children of Survivors in America*. New York: Bloch, pp. 157-167.

1777 Pines, Dinora (1986). Working with women survivors of the Holocaust: Affective experiences in transference and countertransference. *International Journal of Psycho-Analysis*, 67(3), 295-307.

1778 Pingel, Falk (1991). The destruction of human identity in concentration camps: The contribution of the social sciences to an analysis of behavior under extreme conditions. *Holocaust and Genocide Studies*, 6(2), 167-184.

1779 Piórek, Julian (1976). Kilka spostrzeżeń z pobytu w Gross Rosen [The Gross-Rosen camp: A few observations]. *Przegląd Lekarski*, 33(1), 184-188.

1780 Platz, Werner E., and Oberlaender, Franklin A. (1995). On the problems of expert opinion on Holocaust survivors submitted to the compensation authorities in Germany. *International Journal of Law and Psychiatry*, 18(3), 305-321.

1781 Podietz, Lenore (1975). The Holocaust revisited in the next generation. *Jewish Institute for Policy Studies Bulletin*, 54, 1-5.

1782 Podietz, Lenore; Zwerling, Israel; Ficher, Ilda; Belmont, Herman; Eisenstein, Talia; Shapiro, Marion; and Levick, Myra (1984). Engagement in families of Holocaust survivors. *Journal of Marital and Family Therapy*, 10(1), 43-51.

1783 Podlaha, J., and Zeman, F. (1961). Das Hungerödem und sein Einfluss auf die Arterien der unteren Extremitäten [The edema of famine and its influence on the arteries of the lower extremities]. In: *Die Behandlung der Asthenie und der vorzeitigen Vergreisung bei ehemaligen Widerstandskämpfern und KZ Häftlingen* [Treatment of Asthenia and Premature Aging in Former Resistance Fighters and Concentration Camp Inmates]. Wien: Verlag der FIR, pp. 97-99. [III Internationale Medizinisch Konferenz. Liege, 17-19 März 1961].

1784 Podlaha, J., and Zeman, F. (1964). Dauerfolgen des Hungers in den Konzentrationslagern [Long term sequelae of famine in the concentration camps]. In: *Ätio-Pathogenese und Therapie der Erschöpfung und vorzeitigen Vergreisung* [The Aetiology, Pathogenesis and Therapy of Exhaustion and Premature Aging]. Wien: Verlag der FIR, pp. 114-118. [IV Internationaler Medizinischer Kongress. Bucharest, 22-27 Juni 1964].

1785 Polak, B.S. (1984). De rol van de huisarts bij de signalering en behandeling van psychosomatische klachten van oorlogsgetroffen [The role of the general practitioner in the recognition and treatment of psychosomatic complaints of war victims]. In: Dane, Jan (Ed.), *Keerzijde van de bevrijding: Opstellen over de maatschappelijke, psycho-sociale en medische aspekten van de problematiek van oorlogsgetroffenen* [The Other Side of Liberation: Essays on the Social, Psychosocial and Medical Aspects of the Problems of War Victims]. Deventer: Van Loghum Slaterus, pp. 190-203.

1786 Poliezer, M., and Szokodi, D. (1961). Über Störungen der Schilddrüzenfunktion und deren Beeinflüssung bei den Opfern des Faschismus [Disturbances of the thyroid function in victims of fascism]. In: *Die Behandlung der Asthenie und der vorzeitigen Vergreisung bei ehemaligen Widerstandskämpfern und KZ- Häftlingen* [Treatment of Asthenia and Premature Aging in Former Resistance Fighters and Concentration Camp Inmates]. Wien: Verlag der FIR, pp. 119-125. [III Internationale Medizinische Konferenz. Liege, 17-19 März 1961].

1787 Poller, Walter (1988). *Medical Block, Buchenwald: The Personal Testimony of Inmate 966, Block 36*. London: Grafton. 254 pp.

1788 Poltawska, Wanda (1965). Badania nad "dziećmi oswiecimskimi" (uwagi ogólne) [From the research on the so-called "Auschwitz children," (general considerations)]. *Przegląd Lekarski*, 21(1), 21-24.

1789 Poltawska, Wanda (1971). "Guinea pigs" in the Ravensbrück concentration camp. In: *Auschwitz Anthology. Vol. 1: Inhuman*

Medicine. Part 2. Warsaw: International Auschwitz Committee, pp. 131-162.

1790 Poltawska, Wanda (1971). On examinations of "Auschwitz children." In: *Auschwitz Anthology. Vol. 2: In Hell They Preserved Human Dignity. Part 3*. Warsaw: International Auschwitz Committee, pp. 21-36.

1791 Poltawska, Wanda (1971). States of paroxysmal hypermnesia. In: *Auschwitz Anthology. Vol. 2: In Hell They Preserved Human Dignity. Part 3*. Warsaw: International Auschwitz Committee, pp. 190-218.

1792 Poltawska, Wanda (1978). Stany hipermnezji napadowej u byłych więźniów obserwowane po 30 latach [Paroxysmal hypermnesia states among ex-prisoners observed 30 years after imprisonment]. *Przegląd Lekarski*, 35, 20-24.

1793 Poltawska, Wanda; Jakubik, Andrzej; Sarnecki, Józef; and Gątarski, Julian (1966). Wyniki badań psychiatrycznych osób urodzonych lub więzionych w dzieciństwie w hitlerowskich obozach koncentracyjnych [Results of the psychiatric studies of persons either born or imprisoned in childhood in Hitlerian concentration camps]. *Przegląd Lekarski*, 23, 21-36.

1794 Poltawska, Wanda; Jakubik, Andrzej; Sarnecki, Józef; and Gątarski, Julian (1971). Results of psychiatric examinations of people born in Nazi concentration camps or imprisoned there during their childhood. In: *Auschwitz Anthology. Vol. 2: In Hell They Preserved Human Dignity. Part 3*. Warsaw: International Auschwitz Committee, pp. 37-132.

1795 Pomerantz, B. (1977). *Children of survivors of the Holocaust: Perceptions of their need for social work and community services*. Unpublished master's thesis, School of Social Work, University of Southern California, Los Angeles.

1796 Pomerantz, B. (1980). Group work with children of Holocaust Survivors. In: *The Many Dimensions of Family Practice: Proceedings of the North American Symposium on Family Practice, 1-4 November 1978*. New York: Family Service Association of America, pp. 194-203.

1797 Popek, Walenty (1978). W rewirze obozu w Gross-Rosen [In the sick bay of the concentration camp Gross-Rosen]. *Przegląd Lekarski*, 35, 171-172.

1798 Popou, V.L. (1985). Sudebno-meditsinskaia ekspertiza pro rass ledovanii zlodeianii fashistov v Osventsime [Forensic medical expertise in investigating the crimes of the racists at Auschwitz]. *Sudebno Meditsinskaia Ekspertiza*, 28(2), 14-16.

1799 Popper, Ludwig (1955). Ärztliche Erfahrungen bei Untersuchungen nach dem österreichischen Opferfürsorgegesetz [Medical experience in investigations according to the Austrian law of compensation]. In: Michel, Max (Ed.), *Gesundheitsschäden durch Verfolgung und Gefangenschaft und ihre Spätfolgen: Zusammenstellung der Referate und Ergebnisse der Internationalen Sozialmedizinischen Konferenz über die Pathologie der Ehemaligen Deportierten und Internierten, 5-7 Juni 1954 in Kopenhagen* [Health Damages Caused by Persecution and Captivity and the Late Effects: Compilation of the Papers and Results of the International Conference of Social Medicine on the Pathology of Former Deported and Interned Persons, 5-7 June 1954 in Copenhagen]. Frankfurt am Main: Röderberg, pp. 281-287.

1800 Porot, M.; Couadau, A.; and Plenat, M. (1985). Le syndrome de culpabilité du survivant [The survivor's guilt syndrome]. *Annales Medico Psychologiques*, 143(3), 256-262.

1801 Porter, Jack N. (1979). Social psychological aspects of the Holocaust. In: Sherwin, Byron L.; and Amend, Susan G. (Eds.), *Encountering the Holocaust*. Chicago, IL: Impact, pp. 189-222.

1802 Porter, Jack N. (1981). Is there a survivor syndrome? Psychological and socio-political implications. *Journal of Psychology and Judaism*, 6(1), 33-52.

1803 Post, Stephen G. (1991). The echo of Nuremberg: Nazi data and ethics. *Journal of Medical Ethics*, 17(1), 42-44.

1804 Poznaniak, W. (1972). The stress mechanism of the desocialization of the personality of a concentration camp prisoner. Introductory psychological analysis. *Przegląd Psychologiczny*, 15(2), 29-44.

1805 Prakken, Han G.; Laden, Antonie; and Stufkens, Antonius (Eds.) (1995). *The Dutch Annual of Psychoanalysis: 1995-1996. Vol. 2: Traumatisation and War*. Amsterdam: Swetz and Zeitlinger.

1806 Prince, Robert M. (1975). *Psychohistorical themes in the lives of young adult children of concentration camp survivors*. Unpublished doctoral dissertation, Columbia University, New York, 339 pp. *Dissertation Abstracts International*, 36(3-B), p. 1453. (University Microfilms no. AAC 75-18431)

1807 Prince, Robert M. (1980). A case study of a psychohistorical figure: The influence of the Holocaust on identity. In: Quaytman, Wilfred (Ed.), *Holocaust Survivors: Psychological and Social Sequelae*. New York: Human Sciences Press, pp. 44-60. [Published as a special issue of *Journal of Contemporary Psychotherapy*, 11(1)].

1808 Prince, Robert M. (1985). Knowing the Holocaust. *Psychoanalytic Inquiry*, 5(1), 51-61.

1809 Prince, Robert M. (1985). Second generation effects of historical trauma. *Psychoanalytic Review*, 72(1), 9-29.

1810 Proctor, Robert N. (1988). *Racial Hygiene: Medicine Under the Nazis*. Cambridge, MA: Harvard University Press. 414 p.

1811 Proctor, Robert N. (1994). Racial hygiene: The collaboration of medicine and Nazism. In: Michalcyzk, John J. (Ed.), *Medicine, Ethics, and the Third Reich: Historical and Contemporary Issues*. Kansas City, MO: Sheed & Ward, pp. 35-41.

1812 Pross, Christian (1988). *Wiedergutmachung: Der Kleinkrieg gegen die Opfer* [Compensation: The Small War Against the Victim]. Frankfurt am Main: Athenäum. 384 pp.

1813 Pross, Christian (1991). Breaking through the post-war coverup of Nazi doctors in Germany. *Journal of Medical Ethics*, 17(supplement), 13-16.

1814 Pross, Christian (1992). German medicine and historical truth. In: Annas, George J., and Grodin, Michael A. (Eds.), *The Nazi Doctors and the Nuremberg Code: Human Rights in Human Experimentation*. New York: Oxford University Press, pp. 32-52.

1815 Prozozorovskii, V.I., and Panfilenko, O.A. (1985). Rol' sovetskoi sudebno-meditsinskoi ekspertizy v rassledovanii Rashistskikh prestuplenii, sovershennykh v period Velikoi Otechesvennoi voiny [The role of Soviet forensic medical expertise in investigating the fascist crimes committed during World War II]. *Sudebno Meditsinskaia Ekspertiza*, 28(2), 11-13.

1816 Przychodzki, Michał (1978). Martyrologia lekarzy wielkopolskich podczas okupacji hitlerowskie [Physicians from the "greater Poland" region during the Nazi occupation - a martyrdom]. *Przegląd Lekarski*, 35(1), 116-131.

1817 Quaytman, Wilfred (Ed.) (1980). *Holocaust Survivors: Psychological and Social Sequelae*. New York: Human Sciences Press. 85 pp. [Published as a special issue of *Journal of Contemporary Psychotherapy*, 11(1)].

1818 Quindeau, Illka, and Hughes, Jula (1994). Narration as a construction of identity. In: Kestenberg, Judith S., and Fogelman, Eva (Eds.), *Children during the Nazi Reign: Psychological Perspective on the Interview Process*. Westport, CT: Praeger, pp. 35-53.

1819 Rabinowitz, Dorothy (1976). *New Lives: Survivors of the Holocaust Living in America*. New York: Alfred A. Knopf. 242 pp.

1820 Rabkin, Leslie (1975). Countertransference in the extreme situation: The family therapy of survivor families. In: Wolberg, Lewis R., and Aronson, Marvin L. (Eds.), *Group Therapy, 1975: An Overview*. New York: Stratton Intercontinental.

1821 Radil-Weiss, Tomas (1983). Men in extreme conditions: Some medical and psychological aspects of the Auschwitz concentration camp. *Psychiatry*, 46(3), 259-269.

1822 Radil-Weiss, Tomas (1985). Po 40 letech: Psychologicke aspekty demoralizace a dehumanizace za fasismu a pouceni dnesek [After 40 years: Psychological aspects of demoralization and dehumanism during fascism and instructions for today]. *Ceskoslovenska Psychologie*, 29(1), 1-9.

1823 Radujkat-Faist, Z. (1984). Prva godina lekarskog rade u logoru. I Medicinski aspekti zivota u Staroj Gradiski [The first year's medical activity in a concentration camp: Medical aspects of life in Stara-Gradiska]. *Medicinski Pregled*, 37(11-12), 573-576.

1824 Radzynski, Annie (1988). Auschwitz, un signifiant sans representation: Transmission et structuration symbolique [Auschwitz, a signifier without representation: Transmission and symbolic structuring]. *Patio*, 11, 105-114.

1825 Rakoff, Vivian (1966). Long-term effects of the concentration camp experience. *Viewpoints: Labor Zionist Movement of Canada*, 1, 17-22.

1826 Rakoff, Vivian; Sigal, John J.; and Epstein, Nathan (1966). Children and families of concentration camp survivors. *Canada's Mental Health*, 14, 24-26.

1827 Rappaport, Ernest A. (1968). Beyond traumatic neurosis: A psychoanalytic study of late reactions to concentration camp trauma. *International Journal of Psycho-Analysis*, 49, 719-731.

1828 Rappaport, Ernest A. (1971). Survivor guilt. *Midstream*, 17(7), 41-47.

1829 Rappoport, Leon, and Kren, George (1993). Amoral rescuers: The ambiguities of altruism. *Creativity Research Journal*, 6(1-2), 129-136.

1830 Rappaport, Sandra (1991). *Coping and adaptation to massive psychic trauma: Case studies of Nazi Holocaust survivors*. Unpublished doctoral dissertation, The Union Institute, Cincinnati, Ohio, 295 pp. *Dissertation Abstracts International*, 52(8-B), p. 4479. (University Microfilms no. AAC 9202325).

1831 Raveau, François (1960). Neuropsychiatric data on the state of health of former deportees fifteen years after their liberation. In: *Experts Meeting on the Effects of Imprisonment and Deportation, Oslo*. Paris: World Veterans Federation, pp. 79-88.

1832 Reich, Stéphane (1955). Ohrenkrankheitsfolgen. Einige Aspekte der durch Verletzung entstandenen Taubheit bei den ehemaligen Deportierten [Sequelae of ear diseases. Some aspects of deafness caused by trauma in ex-deportees]. In: Michel, Max (Ed.), *Gesundheitsschäden durch Verfolgung und Gefangenschaft und ihre Spätfolgen: Zusammenstellung der Referate und Ergebnisse der Internationalen Sozialmedizinischen Konferenz über die Pathologie der Ehemaligen Deportierten und Internierten, 5-7 Juni 1954 in Kopenhagen* [Health Damages Caused by Persecution and Captivity and the Late Effects: Compilation of the Papers and Results of the International Conference of Social Medicine on the Pathology of Former Deported and Interned Persons, 5-7 June 1954 in Copenhagen]. Frankfurt am Main: Röderberg, pp. 216-224.

1833 Reijzer, Hans M. (1995). On having been in hiding. In: Groen-Prakken, Han; Ladan, Antoine; and Stufkens, Antonius (Eds.), *The Dutch Annual of Psychoanalysis: 1995-1996. Vol. 2: Traumatisation and War*. Amsterdam: Swets & Zeitlinger, pp. 96-117.

1834 Reinhardt, Olaf (1990). The "Nazi doctors" debate. *Medical Journal of Australia*, 153(11-12), 645-647.

1835 Reitoft, E. (1990). Concentration camp syndrome. *Sygeplejersken*, 90(14), 4-8.

1836 Rewerts, G. (1959). Die akuten neurologischen Syndrome bein Hungernden [The acute neurological syndromes of the starving individual]. In: Schench, E.G., and Nathusius, W. von (Eds.), *Extrem Lebensverhältnisse und ihre Folgen. Bericht über den 4. Ärztekongress für Pathologie, Therapie und Begutachtung der Heimkehrerkrankheiten in Düsseldorf, 1959* [Extreme Life Conditions and Their Effects. Report on the 4th Physicians Conference on Pathology, Therapy and Survey of Returnees' Diseases in Dusseldorf, 1959]. Verband der Heimkehrer, pp. 128-172.

1837 Rexer, Martin, and Rüdenburg, Bodo (1992). Zwiefalten as "halfway house" on the road to Grafeneck. In: Jockush, Ulrich, and Scholz, Lothar (Eds.), *Administered Killings at the Time of National Socialism: Involvement, Suppression, Responsibility of Psychiatry and Judicial System*. Regensburg: Roderer, pp. 110-146.

1838 Rexer, Martin, and Rüdenburg, Bodo (1992). Zwiefalten als Zwischenanstalt auf dem Weg nach Grafeneck [Zwiefalten as "halfway house" on the road to Grafeneck]. In: Jockush, Ulrich, and Scholz, Lothar (Eds.), *Verwaltetes Morden im Nationalsozialismus: Verstrickung, Verdrängung, Verantwortung von Psychiatrie und Justiz* [Administered Killings at the Time of National Socialism: Involvement, Suppression, Responsibility of Psychiatry and Judicial System]. Regensburg: Roderer, pp. 119-156.

1839 Rich, Melina S. (1982). *Children of Holocaust survivors: A concurrent validity study of a survivor family typology*. Unpublished doctoral dissertation, California School of Professional Psychology, Berkeley, 133 pp. *Dissertation Abstracts International*, 43(5-B), p. 1626. (University Microfilms no. AAC 822353).

1840 Richartz, M. (1978). Zur Frage der wesentlichen Mitverursachung schizophrener Psychosen durch verfolgungsbedingte Extrembelastungen [The question of contribution to schizophrenia psychoses by extreme stress caused by persecution]. In: *Medizinische Untersuchungen der Spätfolgen des Krieges und des NS-Regimes bei Jugendlichen und Kindern von ehemaligen KZ-Häftlingen und Verfolgten* [Medical Research of the Late Effects of the War and National Socialism Regime on Youth and Children of Former Concentration Camp Inmates and Persecuted Persons]. Wien: Internationale Föderation der Widerstandskämpfer. [VI Internationaler Medizinischer Kongress der FIR. Prague, 1976].

1841 Richet, Charles (1945). Notes médicales sur le camp de Buchenwald en 1944-1945 [Medical notes on the Buchenwald camp]. *Bulletin de l'Academie de Médecine*, 129, 377-388.

1842 Richet, Charles (1960). Introduction. In: *Experts Meeting on the Later Effects of Imprisonment and Deportation, Oslo*. Paris: World Veterans Federation, pp. 7-11.

1843 Richet, Charles (1961). Opening session: Introduction. In: *International Conference on the Later Effects of Imprisonment and Deportation Organized by the World Veterans Federation. The Hague, November 20-25, 1961*. The Hague: World Veterans Federation, pp. 23-26.

1844 Richet, Charles; Gilbert-Dreyfuss, H.; Fichez, Louis F.; and Uzan, H. (1955). Die Folgeerscheinungen des physiologischen Elendszustandes [The sequelae of physiological suffering]. In: Michel, Max (Ed.), *Gesundheitsschäden durch Verfolgung und Gefangenschaft und ihre Spätfolgen: Zusammenstellung der Referate und Ergebnisse der Internationalen Sozialmedizinischen Konferenz über die Pathologie der Ehemaligen Deportierten und Internierten, 5-7 Juni 1954 in Kopenhagen* [Health Damages Caused by Persecution and Captivity and the Late Effects: Compilation of the Papers and Results of the International Conference of Social Medicine on the Pathology of Former Deported and Interned Persons, 5-7 June 1954 in Copenhagen]. Frankfurt am Main: Röderberg, pp. 73-81.

1845 Richet, Charles, and Mans, Antonin (1956). *Pathologie de la déportation* [The Pathology of Deportation]. Paris: Plon. 288 pp.

1846 Richet, Charles, and Mans, Antonin (1960). Delayed cardiovascular aftereffects among former deportees. In: *Experts Meeting on the Later Effects of Imprisonment and Deportation, Oslo*. Paris: World Veterans Federation, pp. 13-19.

1847 Richet, Charles; Parisot; Desoille, Henri; Ellenbogen, Raphael; Fichez, Louis F.; Gallet; Gilbert-Dreyfuss, H.; Mans, Antonin; Segelle; and Uzan, H. (1955). Les séquelles de la misère chez l'adulte [The effects of misery in adults]. *Bulletin de l'Academie de Médecine*, 139, 245-250.

1848 Richman, Liliane (1975). From the family album. In: Steinitz, Lucy Y., and Szonyi, David M. (Eds.), *Living After the Holocaust: Reflections by the Post-War Generation*. New York: Bloch, pp. 131-135.

1849 Rieck, Miriam (1994). The psychological state of Holocaust survivors' offspring: An epidemiological and psychodiagnostic study. *International Journal of Behavioral Development*, 17(4), 649-667.

1850 Rieck, Miriam, and Eitinger, Leo (1983). Controlled psychodiagnostic studies of survivors of the Holocaust and their children. *Israel Journal of Psychiatry and Related Disciplines*, 20(4), 312-324.

1851 Riis, Povl (1980). The many faces of inhumanity - and the few faces of its psychic and somatic sequelae. *Danish Medical Bulletin*, 27(5), 213-214.

1852 Rim, Yeshayahu (1991). Coping styles of (first- and second-generation) Holocaust survivors. *Personality and Individual Differences*, 12(12), 1315-1317.

1853 Ringelheim, Joan M. (1991). Women and the Holocaust: A reconsideration of research. In: Baskin, Judith R. (Ed.), *Jewish Women in Historical Perspective*. Detroit, MI: Wayne State University Press, pp. 243-264.

1854 Rittner, Carol, and Myers, Sondra (Eds.). (1986). *The Courage to Care: Rescuers of Jews during the Holocaust*. New York: New York University Press. 158 pp.

1855 Rittner, Carol, and Roth, John K. (Eds.) (1993). *Different Voices: Women and the Holocaust*. New York: Paragon House. 435 pp.

1856 Robinson, Shalom (1979). Holocaust survivors' attitudes toward death. In: de Vries, Andre, and Carmi, Amnon (Eds.), *The Dying Human*. Ramat Gan, Israel: Turtledove, pp. 1-8.

1857 Robinson, Shalom (1979). Late effects of persecution in persons who as young children or young adolescents survived Nazi occupation in Europe. *Israel Annals of Psychiatry and Related Disciplines*, 17(3), 209-214.

1858 Robinson, Shalom (1990). Psychology of survivors in Israel. In: Gutman, Israel (Ed.), *Encyclopedia of the Holocaust. Vol. 4*. New York: Macmillan, pp. 1431-1432.

1859 Robinson, Shalom (Ed.) (1992-1995). *Echoes of the Holocaust*, 1-4, [Published irregularly by Center for Research into the Late Effects of the Holocaust, Talbieh Mental Health Center. Jerusalem, Israel].

1860 Robinson, Shalom; Adler, I.; and Metzer, Sara (1995). A comparison between elderly Holocaust survivors and people who survived the Holocaust as children. *Echoes of the Holocaust*, 4, 22-29. [Bulletin of the Jerusalem Center for Research into the Late

Effects of the Holocaust, Talbieh Mental Health Center. Jerusalem, Israel].

1861 Robinson, Shalom, and Dasberg, Haim (1988). Tguvot l'mishpat Demyanyuk etzel psychoterapistism ou'metupaleihem [Therapists' and patients' reactions to the Demjanjuk trial]. *Sihot: Israel Journal of Psychotherapy*, 4, 21-25.

1862 Robinson, Shalom, and Dasberg, Haim (1992). The effect of the Treblinka testimonies in Jerusalem 1987 on patients and therapists. *Echoes of the Holocaust*, 1, 13-26. [Bulletin of the Jerusalem Center for Research into the Late Effects of the Holocaust. Talbieh Mental Health Center, Jerusalem, Israel].

1863 Robinson, Shalom, and Hemmendinger, Judith (1982). Psychosocial adjustment 30 years later of people who were in Nazi concentration camps as children. In: Spielberger, Charles D.; Sarason, Irwin G; and Milgram, Norman (Eds.), *Stress and Anxiety. Vol. 8.* Washington, D.C.: Hemisphere, pp. 397-399.

1864 Robinson, Shalom; Hemmendinger, Judith; Netanel, R.; Rapaport, Michal; Zilberman, L.; and Gal, A. (1994). Retraumatization of Holocaust survivors during the Gulf War and SCUD missile attacks on Israel. *British Journal of Medical Psychology*, 67(4), 353-362.

1865 Robinson, Shalom; Netanel, R.; and Rapaport, Judith (1992). Reactions of Holocaust survivors to the Gulf war and SCUD missile attacks on Israel. *Echoes of the Holocaust*, 1, 1-12. [Bulletin of the Jerusalem Center for Research into the Late Effects of the Holocaust. Talbieh Mental Health Center. Jerusalem, Israel].

1866 Robinson, Shalom; Rapaport, Judith; Durst, Natan; and Rapaport, Michal (1990). The late effects of Nazi persecution among elderly Holocaust survivors. *Acta Psychiatrica Scandinavica*, 82(4), 311-315.

1867 Robinson, Shalom; Rapaport-Bar-Sever, Michal; and Metzer, Sara (1994). The feelings of Holocaust survivors towards their persecutors. *Echoes of the Holocaust*, 3, 9-20. [Bulletin of the Jerusalem Center for Research into the Late Effects of the Holocaust, Talbieh Mental Health Center, Jerusalem, Israel].

1868 Robinson, Shalom; Rapaport-Bar-Sever, Michal; and Rapaport, Judith (1993). Child survivors of the Holocaust: Their present mental state and coping. A preliminary report. *Echoes of the Holocaust*, 2, 24-30. [Bulletin of the Jerusalem Center for Research into the Late Effects of the Holocaust. Talbieh Mental Health Center, Jerusalem, Israel].

1869 Robinson, Shalom; Rapaport-Bar-Sever, Michal; and Rapaport, Judith (1994). The present state of people who survived the Holocaust as children. *Acta Psychiatrica Scandinavica*, 89(4), 242-245.

1870 Robinson, Shalom; Rebaudengo-Rosco, P.; and Rapaport, Michal (1993). Effetti tardivi del trauma psichico massivo. I sopravvissut; all'Olocausto 50 anni dopo [Late effects of massive psychic trauma: Holocaust survivors 50 years later]. *Minerva Psichiatrica*, 34(1), 57-63.

1871 Robinson, Shalom, and Winnik, Heinrich Z. (1981). Second generation of the Holocaust. Holocaust survivors' communication of experience to their children and its effects. *Israel Journal of Psychiatry and Related Sciences*, 18(2), 99-107.

1872 Roden, Rudolph G. (1982). Suicide and Holocaust survivors. *Israel Journal of Psychiatry and Related Sciences*, 19(2), 129-135.

1873 Roden, Rudolph G. (1985). Sexuality and the Holocaust survivor. *Israel Journal of Psychiatry and Related Sciences*, 22(3), 211-220.

1874 Roden, Rudolph G., and Roden, M.M. (1982). Children of Holocaust survivors. *Adolescent Psychiatry*, 10, 66-72.

1875 Rogan, Bjorn (1960). Criteria to be considered for the evaluation of disability. In: *Experts Meetings on the Later Effects of Imprisonment and Deportation, Oslo*. Paris: World Veterans Federation.

1876 Rogan, Bjorn (1960). Short survey of an investigation carried out in Norway on medical problems of camp survivors. In: *Experts Meeting on the Later Effects of Imprisonment and Deportation, Oslo*. Paris: World Veterans Federation, pp. 99-106.

1877 Rogan, Bjorn (1961). Sosiale og yrkesmessige forhold hos tidligere konsentrasjonsleirfanger [Social and professional problems of ex-concentration camp prisoners]. *Tidsskrift for den Norske Laegeforening. Journal of the Norwegian Medical Association*, 81, 812-815.

1878 Rogan, Bjorn (1961). Study of a group of former Norwegian deportees. Part 6: Social and vocational problems of ex-concentration camp prisoners. In: *International Conference on the Later Effects of Imprisonment and Deportation Organized by the World Veterans Federation*. The Hague, November 20-25, 1961. The Hague: World Veterans Federation, pp. 162-166.

1879 Roland, Charles (1992). *Courage Under Siege: Starvation, Disease and Death in the Warsaw Ghetto*. Oxford: Oxford University Press. 310 pp.

1880 Roland, Charles (1992). An underground medical school in the Warsaw ghetto, 1941-1942. *Medical History*, 33, 399-419.

1881 Roland, Charles (1994). Creativity in the face of disaster: Medicine in the Warsaw ghetto. In: Michalczyk, John J. (Ed.), *Medicine, Ethics, and the Third Reich: Historical and Contemporary Issues*. Kansas City, MO: Sheed & Ward, pp. 153-160.

1882 Rose, H.K. (1978). Zur Frage der wesentlichen Mitverursachung schizophrener Psychosen durch verfolgungsbedingte Extrembelastungen [The problem of causal relationship between schizophrenic psychoses and extreme stress caused by persecution]. In: *Medizinische Untersuchungen der Spätfolgen des Krieges und des NS-Regimes bei Jugendlichen und Kindern von ehemaligen KZ-Häftlingen und Verfolgten* [Medical Research of the Late Effects of the War and National Socialism Regime on Youth and Children of Former Concentration Camp Inmates and Persecuted Persons]. Wien: Internationale Föderation der Widerstandskämpfer. [VI Internationaler Medizinischer Kongress der FIR. Prague, 1976].

1883 Rose, Susan L. (1983). *Adaptive behavior and coping among children of Holocaust survivors: Controlled comparative investigation*. Unpublished doctoral dissertation, Ohio University, Athens, 266 pp. *Dissertation Abstracts International*, 44(9-B), p. 2905. (University Microfilms no. AAC 8329150).

1884 Rose, Susan L., and Garske, John (1987). Family environment, adjustment, and coping among children of Holocaust survivors: A comparative investigation. *American Journal of Orthopsychiatry*, 57(3), 332-344.

1885 Rosen, Jules; Reynolds, Charles F.; Yeager, Amy L.; Houck, Patricia R.; and Hurwitz, Linda F. (1991). Sleep disturbances in survivors of the Nazi Holocaust. *American Journal of Psychiatry*, 148(1), 62-66.

1886 Rosenbaum, Julie F. (1993). *Female experiences during the Holocaust*. Unpublished master's thesis, Boston College, Chestnut Hill, Massachusetts, 204 pp. *Masters Abstracts International*, 31(4), p. 1618. (University Microfilms no. ACC 1353166).

1887 Rosenberg, Jerome (1984). Holocaust survivors and post-traumatic stress disorders: The need for conceptual reassessment and development. *Journal of Sociology and Social Welfare*, 11(4), 930-938.

1888 Rosenberger, L. (1973). Children of survivors. In: Anthony, E. James, and Koupernik, Cyrille (Eds.), *The Child in His Family. Vol. 2: The Impact of Disease and Death*. New York: John Wiley & Sons, pp. 375-377.

1889 Rosenbloom, Maria (1983). Implications of the Holocaust for social work. *Social Casework*, 65(4), 205-213.

1890 Rosenbloom, Maria (1985). The Holocaust survivor in late life. *Journal of Gerontological Social Work*, 8(3-4), 181-191.

1891 Rosenbloom, Maria (1988). Lessons of the Holocaust for mental health practice. In: Braham, Randolph L. (Ed.), *The Psychological Perspectives of the Holocaust and of its Aftermath*. Boulder, CO: Social Sciences Monographs; and New York: Csengeri Institute for Holocaust Studies of the Graduate School of the City University of New York, pp. 145-159.

1892 Rosenbloom, Maria (1991). Bearing witness by Holocaust survivors: Implications for mental health theory and practice. In: Berger, Alan L. (Ed.), *Bearing Witness to the Holocaust, 1939-1989*. Lewiston, NY: Edwin Mellen, pp. 341-352.

1893 Rosenbloom, Maria (1995). Implications of the Holocaust for social work. *Families in Society*, 76(9), 567-576.

1894 Rosenfeld, David (1985). Identificacion y sus vicisitudes en relacion con el fenomeno nazi [Identification and its vicissitudes in connection with the Nazi phenomenon]. *Revista de Psicoanalisis*, 42(4), 767-780.

1895 Rosenfeld, David (1986). Identification and its vicissitudes in relation to the Nazi phenomenon. *International Journal of Psycho-Analysis*, 67(1), 53-64.

1896 Rosenkotter, Lutz (1979). Schatten der Zeitgeschichte auf psychoanalytischen Behandlungen [Shadow of history upon psychoanalytic therapy]. *Psyche: Zeitschrift für Psychoanalyse und ihre Anwendungen*, 33(11), 1024-1028.

1897 Rosenman, Stanley (1982). Compassion versus contempt toward Holocaust victims: Difficulties in attaining an adaptive identity in an annihilative world. *Israel Journal of Psychiatry and Related Sciences*, 19(1), 39-73.

1898 Rosenman, Stanley (1984). Out of the Holocaust: Children as scarred souls and tempered redeemers. *Journal of Psychohistory*, 11(4), 555-567.

1899 Rosenman, Stanley (1984). The psychoanalytic writer on the Holocaust and Bettelheim. *American Journal of Social Psychiatry*, 4(2), 62-71.

1900 Rosenman, Stanley, and Handelsman, Irving (1990). The collective past, group psychology and personal narrative: Shaping Jewish identity by memoirs of the Holocaust. *American Journal of Psychoanalysis*, 50(2), 151-170.

1901 Rosenman, Stanley, and Handelsman, Irving (1990). Identity as legacy of the Holocaust: Encountering a survivor's narrative. *Journal of Psychohistory*, 18(1), 35-69.

1902 Rosenman, Stanley, and Handelsman, Irving (1992). Rising from the ashes: Modelling resiliency in a community devastated by man-made catastrophe. *American Imago*, 49(2), 185-226.

1903 Rosenthal, Gabriele, and Bar-On, Dan (1992). A biographical case study of a victimizer's daughter's strategy. *Journal of Narrative and Life History*, 2(2), 105-127.

1904 Rosenthal, Perihan A., and Rosenthal, Stuart (1980). Holocaust effect in the third generation: Child of another time. *American Journal of Psychotherapy*, 34(4), 572-580.

1905 Rosenwald, George C., and Ochberg, Richard L. (Eds.) (1992). *Storied Lives: The Cultural Politics of Self-Understanding*. New Haven, CT: Yale University Press. 304 pp.

1906 Rotenberg, Larry (1985). A child survivor/psychiatrist's personal adaptation. *Journal of the American Academy of Child Psychiatry*, 24(4), 385-389.

1907 Roth, Sheldon (1993). The shadow of the Holocaust. In: Moses, Rafael (Ed.), *Persistent Shadows of the Holocaust: The Meaning to Those Not Directly Affected*. Madison, CT: International Universities Press, pp. 37-64.

1908 Rothman, David J. (1995). Medicine and the Holocaust: Learning more of the lessons. *Annals of Internal Medicine*, 122(10), 793-794.

1909 Rozen, Roland (1983). *Depression and anxiety in Holocaust survivors*. Unpublished doctoral dissertation, California School of Professional Psychology, Los Angeles, 136 pp. *Dissertation Abstracts International*, 44(11-B), p. 3540. (University Microfilms no. AAC 8400528).

1910 Rubenstein, Richard L. (1984). The victim as a non-person. *Journal of Psychohistory*, 11(4), 545-554.

1911 Rubinstein, Israel (1981). *Multigenerational occurrence of survivor syndrome symptoms in the families of Holocaust survivors*. Unpublished doctoral dissertation, California School of Professional Psychology, Fresno, 159 pp. *Dissertation Abstracts International*, 42(10-B), p. 4209. (University Microfilms no. AAC 8207545).

1912 Rubinstein, Israel; Cutter, Fred; and Templer, Donald I. (1990). Multigenerational occurrence of survivors syndrome symptoms in families of Holocaust survivors. *Omega Journal of Death and Dying*, 20(3), 239-244.

1913 Rudowski, W. (1983). The last illness of General Stefan Grot-Rowecki (1895-1944). *Archiwum Historii Medycyny*, 46(4), 475-480.

1914 Rumke, H.C. (1951). Late werkingen van psychotraumata [Late consequences of psychic trauma]. *Nederlands Tijdschrift voor Geneeskunde*, 95, 2928-2937.

1915 Rusinek, Kazimierz (1979). Uroczystości w Mauthausen ku czci lekarzy. Dr. Wladyslaw Czapliński [Ceremony at Mauthausen in honor of interred physicians. Dr. Wladyslaw Czaplinski]. *Przegląd Lekarski*, 36(1), 124-131.

1916 Russell, Axel (1974). Late psychosocial consequences in concentration camp survivors families. *American Journal of Orthopsychiatry*, 44(4), 611-619.

1917 Russell, Axel (1980). Late effects - influence on children of concentration camp survivors. In: Dimsdale, Joel E. (Ed.), *Survivors, Victims, and Perpetrators: Essays on the Nazi Holocaust*. Washington, D.C.: Hemisphere, pp. 175-204.

1918 Russell, Axel (1982). Family/marital therapy with second generation Holocaust survivor families, questions and answers. In: Gurman,

Alan S. (Ed.), *The Practice of Family Therapy. Vol. 2*. New York: Brunner/Mazel, pp. 233-237.

1919 Russell, Axel (1982). Late psychosocial consequences of the Holocaust experience on survivor families: The second generation. *International Journal of Family Psychiatry*, 3(3), 375-402.

1920 Russell, Axel (1983). Effects of extreme stress: reflections on some long-term consequences of the Holocaust on second generation survivor families. In: *Abstracts: VII World Congress of Psychiatry*. Switzerland: Ciba-Geigy, pp. 546-550.

1921 Russell, Axel (1983). Some late psychosocial effects of the Holocaust on survivor families: The second generation. In: Charny, Israel W., and Davidson, Shamai (Eds.), *The Book of the International Conference on the Holocaust and Genocide. Book One: The Conference Program and Crisis*. Tel Aviv: The Institute of the International Conference on the Holocaust and Genocide, p. 232.

1922 Russell, Axel; Plotkin, Donna; and Heapy, Nelson (1985). Adaptive abilities in nonclinical second-generation Holocaust survivors and controls: A comparison. *American Journal of Psychotherapy*, 39(4), 564-579.

1923 Rustin, Stanley L. (1971). *Guilt, hostility and Jewish identification among a self-selected sample of adolescent children of Jewish concentration camp survivors: A descriptive study*. Unpublished doctoral dissertation, City University of New York. *Dissertation Abstracts International*, 32(3-B), p. 1859. (University Microfilms no. AAC 72-24810).

1924 Rustin, Stanley L. (1980). The legacy is loss. In: Quaytman, Wilfred (Ed.), *Holocaust Survivors: Psychological and Social Sequelae*. New York: Human Sciences Press, pp. 32-43. [Published as a special issue of *Journal of Contemporary Psychotherapy*, 11(1)].

1925 Rustin, Stanley L. (1988). A psychological examination of the survivors of the Holocaust and the generation after. In: Braham, Randolph L. (Ed.), *The Psychological Perspectives of the Holocaust and of its Aftermath*. Boulder, CO: Social Science Monographs; and New York: Csengeri Institute for Holocaust Studies of the Graduate School of the City University of New York, pp. 161-173.

1926 Rustin, Stanley L., and Lipsig, Florence (1972). Psychotherapy with the adolescent children of concentration camp survivors. *Journal of Contemporary Psychotherapy*, 4(2), 87-94.

1927 Rustow, Margrit (1989). From Jew to Catholic and back: Psychodynamics of child survivors. In: Marcus, Paul, and Rosenberg, Alan (Eds.), *Healing Their Wounds: Psychotherapy with Holocaust Survivors and Their Families*. New York: Praeger, pp. 271-286.

1928 Rybnicki, Abraham (1984). *Ify'unim psychologim b'kerev dor sheyni l'nitzoley shoah k'functziah shel midat hadimion hanitfas im hahorim* [Psychological characteristics of second generation Holocaust survivors as a function of perceived similarity with their parents]. Unpublished master's thesis, Department of Psychology, Tel Aviv University, Tel Aviv, Israel. 52 pp.

1929 Ryn, Zdzisław (1972). Czy Oświęcium jest nadal rzeczywistością? Refleksje psychiatrycne [Is Auschwitz far from reality? Psychiatric reflections]. *Przegląd Lekarski*, 29(1), 206-210.

1930 Ryn, Zdzisław (1977). Z badań nad zachorowalnością i śmiertelnością byłych wiezniów obozów koncentracyjnych [Research in mortality and morbidity of ex-concentration camp survivors]. *Przegląd Lekarski*, 34(1), 1-15.

1931 Ryn, Zdzisław (1978). Antoni Kepinski w obozie Miranda de Ebro [Antoni Kepinski at the Miranda de Ebro concentration camp]. *Przegląd Lekarski*, 35(1), 95-115.

1932 Ryn, Zdzisław (1978). Z psychologii i psychopatologii obozów koncentracyjnych i jenieckich. Przegląd piśmiennictwa zachodniego [On the psychology and psychopathology of the concentration camps: A survey of the Western literature]. *Przegląd Lekarski*, 35, 231-237.

1933 Ryn, Zdzisław (1981). Uwagi psychiatryczne o tzw KZ-syndromie [A psychiatrist's remarks on the so-called concentration camp syndrome]. *Przegląd Lekarski*, 38(10), 26-29.

1934 Ryn, Zdzisław (1983). Death and dying in the concentration camp. *American Journal of Social Psychiatry*, 3(3), 32-38.

1935 Ryn, Zdzisław (1983). The evolution of mental disturbances in the concentration camp syndrome. *Cahiers d'Informations Médicine, Sociales et Juridiques*, 19, 209-223.

1936 Ryn, Zdzisław (1985). Medycyna obozów koncentracyjnych i jenieckich w piśmiennictwie zachodnim [Medical aspects of concentration camps and prisoner of war camps in Western literature]. *Przegląd Lekarski*, 42(1), 196-201.

1937 Ryn, Zdzisław (1985). Psychopatologia głodu w obozie koncentracyjnym [Psychopathology of hunger in concentration camps]. *Przegląd Lekarski*, 42(1), 41-55.

1938 Ryn, Zdzisław (1986). Suicides in the Nazi concentration camps. *Suicide and Life Threatening Behavior*, 16(4), 419-433.

1939 Ryn, Zdzisław (1987). Die Dynamik der psychischen Störungen beim KZ-Syndrom [The dynamics of psychic disturbances in the concentration camp syndrome]. In: Hamburger Institut für Sozialforschung (Eds.), *Die Auschwitz-Hefte. Texte der polnischen Zeitschrift "Przegląd Lekarski" über historische, psychische und medizinische Aspekte des Lebens und Sterbens in Auschwitz. Band 2* [The Auschwitz Journal. Text of the Polish Journal "Medical Review" on Historical, Psychic and Medical Aspects of Life and Death in Auschwitz. Volume 2]. Weinheim and Basel: Beltz, pp. 69-74.

1940 Ryn, Zdzisław (1987). Drei Geschwister im Lager: Eine klinische Analyse [Three sisters in a camp: A clinical analysis]. In: Hamburger Institut für Sozialforschung (Eds.), *Die Auschwitz-Hefte. Texte der polnischen Zeitschrift "Przegląd Lekarski" über historische, psychische und medizinische Aspekte des Lebens und Sterbens in Auschwitz. Band 2* [The Auschwitz Journal. Text of the Polish Journal "Medical Review" on Historical, Psychic and Medical Aspects of Life and Death in Auschwitz. Volume 2]. Weinheim and Basel: Beltz, pp. 89-96.

1941 Ryn, Zdzisław (1987). KZ syndrom u więźniów obozu koncentracynego Miranda de Ebro [The KZ syndrome (concentration camp syndrome) in prisoners of the Miranda de Ebro concentration camp]. *Przegląd Lekarski*, 44(1), 34-44.

1942 Ryn, Zdzisław (1987). Wdowy po więźniach obozów koncentracyjnych. Studium psychologiczne i społeczne [Widows of prisoners in concentration camps: Psychological and social studies]. *Przegląd Lekarski*, 44(1), 14-34.

1943 Ryn, Zdzisław (1990). Der Alptraum geht weiter. Das Nachleben der Okkupationszeit in den überlebenden und ihren Nachkommen [The nightmares continue: Life after the German occupation as lived by concentration camp survivors and their descendants]. *Psyche: Zeitschrift für Psychoanalyse und ihre Anwendungen*, 44(2), 101-117.

1944 Ryn, Zdzisław (1990). Between life and death: Experiences of concentration camp mussulmen during the Holocaust. *Genetic, Social, and General Psychology Monographs*, 116(1), 5-19.

1945 Ryn, Zdzisław (1990). The evolution of mental disturbances in the concentration camp syndrome. *Social and General Psychology Monographs*, 116(1), 21-36.

1946 Ryn, Zdzisław (1992). Widows of victims of Nazi concentration camps: Their pathology. *Acta Psiquiatrica y Psicologica de America Latina*, 38(3), 223-228.

1947 Ryn, Zdzisław, and Kłodziński, Stanisław (1974). Patologia sportu w obozie koncentracyjnym Oświęcim-Brzezinka [Pathology of sport at the Auschwitz-Birkenau concentration camp]. *Przegląd Lekarski*, 31(1), 46-48.

1948 Ryn, Zdzisław, and Kłodziński, Stanisław (1976). Z problematyki samobójstwa w hitlerowskich obozach koncentracyjnych [The problem of suicides in Nazi concentration camps]. *Przegląd Lekarski*, 33(1), 25-46.

1949 Ryn, Zdzislaw, and Kłodziński, Stanisław (1984). Głod w obozie koncentracyjnym [Hunger in the concentration camp]. *Przegląd Lekarski*, 41(1), 21-37.

1950 Ryn, Zdzislaw, and Kłodziński, Stanisław (1986). Postawy i czyny heroiczne w obozach koncentracyjnych [Attitudes and heroic actions in concentration camps]. *Przegląd Lekarski*, 43(1), 28-45.

1951 Ryn, Zdzisław, and Kłodziński, Stanisław (1987). An der Grenze zwischen Leben und Tod. Eine Studie über die Erscheinung des "Muselmanns" im Konzentrationslager [At the border between life and death. A study of the appearance of "musselman" in concentration camps]. In: Hamburger Institut für Sozialforschung (Eds.), *Die Auschwitz-Hefte. Texte der polnischen Zeitschrift "Przegląd Lekarski" über historische, psychische und medizinische Aspekte des Lebens und Sterbens in Auschwitz. Band 1* [The Auschwitz Journal. Text of the Polish Journal "Medical Review" on Historical, Psychic and Medical Aspects of Life and Death in Auschwitz. Volume 1]. Weinheim and Basel: Beltz, pp. 89-154.

1952 Ryn, Zdzisław, and Kłodziński, Stanisław (1987). Hunger im Konzentrationslager [Hunger in concentration camps]. In: Hamburger Institut für Sozialforschung (Eds.), *Die Auschwitz-Hefte. Texte der polnischen Zeitschrift "Przegląd Lekarski" über historische, psychische und medizinische Aspekte des Lebens und Sterbens in Auschwitz. Band 1* [The Auschwitz Journal. Text of the Polish Journal "Medical Review" on Historical, Psychic and Medical Aspects of Life and Death in Auschwitz. Volume 1]. Weinheim and Basel: Beltz, pp. 241-260.

1953 Ryn, Zdzisław, and Kłodziński, Stanisław (1987). Zur Psychopathologie von Hunger und Hungererleben im Konzentrationslager [The psychopathology of hunger and its experience in concentration camps]. In: Hamburger Institut für Sozialforschung (Eds.), *Die Auschwitz-Hefte. Texte der polnischen Zeitschrift "Przegląd Lekarski" über historische, psychische und medizinische Aspekte des Lebens und Sterbens in Auschwitz. Band 2* [The Auschwitz Journal. Text of the Polish Journal "Medical Review" on Historical, Psychic and Medical Aspects of Life and Death in Auschwitz. Volume 2]. Weinheim and Basel: Beltz, pp. 113-133.

1954 Ryn, Zdzisław, and Kłodziński, Stanisław (1987). Tod und Sterben im Konzentrationslager [Death and dying in concentration camps]. In: Hamburger Institut für Sozialforschung (Eds.), *Die Auschwitz-Hefte. Texte der polnischen Zeitschrift "Przegląd Lekarski" über historische, psychische und medizinische Aspekte des Lebens und Sterbens in Auschwitz. Band 1* [The Auschwitz Journal. Text of the Polish Journal "Medical Review" on Historical, Psychic and Medical Aspects of Life and Death in Auschwitz. Volume 1]. Weinheim and Basel: Beltz, pp. 281-328.

1955 Sachs, Hagai (1988). *Hakesher beyn hahistaglut v'halechidut hamishpachtit l'beyn haharada v'hadic'aon b'kerev tze'atzey nitzoley shoah* [The relationship between family adaptability and cohesion levels, and anxiety and depression levels in Holocaust survivor's offspring]. Unpublished master's thesis, Department of Psychology, Tel Aviv University, Tel Aviv, Israel. 89 pp.

1956 Sachs, Lisbeth J., and Titievsky, Jaime (1967). On identification with the aggressor: A clinical note. *Israel Annals of Psychiatry and Related Disciplines*, 5, 181-184.

1957 Safford, Florence (1995). Aging stressors for Holocaust survivors and their families. *Journal of Gerontological Social Work*, 24(1-2), 131-153.

1958 Sagy, Shifa, and Antonovsky, Helen (1996). Structural sources of the sense of coherence: Two life stories of Holocaust survivors in Israel. *Israel Journal of Medical Sciences*, 32(3-4), 200-205.

1959 Salamon, Michael J. (1994). Denial and acceptance: Coping and defense mechanisms. In: Brink, Terry L. (Ed.), *Holocaust Survivors' Mental Health*. New York: Haworth, pp. 17-25. [Published as a special issue of *Clinical Gerontologist*, 14(3).]

1960 Saller, Karl (1964). Gutachten über vorzeitige Entpflichtung Verfolgter des Naziregimes [Expert statement on premature retirement of Nazi persecutees]. In: *Ätio-Pathogenese und Therapie der Erschöpfung und vorzeitigen Vergreisung* [The Aetiology, Pathogenesis and Therapy of Exhaustion and Premature Aging]. Wien: Verlag der FIR, pp. 568-572. [IV Internationaler Medizinischer Kongress. Bucharest, 22-27 Juni 1964].

1961 Saller, Karl (1970). Racial murder and the mad hero-worship of National Socialism. In: *Auschwitz Anthology. Vol. 1: Inhumane Medicine. Part 1*. Warsaw: International Auschwitz Committee, pp. 85-122.

1962 Saller, Karl (1971). Erb- und Umwelteinflüsse bei "Anlageleiden" [The influence of genetics and environment in diseases "caused by" disposition]. In: Herberg, Hans-Joachim (Ed.), *Spätschäden nach Extrembelastungen* [Late Damage After Extreme Stress]. Herford: Nicolai, pp. 13-20. [II Internationalen Medizinisch-Juristischen Konferenz. Dusseldorf, 1969].

1963 Sandler, Joseph (1967). Trauma, strain and development. In: Furst, Sidney S. (Ed.), *Psychic Trauma*. New York: Basic Books, pp. 154-174.

1964 Sarid, Orly (1990). *Hitachasut shel yisraelim-yehudim l'kvutzot miyutim: Arachim mool pragmatiyut* [Attitudes of Jewish Israelis to minority groups: Values versus pragmatism]. Unpublished master's thesis, Bob Shapell School of Social Work, Tel Aviv University, Tel Aviv, Israel. 183 pp.

1965 Sarnecki, Józef (1966). Konflikty emocjonalne osób urodzonych lub więźnionych w dziecinstwie w hitlerowskich obozach koncentracyjnych [Emotional conflicts in persons born in Hitlerian concentration camps or arrested in their earliest childhood]. *Przegląd Lekarski*, 23, 39-46.

1966 Sarnecki, Józef (1971). Emotional conflicts of people born in Nazi concentration camps or imprisoned there during their childhood. In: *Auschwitz Anthology. Vol. 2: In Hell They Preserved Human Dignity. Part 3*. Warsaw: International Auschwitz Committee, pp. 143-189.

1967 Savran, Bella, and Fogelman, Eva (1979). Therapeutic groups for children of Holocaust survivors. *International Journal of Group Psychotherapy*, 29, 211-215.

1968 Scagnet, E. (1992). Work and life of the nurse Elisabeth Kasser, the angel of Gurs. *Krankenpflege*, 85(9), 15-20.

1969 Schachter, M. (1965). Le syndrome neuro-psychiatrique séquellaire des anciens deportés et persecutés non-deportés à la lumière du test de Rorschach [Late neuro-psychiatric problems in ex-deportees and non-deported persecutees as demonstrated in the Rorschach Test]. *Giornale di Psichiatria e di Neuropatologia*, 93, 153-186.

1970 Schappes, Morris U. (1980). Holocaust and resistance: A response on receiving the Holocaust Memorial Award of the New York Society of Clinical Psychologists. In: Quaytman, Wilfred (Ed.), *Holocaust Survivors: Psychological and Social Sequelae*. New York: Human Sciences Press, pp. 61-69. [Published as a special issue of *Journal of Contemporary Psychotherapy*, 11(1)].

1971 Scharfenberg, Joachim (1990). Der Mythos des 20. Jahrhunderts als Hindernis der Friedensfagkeit [Twentieth century myth as obstacle to inner peace]. *Zeitschrift für Psychoanalytische Theorie und Praxis*, 5(3), 228-237.

1972 Schatzker, Chaim (1981). The teaching of the Holocaust-dilemmas and considerations. In: *Israel-Netherlands Symposium on the Impact of Persecution. Dalfsen, Amsterdam, 14-18 April 1980*. Rijswijk, The Netherlands: Ministry of Cultural Affairs, Recreation and Social Welfare, pp. 79-84.

1973 Schellekes, S. (1968). *Effects of concentration camp internment on marriage and interpersonal characteristics of the second generation*. Unpublished master's thesis, Bar Ilan University, Ramat Gan, Israel.

1974 Schenck, E.G. (1977). Verälterung als Folge exogener Einflüsse auf eine endogene Bereitschaft [Premature aging resulting from exogenous factors and endogenous predisposition]. *Therapie die Gegenwart*, 166(3), 446-450, 455-470.

1975 Schenck, E.G., and Scheid, G. (1965). Die Folgen extremer Lebensverhältnisse bei Gefangener und Internierten und ihre Beurteilung [The sequelae of extreme life situations in prisoners and internees, and their evaluation]. *Internist*, 6, 276-284.

1976 Schiffer, Irvine (1978). *The Trauma of Time: A Psychoanalytic Investigation*. New York: International Universities Press. 279 pp.

1977 Schindler, Ruben (1992). Introduction: The impact of the Holocaust on the second generation. *Journal of Social Work and Policy in Israel*, 5-6, 11-15.

1978 Schindler, Ruben; Spiegel, Chya; and Malachi, Esther (1992). Silences: Helping elderly Holocaust victims deal with the past.

International Journal of Aging and Human Development, 35(4), 243-252.

1979 Schleuderer, Claude G. (1991). *Issues of the Phoenix: Personality characteristics of children of Holocaust survivors*. Unpublished doctoral dissertation, University of Georgia, Athens, 224 pp. *Dissertations Abstracts International*, 51(8-B), p. 4066. (University Microfilms no. ACC 9100723).

1980 Schmale, Arthur H. (1970). Psychic trauma during bereavement. In: Krystal, Henry, and Niederland, William G. (Eds.), *Psychic Traumatization: Aftereffects in Individuals and Communities*. Boston, MA: Little, Brown, pp. 147-168.

1981 Schmidt, D. (1978). Probleme der zweiten Generation aus internistischer Sicht [Problems of the second generation as seen in internal medicine]. In: *Medizinische Untersuchungen der Spätfolgen des Krieges und des NS-Regimes bei Jugendlichen und Kindern von ehemaligen KZ-Häftlingen und Verfolgten* [Medical Research of the Late Effects of the War and National Socialism Regime on Youth and Children of Former Concentration Camp Inmates and Persecuted Persons]. Wien: Internationale Föderation der Widerstandskämpfer. [VI Internationaler Medizinischer Kongress der FIR. Prague, 1976].

1982 Schmidt, Stefan (1977). Wspomnienia z bloku 46 w Sachsenhausen [Memoirs from Barrack 46 in Sachsenhausen]. *Przegląd Lekarski*, 34(1), 191-193.

1983 Schmidt-Hellerau, Cordelia (1990). Über Berufsethos und personliche Integrität: Zur Geschichte der deutschen Psychoanalyse im Dritten Reich [On professional ethics and personal integrity: The history of German psychoanalysis in the Third Reich]. *Zeitschrift für Psychoanalytische Theorie und Praxis*, 5(3), 262-272.

1984 Schmolling, Paul (1984). Human reactions to the Nazi concentration camps: A summing up. *Journal of Human Stress*, 10(3), 108-120.

1985 Schnaper, Nathan (1995). Medicine and the Holocaust. *Annals of Internal Medicine*, 123(12), 964-965.

1986 Schneider, Gertrude (1975). Survival and guilt feelings of Jewish concentration camp victims. *Jewish Social Studies*, 37, 74-83.

1987 Schneider, Stanley (1978). Attitudes toward death in adolescent offspring of Holocaust survivors. *Adolescence*, 13(52), 575-584.

1988 Schneider, Stanley (1981). A proposal for treating adolescent offspring of Holocaust survivors. *Journal of Psychology and Judaism*, 6(1), 68-76.

1989 Schneider, Stanley (1988). Attitudes toward death in adolescent offspring of Holocaust survivors: A comparison of Israeli and American adolescents. *Adolescence*, 23(91), 703-710.

1990 Schreuder, J.N. (1993). Psychische klachten en kenmerken bij polyklinische patienten van de naaroorlogse generatie [Psychiatric complaints and symptoms of clinical patients of the post-war generation]. *Tijdschrift voor Psychiatrie*, 35(4), 227-241.

1991 Schreuder, J.N., and Van Tiel-Kadiks, G.W. (1994). Psychopathological symptoms in children of war victims. *Nederlands Tijdschrift voor Geneeskunde*, 138(13), 641-644.

1992 Schroder, A. (1978). Betrifft Kriegskörperschäden [On body damage due to war]. In: *Medizinische Untersuchungen der Spätfolgen des Krieges und des NS-Regimes bei Jugendlichen und Kindern von ehemaligen KZ-Häftlingen und Verfolgten* [Medical Research of the Late Effects of the War and National Socialism Regime on Youth and Children of Former Concentration Camp Inmates and Persecuted Persons]. Wien: Internationale Föderation der Widerstandskämpfer. [VI Internationaler Medizinischer Kongress der FIR. Prague, 1976].

1993 Schulman, Michelle D. (1987). *Factors related to experiences of depression among children of Holocaust survivors*. Unpublished doctoral dissertation, City University of New York, 129 pp. *Dissertation Abstracts International*, 48(6-B), p. 1820. (University Microfilms no. ACC 8713794).

1994 Schwann-Pawłowska, Jadwiga (1967). Wstępne wyniki badań lekarskich byłych wiezniow hitlerowskich obozow koncentracyjnch [Preliminary results of a medical investigation of ex-concentration camp prisoners]. *Przegląd Lekarski*, 24, 98-101.

1995 Schwann-Pawłowska, Jadwiga (1971). The Szczecin environment. In: *Auschwitz Anthology. Vol. 3: It Did Not End in Forty-Five. Part 1*. Warsaw: International Auschwitz Committee, pp. 171-179.

1996 Schwarberg, Günter (1984). *The Murders at Bullenhuser Damm: The SS Doctor and the Children*. Bloomington, IN: Indiana University Press. 178 pp.

1997 Schwartz, Harvey J. (1984). Conscious and unconscious guilt in patients with traumatic neuroses [letter]. *American Journal of Psychiatry*, 141(12), 1638-1639.

1998 Schwartz, Jack (1994). Holocaust survivors and their children: An evolving understanding. *Jewish Social Work Forum*, 30, 56-70.

1999 Schwartz, Sharon; Dohrenwend, Bruce P.; and Levav, Itzhak (1994). Nongenetic familial transmission of psychiatric disorders? Evidence from children of Holocaust survivors. *Journal of Health and Social Behavior*, 35(4), 385-402.

2000 Schwarz, Regina P. (1986). *The effect of parental communication of trauma on offspring of Holocaust survivors*. Unpublished doctoral dissertation, Columbia University, New York, 152 pp. *Dissertation Abstracts International*, 47(10-B), p. 4314. (University Microfilms no. AAC 8703083).

2001 Sedan, J. (1965). Sequelae of oculary lesions in deportees to the concentration camps of 1943-1944. *Bulletin de la Societé Ophtalmologique Française*, 9, 728-733.

2002 Segal, Julius (1973). *Long-Term Psychological and Physical Effects of the POW Experience: A Review of the Literature*. San Diego, CA: Naval Health Research Center. 29 pp.

2003 Segal, Julius; Hunter, Edner J.; and Segal, Zelda (1976). Universal consequences of captivity: Stress reactions among divergent populations of prisoners of war and their families. *International Social Sciences Journal*, 28(3), 593-609.

2004 Segall, A. (1971). Spätreaktion auf Konzentrationslagererlebnisse [Late reaction to experiences of concentration camps]. *Psyche: Zeitschrift für Psychoanalyse und ihre Anwendungen*, 28, 221-230.

2005 Segev, Tom (1988). *Soldiers of Evil: The Commandants of the Nazi Concentration Camps*. New York: McGraw-Hill. 240 pp.

2006 Segev, Tom (1994). *The Seventh Million: The Israelis and the Holocaust*. New York: Hill and Wang. 593 pp.

2007 Sehn, Jan (1970). The case of the Auschwitz physician, J.P.Kremer. In: *Auschwitz Anthology. Vol. 1: Inhuman Medicine. Part 1*. Warsaw: International Auschwitz Committee, pp. 206-258.

2008 Sehn, Jan (1970). Some of the legal aspects of the so-called experiments carried out by SS physicians in concentration camps. In: *Auschwitz Anthology. Vol. 1: Inhuman Medicine. Part 1*. Warsaw: International Auschwitz Committee, pp. 43-84.

2009 Seidel, K. (1978). Über psychische Spätschäden bei ehemaligen KZ-Häftlingen [Late psychic sequelae in ex-concentration camp prisoners]. In: *Medizinische Untersuchungen der Spätfolgen des Krieges und des NS-Regimes bei Jugendlichen und Kindern von ehemaligen KZ-Häftlingen und Verfolgten* [Medical Research of the Late Effects of the War and National Socialism Regime on Youth and Children of Former Concentration Camp Inmates and Persecuted Persons]. Wien: Internationale Föderation der Widerstandskämpfer. [VI Internationaler Medizinischer Kongress der FIR. Prague, 1976].

2010 Seidel, Ralf (1983). Psychiatrie und Nationalsozialismus [Psychiatry and Nazism]. *Sozialpsychiatrische Informationen*, 13, 26-43.

2011 Seidel, Ralf (1992). Everyday psychiatry and human dignity. In: Jockush, Ulrich, and Scholz, Lothar (Eds.), *Administered Killings at the Time of National Socialism: Involvement, Suppression, Responsibility of Psychiatry and Judicial System*. Regensburg: Roderer, pp. 1-17.

2012 Seidel, Ralf (1992). Psychiatrischer Alltag und Menschenwürde [Everyday psychiatry and human dignity]. In: Jockush, Ulrich, and Scholz, Lothar (Eds.), *Verwaltetes Morden im Nationalsozialismus: Verstrickung, Verdrängung, Verantwortung von Psychiatrie und Justiz* [Administered Killings at the Time of National Socialism: Involvement, Suppression, Responsibility of Psychiatry and Judicial System]. Regensburg: Roderer, pp. 1-17.

2013 Seidelman, William E. (1988). Mengele medicus: Medicine's Nazi heritage. *Millbank Quarterly*, 66(2), 221-239.

2014 Seidelman, William E. (1989). Medical selection: Auschwitz antecedents and effluent. *Holocaust and Genocide Studies*, 4(4), 435-448.

2015 Seidelman, William E. (1991). Medical selection: Auschwitz antecedents and effluent. *International Journal of Health Services*, 21, 401-415.

2016 Seidelman, William E. (1995). Whither Nuremberg?: Medicine's continuing Nazi heritage. *Medicine and Global Survival*, 2(3), 148-157.

2017 Seifert, W. (1980). "Holocaust" und Kulturpsychologie Sigmund Freud [The Holocaust and the cultural psychology of Sigmund Freud]. *Zeitschrift für Klinische Psychologie und Psychotherapie*, 28(4), 292-301.

2018 Selavan, Ida C. (1979). Behavior disorders of Jews: A review of the literature. *Journal of Psychology and Judaism*, 42(2), 117-124.

2019 Selga, E. (1948). Tatspiyot r'fuiyot-psichologiyot bitkufat hashoa [Medical-psychological observations in the time of the Shoah]. *Higena Ruhanit*, 5, 103-108.

2020 Seligman, Zivya (1995). Trauma and drama: A lesson from the concentration camps. *Arts in Psychotherapy*, 22(2), 119-132.

2021 Serok, Shraga (1985). Implications of Gestalt therapy with post-traumatic patients. *Gestalt Journal*, 8(1), 78-89.

2022 Severino, Sally K. (1986). Use of a Holocaust fantasy for the consolidation of identity. *Journal of the American Academy of Psychoanalysis*, 14(2), 227-239.

2023 Shafir, Abraham; Hirsch, Malka; and Shepps, Shmr'yahu (1975). *Hahashpa'ah hanaphshit ham'oocheret shel havayat hashoah k'phi sh'mishtakefet b'ma'arechet mivchanim psychodyagnostim* [The Delayed Mental Influence of the Holocaust Experience as Projected in a Psychodiagnostic Battery]. Ramat Chen: Mental Health Clinic, Tel Aviv: Tel Aviv University and Kupat Cholim. 75 pp.

2024 Shampi, M.A., and Kyle, R.A. (1975). Henryk Goldszmit (1879-1942). *Journal of the American Medical Association*, 234(10), 1042.

2025 Shanan, Joel (1989). Surviving the survivors: Late personality development of Jewish Holocaust survivors. *International Journal of Mental Health*, 17(4), 42-71.

2026 Shanan, Joel, and Shahar, Orna (1983). Cognitive and personality functioning of Jewish Holocaust survivors during the midlife transition (46-55) in Israel. *Archiv für Psychologie*, 135(4), 275-294.

2027 Shanon, Jacob (1962). The subconscious motivation for the appearance of psychosomatic skin disorders in concentration camp survivors and their rehabilitation. *Psychosomatics*, 3, 178-182.

2028 Shanon, Jacob (1969). Stress and conflict as criteria for the classification of psychosomatic skin disorders. *Archives Belges de Dermatologie et de Syphiligraphie*, 25, 429-437.

2029 Shanon, Jacob (1970). Delayed psychosomatic skin disorders in survivors of concentration camps. *British Journal of Dermatology*, 83, 536-542.

2030 Shanon, Jacob (1970). Psychosomatic skin disorders in survivors of Nazi concentration camps. *Psychosomatics*, 2, 95-98.

2031 Shanon, Jacob (1979). Psychogenic pruritus in concentration camp survivors. *Dynamische Psychiatrie*, 12(3), 232-241.

2032 Shapiro, Moshe H. (1980). Psychophysiological sequelae of Holocaust trauma in a Jewish child. *American Journal of Psychoanalysis*, 40(1), 53-66.

2033 Shelley, Lore (1983). *Jewish Holocaust survivors' attitudes toward contemporary beliefs about themselves*. Unpublished doctoral dissertation, The Fielding Institute, Santa Barbara, California, 504 pp. *Dissertation Abstracts International*, 44(6), p. 2016. (University Microfilms no. 8322603).

2034 Shelley, Lore (Ed.) (1991). *Criminal Experiments on Human Beings in Auschwitz and War Research Laboratories*. San Francisco, CA: Mellen Research University Press. 402 pp.

2035 Sheps, J. (1971). Organische Hirnschäden bei Überlebenden aus Konzentrationslagern in den Vereinigten Staaten-langfristige Reaktion auf extrem Unweltbelastungen [Organic brain damages in concentration camp survivors in the United States: Late sequelae of extreme distress]. In: Herberg, Hans-Joachim (Ed.), *Spätschäden nach Extrembelastungen* [Late Damage After Extreme Stress]. Herford: Nicolai, pp. 165-175. [II Internationalen Medizinisch-Juristischen Konferenz. Dusseldorf, 1969].

2036 Shibolet, R. (1982). *Kiezen of delen, een visie over de ontwikkeling van de na-oorlogse joodse generatie in Nederland* [Taking it or leaving it: A vision on the development of the post-war Jewish generation in the Netherlands]. Unpublished doctoral dissertation, University of Amsterdam, Netherlands.

2037 Shiloh, Roni; Schwartz, Bruria; Weizman, Abraham; and Radwan, Marguerite (1995). Catatonia as an unusual presentation of post-tramautic stress disorder. *Psychopathology*, 28(6), 285-290.

2038 Shiryon, Sarah (1982). *The second generation leaves home: The function of the sibling subgroup in the separation-individuation process of the survivor family*. Unpublished doctoral dissertation, The

Wright Institute, Berkeley, California, 146 pp. *Dissertation Abstracts International*, 43(10-B), p. 3376. (University Microfilms no. AAC 8305602).

2039 Shiryon, Sarah (1988). The second generation leaves home: The function of the sibling subgroup in the separation-individuation process of the survivor family. *Family Therapy*, 15(3), 239-253.

2040 Shiryon, Sarah (1990). De tweede generatie verlaat het huis, de functie van de siblings [The second generation leaves home: The function of the sibling subgroup in the separation-individuation process of the survivor family]. *Psychother Pasp*, 7, 7-27.

2041 Shortt, Joann W., and Pennebaker, James W. (1992). Talking versus hearing about Holocaust experiences. *Basic and Applied Social Psychology*, 13(2), 165-179.

2042 Shoshan, Tamar (1989). Mourning and longing from generation to generation. *American Journal of Psychotherapy*, 43(2), 193-207.

2043 Shour, April (1990). The aging Holocaust survivor in the institution. *Journal of Aging and Judaism*, 4(3), 141-160.

2044 Shuval, Judith T. (1957-1958). Some persistent effects of trauma: Five years after the Nazi concentration camps. *Social Problems*, 5(3), 230-243.

2045 Siegel, Lloyd M. (1980). Holocaust survivors in Hasidic and ultra-orthodox Jewish population. In: Quaytman, Wilfred (Ed.), *Holocaust Survivors: Psychological and Social Sequelae*. New York: Human Sciences Press, pp. 15-31. [Published as a special issue of *Journal of Contemporary Psychotherapy*, 11(1)].

2046 Siegel, Lloyd M. (1980). Holocaust survivors in Hasidic and ultra-orthodox Jewish populations. *Journal of Contemporary Psychotherapy*, 11(1), 15-31.

2047 Sigal, John J. (1970). Second generation effects of massive psychic trauma. In: Krystal, Henry, and Niederland, William G. (Eds.), *Psychic Traumatization: Aftereffects in Individuals and Communities*. Boston, MA: Little, Brown, pp. 55-65.

2048 Sigal, John J. (1973). Hypotheses and methodology in the families of Holocaust survivors. In: Anthony, E. James, and Koupernik, Cyrille (Ed.), *Yearbook of the International Association for Child Psychiatry and Allied Professions. Vol 2*. New York: John Wiley & Sons, pp. 411-416.

2049 Sigal, John J. (1976). Effects of paternal exposure to prolonged stress on the mental health of the spouse and children: Families of Canadian survivors of the Japanese World War II camps. *Canadian Journal of Psychiatry*, 21(3), 166-170.

2050 Sigal, John J. (1986). The nature of evidence for intergenerational effects of the Holocaust. *Simon Wiesenthal Center Annual*, 3, 363-376.

2051 Sigal, John J. (1993). Concentration camps. In: Ghadirian, Abdul-Missagh A., and Lehmann, Heinz E. (Eds.), *Environment and Psychopathology*. New York: Springer, pp. 158-171.

2052 Sigal, John J. (1995). Resilience in survivors, their children and their grandchildren. *Echoes of the Holocaust*, 4, 9-13. [Bulletin of the Jerusalem Center for Research into the Late Effects of the Holocaust. Talbieh Mental Health Center, Jerusalem, Israel].

2053 Sigal, John J.; DiNicola, Vincenzo E.; and Buonvino, Michael (1988). Grandchildren of survivors: Can negative effects of prolonged exposure to excessive stress be observed two generations later? *Canadian Journal of Psychiatry*, 33(3), 207-212.

2054 Sigal, John J., and Rakoff, Vivian (1971). Concentration camp survival: A pilot study of the effects on the second generation. *Canadian Psychiatric Association Journal*, 16, 393-397.

2055 Sigal, John J.; Silver, D.; Rakoff, Vivian; and Ellin, B. (1973). Some second generation effects of survival of the Nazi persecution. *American Journal of Orthopsychiatry*, 43(3), 320-327.

2056 Sigal, John J., and Weinfeld, Morton (1985). Control of aggression in adult children of survivors of the Nazi persecution. *Journal of Abnormal Psychology*, 94(4), 556-564.

2057 Sigal, John J., and Weinfeld, Morton (1987). Mutual involvement and alienation in families of Holocaust survivors. *Psychiatry*, 50(3), 280-288.

2058 Sigal, John J., and Weinfeld, Morton (1989). *Trauma and Rebirth: Intergenerational Effects of the Holocaust*. New York: Praeger. 204 pp.

2059 Sigal, John J.; Weinfeld, Morton; and Eaton, William W. (1985). Stability of coping style 33 years after prolonged exposure to extreme stress. *Acta Psychiatrica Scandinavica*, 71(6), 554-566.

2060 Signorini, Franca M. (1993). L'uomo in rivolta [The rebellion of the individual]. *Giornale Storico di Psicologia Dinamica*, 17(34), 97-113.

2061 Sikorski, Jan (1975). Zaopatrzenie farmaceutyczno-sanitarne w obozie koncentracyjnym Oświęcim-Brzezinka 1940-1945. [Phamaceutical and sanitary supplies and facilities in the concentration camps of Oswiecim-Brzezinka in 1940-1945)]. *Archiwum Historii Medycyny*, 38(3-4), 283-298.

2062 Sikorski, Jan (1989). Więźniowie porządkowi izby chorych SS [Prisoner-cleaners in the concentration camp hospital for the SS personnel]. *Przegląd Lekarski*, 46(1), 92-95.

2063 Silow, Charles J. (1993). *Holocaust survivors: A study of the long-term effects of post-traumatic stress and its relationship to parenting attitudes and behaviors*. Unpublished doctoral dissertation, University of Detroit, Michigan, 207 pp. *Dissertations Abstracts International*, 54(3-B), p. 1684. (University Microfilms no. AAC 9318337).

2064 Silverman, Wendy K. (1987). Methodological issues in the study of transgenerational effects of the Holocaust: Comment on Nadler, Kav-Venaki, and Gleitman. *Journal of Consulting and Clinical Psychology*, 55(1), 125-126.

2065 Simenauer, Erich (1968). Late psychic sequelae of man-made disasters. *International Journal of Psycho-Analysis*, 49(2-3), 306-309.

2066 Simenauer, Erich (1978). A double helix: Some determinants of self-perpetuation of Nazism. In: Eissler, Ruth S.; Freud, Anna; Kris, Marianne; and Neubauer, Peter B. (Eds.), *Psychoanalytic Study of the Child. Vol. 33*. New Haven: Yale University Press, pp. 411-425.

2067 Simenauer, Erich (1981). Die zweite Generation-danach die Wiederkehr der Verfolgermentalität in Psychoanalysen [The second generation: The subsequent return of the persecution mentality in psychoanalysis]. *Jahrbuch der Psychoanalyse*, 12, 8-17.

2068 Simmedinger, A.N. (1955). Neue wege zur Bestimmung verfolgungsbedingter Schäden an Körper und bei Naziopfern, Kriegsbeschädigten und Sozialrentnern [New approaches to finding physical and health damages caused by persecution in Nazi victims, war-disabled and social pensioners]. In: Michel, Max (Ed.), *Gesundheitsschäden durch Verfolgung und Gefangenschaft und ihre Spätfolgen: Zusammenstellung der Referate und Ergebnisse der Internationalen Sozialmedizinischen Konferenz über die Pathologie der Ehemaligen Deportierten und Internierten, 5-7 Juni 1954 in*

Kopenhagen [Health Damages Caused by Persecution and Captivity and the Late Effects: Compilation of the Papers and Results of the International Conference of Social Medicine on the Pathology of Former Deported and Interned Persons, 5-7 June 1954 in Copenhagen]. Frankfurt am Main: Röderberg, pp. 246-250.

2069 Siniecki, Bogdan (1975). Z historii szpitala obozowego w Stuffhofie [The hospital at Stutthof camp: An outline of history]. *Przegląd Lekarski*, 32(1), 85-89.

2070 Skokna, D., and Korhon, M. (1978). Spätfolgen der Tuberkulose und posttuberkulöser Pneumopathien bei Mitgliedern des ZPB (Verband antifachistischer Widerstandskämpfer) [Late sequelae of tuberculosis and post-tuberculosis in members of the ZPB (Union of Antifascist Fighters)]. In: *Medizinische Untersuchungen der Spätfolgen des Krieges und des NS-Regimes bei Jugendlichen und Kindern von ehemaligen KZ-Häftlingen und Verfolgten* [Medical Research of the Late Effects of the War and National Socialism Regime on Youth and Children of Former Concentration Camp Inmates and Persecuted Persons]. Wien: Internationale Föderation der Widerstandskämpfer. [VI Internationaler Medizinischer Kongress der FIR. Prague, 1976].

2071 Skolnick, Andrew A. (1992). Museum scholars to apply Holocaust experience to 1990s biomedical issues. *Journal of the American Medical Association*, 268(5), 575-576.

2072 Skolnik, Gerald L. (1989). The Holocaust survivor in the synagogue community: Issues and perspectives on pastoral care. In: Marcus, Paul, and Rosenberg, Alan (Eds.), *Healing Their Wounds: Psychotherapy with Holocaust Survivors and Their Families*. New York: Praeger, pp. 155-166.

2073 Skulimowski, M.M. (1972). Ludwik Bolesław Kotulski MD (1988-1964): Członek polskiego oporu podziemnego, więzień w Pawiaku i w Oseięcimiu [Ludwik Boleslaw Kotulski, MD (1888-1964) - Member of the Polish underground, inmate of the Pawiak prison and Auschwitz concentration camp]. *Archiwum Historii Medycyny*, 35(1), 181-184.

2074 Slipp, Samuel (1978). The children of survivors of Nazi concentration camps: A pilot study of the transmission of psychic trauma. In: Wolberg, Lewis R., and Aronson, Marvin L. (Eds.), *Group Therapy*. New York: Stratton International.

2075 Slisz-Oryzyńska, Maria (1978). Relacja z bloku nr 17 obozu kobiecego w Brzezince [A report from Barrack No. 17 at the

Women's concentration camp at Birkenau]. *Przegląd Lekarski*, 35(1), 160-166.

2076 Ślizowska, H., and Matuszewski, H. (1990). Stan zdrowia więźniów obozów hitlerowskich [Status of health of former prisoners of the Nazi concentration camps]. *Przegląd Lekarski*, 47(1), 15-17.

2077 Smolenska, Zuzanna M., and Reykowski, Janusz (1992). Motivation of people who helped Jews survive the Nazi occupation. In: Oliner, Pearl M.; Oliner, Samuel P.; Baron, Lawrence; Blum, Lawrence A.; Krebs, Dennis L.; and Smolenska, Zuzanna M. (Eds.), *Embracing the Other: Philosophical, Psychological, and Historical Perspectives on Altruism*. New York: New York University Press.

2078 Snider, Faye L. (1990). Holocaust trauma and imagery: The systematic transmission into the second generation. In: Mirkin, Marsha P. (Ed.), *The Social and Political Contexts of Family Therapy*. Boston, MA: Allyn & Bacon, pp. 307-329.

2079 Sobczyk, Piotr (1980). Trudności psychiatryczne orzecznictwa inwalidzkiego odległych skutków działań wojennych [Difficulties of psychiatry in handling the invalids' claims for compensation with regard to wartime damages]. *Przegląd Lekarski*, 37(1), 86-89.

2080 Sobczyk, Piotr; Cielecki, Andrzej; Zembrzycka-Cielecki, Maryla; Krupka-Matuszczyk, Irena; Kaźmierczak, Barbara; and Łukoszek, Danuta (1980). Analiza psychopatologiczna wstępnego materiału orzeczniczego byłych więźniów obozów koncentracyjnych [Psychopathological analysis of prelimary expert testimony materials with regard to former prisoners of the concentration camps]. *Przegląd Lekarski*, 37(1), 89-91.

2081 Sobolewicz, T. (1984). Z przeżyc w rewirze oswięcimskim [Experiences in the Auschwitz hospital]. *Przegląd Lekarski*, 41(1), 109-110.

2082 Sofletea, A. (1961). Behandlung und weitere Prognose des Erschöpfungssyndrom [Treatment and further prognosis of the exhaustion syndrome]. In: *Die Behandlung der Asthenie und der vorzeitigen Vergreisung bei ehemaligen Widerstandskämpfern und KZ-Häftlingen* [Treatment of Asthenia and Premature Aging in Former Resistance Fighters and Concentration Camp Inmates]. Wien: Verlag der FIR, pp. 69-75. [III Internationale Medizinische Konferenz. Liege, 17-19 März 1961].

2083 Solkoff, Norman (1981). Children of Survivors of the Nazi Holocaust: A critical review of the literature. *American Journal of Orthopsychiatry*, 51, 29-43.

2084 Solkoff, Norman (1982). Survivors of the Holocaust: A critical review of the literature. *Catalog of Selected Documents in Psychology*, 12(4), 47. Ms. 2507.

2085 Solkoff, Norman (1992). Children of Survivors of the Nazi Holocaust: A critical review of the literature. *American Journal of Orthopsychiatry*, 62(3), 342-358.

2086 Solkoff, Norman (1992). The Holocaust: Survivors and their children. In: Basoglu, Metin (Ed.), *Torture and its Consequences: Current Treatment Approaches*. Cambridge: Cambridge University Press, pp. 136-148.

2087 Solladie, R. (1961). Klinische und biologische Ergebnisse der Behandlung von Folgen der Deportation mittels Novokain mit niederem pH-wert und zusätzlichen Medikamenten [Clinical and biological outcomes of treating deportation sequelae with low PH-value novocain and additional drugs]. In: *Die Behandlung der Asthenie und der vorzeitigen Vergreisung bei ehemaligen Widerstandskämpfern und KZ-Häftlingen* [Treatment of Asthenia and Premature Aging in Former Resistance Fighters and Concentration Camp Inmates]. Wien: Verlag der FIR, pp. 221-228. [III Internationale Medizinische Konferenz. Liege, 17-19 März 1961].

2088 Solomon, Zahava (1995). From denial to recognition: Attitudes toward Holocaust survivors from World War II to the present. *Journal of Traumatic Stress*, 8(2), 215-228.

2089 Solomon, Zahava; Kotler, Moshe; and Mikulincer, Mario (1988). Combat related post-traumatic stress disorder among second generation Holocaust survivors: Preliminary findings. *American Journal of Psychiatry*, 145(7), 865-868.

2090 Solomon, Zahava; Kotler, Moshe; and Mikulincer, Mario (1989). Combat related post-traumatic stress disorder among the second generation of Holocaust survivors: Transgenerational effects among Israeli soldiers. *Psychologia: Israel Journal of Psychology*, 1(2), 113-119.

2091 Solomon, Zahava, and Prager, Edward (1992). Elderly Israeli Holocaust survivors during the Persian Gulf War: A study of psychological distress. *American Journal of Psychiatry*, 149(12), 1707-1710.

2092 Somer, Eli (1994). Hypnotherapy and regulated uncovering in the treatment of older survivors of Nazi persecution. In: Brink, Terry L. (Ed.), *Holocaust Survivors' Mental Health*. New York: Haworth, pp. 47-65. [Published as a special issue of *Clinical Gerontologist*, 14(3).]

2093 Sonnenberg, Stephen M. (1972). A special form of survivor syndrome, case report. *Psychoanalytic Quarterly*, 41(1), 58-62.

2094 Sonnenberg, Stephen M. (1974). Children of survivors: Workshop report. *Journal of the American Psychoanalytic Association*, 22(1), 200-204.

2095 Sonnenberg, Stephen M. (1982). A transcultural observation of post-traumatic stress disorders. *Hospital and Community Psychiatry*, 33(1), 58-59.

2096 Sorscher, Nechama L. (1992). *The effects of parental communication of wartime experiences on children of survivors of the Holocaust*. Unpublished doctoral dissertation, Adelphi University, The Institute of Advanced Psychological Studies, Garden City, New York, 311 pp. *Dissertation Abstracts International*, 52(8-B), p. 4482. (University Microfilms no. AAC 9133440).

2097 Spanjaard, J. (1979). Role of self-esteem in concentration camp survivors. *Tijdschrift Psychotherapy*, 5(6), 323-326.

2098 Speier, Sammy (1993). The psychoanalyst without a face: Psychoanalysis without a history. In: Heimannsberg, Barbara, and Schmidt, Christoph J. (Eds.), *The Collective Silence: German Identity and the Legacy of Shame*. San Francisco, CA: Josse Bass.

2099 Spero, Moshe H. (1980). Psychophysiological sequelae of Holocaust trauma in a Jewish child. *American Journal of Psychoanalysis*, 40(1), 53-66.

2100 Spero, Moshe H. (1986). Comments on "Shmuel: Through deaf ears." *Journal of Psychology and Judaism*, 10(1), 39-41.

2101 Spero, Moshe H. (1992). Can psychoanalytic insights reveal the knowability and the aesthetics of the Holocaust? *Journal of Social Work and Policy in Israel*, 5-6, 123-170.

2102 Spiegel, Rose H. (1975). Survival of psychoanalysis in Nazi Germany. *Contemporary Psychoanalysis*, 11, 479-492.

2103 Spiegel, Rose H. (1985). Survival, psychoanalysis and the Third Reich. *Journal of the American Academy of Psychoanalysis*, 13(4), 521-536.

2104 Spiegelman, Art (1986). *Maus I: A Survivor's Tale*. New York: Pantheon. 159 pp.

2105 Spiegelman, Art (1991). *Maus II: A Survivor's Tale*. New York: Pantheon. 135 pp.

2106 Springer, Anna, and Bratini, E. (1976). KZ-Häft und Störungen der Nachfolgegeneration; eine Untersuchung an in Ravensbrück inhäftiert gewesenen Frauen und ihren Kinder [Concentration camp imprisonment and disturbances in the second generation: An investigation of female ex-prisoners from the concentration camp Ravensbrück and their children]. *Mitteilungen der FIR*, 10, 26-29.

2107 Stafford, Florence (1995). Aging stressors for Holocaust survivors and their families. *Journal of Gerontological Social Work*, 24, (1-2), 131-153.

2108 Stastiak, L. (1979). Wspomnienie o prof. Robercie Waitzu [Professor Robert Waitz. Reminiscences]. *Przegląd Lekarski*, 36(1), 152-154.

2109 Staub, Ervin (1985). The psychology of perpetrators and bystanders. *Political Psychology*, 6(1), 61-85.

2110 Staub, Ervin (1989). *The Roots of Evil: The Origins of Genocide and Other Group Violence*. Cambridge: Cambridge University Press. 336 pp.

2111 Staub, Ervin (1993). The psychology of bystanders, perpetrators, and heroic helpers. *International Journal of Intercultural Relations*, 17(3), 315-341.

2112 Steenfeld-Foss, D.W. (1987). Leger som drapsmenn [Physicians as murderers]. *Tidsskrift for den Norske Laegeforening. Journal of the Norwegian Medical Association*, 107(34-360), 3019-3020.

2113 Stefańska-Szymańska, Irena (1977). Medycyna w Oświęcimskiej plastyce obozowej [Health services at the Auschwitz-Birkenau concentration camp as pictured by the inmates]. *Przegląd Lekarski*, 34(1), 108-118.

2114 Stein, André (1993). *Hidden Children: Forgotten Survivors of the Holocaust*. New York: Penguin. 273 pp.

2115 Stein, Howard F. (1984). The Holocaust, the uncanny, and the Jewish sense of history. *Political Psychology*, 5(1), 5-35.

2116 Stein, Howard F. (1993). The Holocaust, the self, and the question of wholeness: A response to Lewin. *Ethos*, 21(4), 485-512.

2117 Stein, Joseph (1979). Pathological anatomy of hunger disease. In: Winick, Myron (Ed.), *Hunger Disease: Studies by the Jewish Physicians in the Warsaw Ghetto*. New York: John Wiley & Sons, pp. 207-234.

2118 Steinberg, Arlene (1986). *Separation-individuation issues among children of Holocaust survivors*. Unpublished doctoral dissertation. Ferkauf Graduate School of Psychology, Yeshiva University, New York.

2119 Steinberg, Arlene (1989). Holocaust survivors and their children: A review of the clinical literature. In: Marcus, Paul, and Rosenberg, Alan (Eds.), *Healing Their Wounds: Psychotherapy with Holocaust Survivors and Their Families*. New York: Praeger, pp. 23-48.

2120 Steiner, George (1971). *In Bluebeard's Castle: Some Notes Toward the Redefinition of Culture*. New Haven, CT: Yale University Press. 141 pp.

2121 Steiner, Riccardo (1989). "It is a new kind of diaspora...." *International Review of Psycho-Analysis*, 16(1), 35-78.

2122 Steinert, Tilman (1992). Reactions in pychiatric institutions to the murder of their patients in Grafeneck. In: Jockush, Ulrich, and Scholz, Lothar (Eds.), *Administered Killings at the Time of National Socialism: Involvement, Suppression, Responsibility of Psychiatry and Judicial System*. Regensburg: Roderer, pp. 1-17.

2123 Steinert, Tilman (1992). Reaktionen in den Psychiatrischen Anstalten auf die Ermordung ihrer Patienten in Grafeneck [Reactions in pychiatric institutions to the murder of their patients in Grafeneck]. In: Jockush, Ulrich, and Scholz, Lothar (Eds.), *Verwaltetes Morden im Nationalsozialismus: Verstrickung, Verdrängung, Verantwortung von Psychiatrie und Justiz* [Administered Killings at the Time of National Socialism: Involvement, Suppression, Responsibility of Psychiatry and Judicial System]. Regensburg: Roderer, pp. 1-17.

2124 Steinfels, Peter (1994). Biomedical ethics and the shadow of Nazism. In: Michalczyk, John J. (Ed.), *Medicine, Ethics, and the Third Reich: Historical and Contemporary Issues*. Kansas City, MO: Sheed & Ward, pp. 13-15.

2125 Steinitz, Lucy Y. (1982). Psychosocial effects of the Holocaust on aging survivors and their families. *Journal of Gerontological Social Work*, 4(3-4), 145-152.

2126 Steinitz, Lucy Y. (1992). A half-century later: Aging Holocaust survivors and their families. In: Kenigsberg, Rositta E., and Lieblich, Cathy M. (Eds.), *The First National Conference on Identification, Treatment and Care of the Aging Holocaust Survivor, March 29-31, 1992: Selected Proceedings*. Miami, FL: Holocaust Documentation and Education Center and Southeast Florida Center on Aging, Florida International University, pp. 75-92.

2127 Steinitz, Lucy Y., and Szonyi, David M. (Eds.) (1976). *Living After the Holocaust: Reflections by the Post-War Generation in America*. New York: Bloch. 175 pp.

2128 Stepak, Sonia (1989). *Tefisat hama'arechet hamishpachtit v'ify'unim ishim b'kerev tze'atzaim l'nitzoley shoah* [Perception of family system and personality characteristics among offspring of Holocaust survivors]. Unpublished master's thesis, Department of Psychology, Tel Aviv University, Israel. 130 pp.

2129 Sterba, Edith (1968). The effects of persecution on adolescents. In: Krystal, Henry (Ed.), *Massive Psychic Trauma*. New York: International Universities Press, pp. 51-59.

2130 Sterboul, J. (1960). Therapie und Diätik der Verdauungskrankheiten bei Kriegsinvaliden, Deportierten und Widerstandskämpfern [Therapy and diet in diseases of the digestive organs of war disabled, deportees and resistance fighters]. In: Fichez, Louis F. (Ed.), *Andere Spätfolgen, auf Grund der Beobachtungen bei den ehemaligen Deportierten und Internierten der nazistischen Gefangnisse und Vernichtungslager* [Other Belated Consequences, Based on the Observations of Former Deportees and Internees of Nazi Prisons and Death Camps]. Wien: Verlag der FIR, pp. 40-49.

2131 Sterboul, J., and Krawiecki, Dr. (1961). Vergleichende Studien der Dyspepsie bei ehemaligen KZ-Häftlingen und bei Greisen [Comparative studies of dyspepsia in ex-concentration camp prisoners and in old people]. In: *Die Behandlung der Asthenie und der vorzeitigen Vergreisung bei ehemaligen Widerstandskämpfern und KZ-Häftlingen* [Treatment of Asthenia and Premature Aging in Former Resistance Fighters and Concentration Camp Inmates]. Wien: Verlag der FIR, pp. 127-135. [III Internationale Medizinische Konferenz. Liege, 17-19 März 1961].

2132 Sterkowicz, Stanisław (1969). Przyczynek do zagadnienia moralności więźniów obozów hitlerowskich [Contribution to the problem of morals among the prisoners in Nazi concentration camps]. *Przegląd Lekarski*, 25(1), 47-52.

2133 Sterkowicz, Stanisław (1977). Pseudomedyczne eksperymenty w obozie Neuengamme [Pseudomedical experiments at Neuengamme concentration camp]. *Przegląd Lekarski*, 34(1), 130-137.

2134 Sterkowicz, Stanisław (1977). Sprawa lekarza SS, Heinricha Schütza [Case of SS physician Heinrich Schutz]. *Przegląd Lekarski*, 34(1), 137-141.

2135 Sterkowicz, Stanisław (1978). Pierwsze tygodnie po wyzwoleniu więźniów Neuengamme [First weeks following the liberation of Neuengamme concentration camps]. *Przegląd Lekarski*, 35(1), 155-157.

2136 Sterkowicz, Stanisław (1987). Lekarz ludobójca, Joachim Mrugowsky [The physician and mass murderer Joachim Mrugowsky]. *Przegląd Lekarski*, 44(1), 126-131.

2137 Sterkowicz, Stanisław (1988). Chorzy więźniowie Dachau w rękach SS, Rudolfa Brachtla [Sick prisoners in Dachau in the hands of the SS physician Rudolf Bracht]. *Przegląd Lekarski*, 45(1), 69-73.

2138 Sterkowicz, Stanisław (1988). Lekarz SS, Kurt Friedrich Plotner, eksperymentator w Dachau [The SS physician Kurt Friedrich Plotner, experimenter at Dachau]. *Przegląd Lekarski*, 45(1), 69-73.

2139 Sterkowicz, Stanisław (1989). Karalność zbrodni lekarzy hitlerowskich [Punishment of Nazi physicians]. *Przegląd Lekarski*, 46(1), 143-149.

2140 Stermer, Edy; Bar, H.; and Levy, Nissim (1991). Chronic functional gastrointestinal symptoms in Holocaust survivors. *American Journal of Gastroenterology*, 86(4), 417-422.

2141 Stern, H. (1948). Observations sur la psychologie collective dans les camps des personnel déplacées [Remarks on collective psychology in the displaced persons camp]. *Psyche: Zeitschrift für Psychoanalyse und ihre Anwendungen*, 3, 891-907.

2142 Stern, Judith (1988). Pet attachment as a delayed mourning process. *Anthrozoos*, 2(1), 18-21.

2143 Stern, Judith (1990). Psychotherapy of loss and grief. *Sante Mentale au Quebec*, 15(2), 221-232.

2144 Stern, Ziva Y. (1995). *The experience of parenthood among children of Holocaust survivors: Reworking a traumatic legacy*. Unpublished doctoral dissertation, Massachusetts School of Professional Psychology, 180 pp. *Dissertation Abstracts International*, 56(6-B), p. 3465. (University Microfilms no. AAC 9536354).

2145 Sternalski, Marek (1978). Przyczynek do psychiatrycznych aspektów tzw KZ-syndromu [A contribution to the psychiatric aspects of the so-called concentration camp syndrome]. *Przegląd Lekarski*, 35, 25-27.

2146 Sternberg, Tamara (1982). Defence mechanisms and the working through of resistance in group therapy. *Group Analysis*, 15(3), 261-277.

2147 Stewart, Sidney (1991). Trauma et realité psychique [Trauma and psychic reality]. *Revue Française de Psychanalyse*, 55(4), 957-975.

2148 Stierlin, Helm (1981). The parents' Nazi past and the dialogue between generations. *Family Process*, 20(4), 379-390.

2149 Stoffels, Hans (1983). Die Gesundheitsutopie der Medizin im Nationalsozialismus [The health utopia of medicine in Nazism]. *Sozialpsychiatrische Informationen*, 13(4), 55-67.

2150 Stoffels, Hans (Ed.) (1991). *Schicksale der Verfolgten: Psychische und Somatische Auswirkungen von Terrorherrschaft* [The Fate of Persecuted Persons: Psychic and Somatic Effects of Terror Reign]. Berlin: Springer. 337 pp.

2151 Stoffels, Hans (Ed.) (1994). *Terrorlandschaften der Seele: Beitrage zur Theorie und Therapie von Extremtraumatisierungen* [Terror Landscapes of the Soul: Articles on the Theory and Therapy of Extreme Traumatization]. Regensburg: Roderer. 237 pp.

2152 Stokvis, Berthold (1951). Observations of an Amsterdam psychiatrist during the Nazi occupation of 1940-1945. *Monatsschrift für Psychologie und Neurologie*, 277-295.

2153 Stokvis, Berthold (1963). Gedanken eines Psychotherapeuten über das Wiedergutmachungsverfahren [A psychotherapist's reflections on the problem of restitution]. *Psyche: Zeitschrift für Psychoanalyse und ihre Anwendungen*, 16, 538-543.

2154 Straker, Manuel (1971). The survivor syndrome: Theoretical and therapeutic dilemmas. *Psychiatry Digest*, 42, 37-41.

2155 Strauss, Herbert A. (1957). Besonderheiten der nichtpsychotischen seelischen Störungen bei Opfern der Nationalsozialistischen Verfolgung und ihre Bedeutung bei der Begutachtung [Peculiarities of non-psychotic psychic disturbances in victims of Nazi-persecution: Their importance for compensation decisions]. *Nervenarzt*, 28, 344-350.

2156 Strauss, Herbert A. (1957). Neuropsychiatric disturbances after national-socialist persecution. *Virchow-Pirquet Medical Society*, 28, 344-350.

2157 Strauss, Herbert A. (1960). Alle Freunde verliessen sie. Eine Angstneurose [All friends deserted her. Anxiety neurosis]. In: March, Hans (Ed.), *Verfolgung und Angst in ihren leib-seelischen Auswirkungen. Dokumente* [Persecution and Anxiety in Their Psychosomatic Forms of Expression. Documentation]. Stuttgart: Klett, pp. 67-76.

2158 Strauss, Herbert A. (1960). Ein entwurzelter Mensch. Eine seelische Entwicklungs- und Anpassungsstörung [An uprooted person: Emotional disturbances and maladaption]. In: March, Hans (Ed.), *Verfolgung und Angst in ihren leib-seelischen Auswirkungen. Dokumente* [Persecution and Anxiety in Their Psychosomatic Forms of Expression. Documentation]. Stuttgart: Klett, pp. 77-83.

2159 Strauss, Herbert A. (1960). Ein neunjähriges Kind im Konzentrationslager. Enuresis und Anpassungsstörungen [A nine year old child in the concentration camp: Enuresis and maladaption]. In: March, Hans (Ed.), *Verfolgung und Angst in ihren leib-seelischen Auswirkungen. Dokumente* [Persecution and Anxiety in Their Psychosomatic Forms of Expression. Documentation]. Stuttgart: Klett, pp. 52-59.

2160 Strauss, Herbert A. (1960). Eine partielle Entmannung. Seelishe Impotenz und depressive Lebenshemmung [A partial demasculation: Mental impotence and depressive inhibition of life]. In: March, Hans (Ed.), *Verfolgung und Angst in ihren leib-seelischen Auswirkungen. Dokumente* [Persecution and Anxiety in Their Psychosomatic Forms of Expression. Documentation]. Stuttgart: Klett, pp. 60-66.

2161 Strauss, Herbert A. (1961). Diskussionsbemerkungen zu vorstehenden Beiträgen [Discussion remarks to the preceeding papers]. *Nervenarzt*, 32, 551-552.

2162 Strauss, Herbert A. (1961). Psychiatric disturbances in victims of racial persecution. In: *Proceedings of the Third World Congress of Psychiatry, Montreal, Canada, 4-10 June 1961*. Toronto, ON: University of Toronto Press, pp. 1207-1212.

2163 Strauss, Herbert A. (1989). *Early Perceptions of Concentration Camp Experience: Autobiographical accounts of Hungarian-Jewish Concentration Camp Survivors 1945/46 as Studied by an Interdisciplinary Team 1948/1951*. [Paper presented at the International Conference on Psychological and Psychiatric Sequelae of the Nazi-Terror in Aging Survivors and their Offspring, Hanover, Germany].

2164 Strauss, Rhona (1995). Group therapy with the second generation of Holocaust survivors. In: Lemberger, John (Ed.), *A Global Perspective on Working with Holocaust Survivors and the Second Generation*. Jerusalem: JDC-Brookdale Institute of Gerontology and Human Development, AMCHA, and JDC-Israel, pp. 401-412.

2165 Strøm, Axel (1961). Study of a group of former Norwegian deportees. Part 1: Purpose and scope of the examination. In: *International Conference on the Later Effects of Imprisonment and Deportation Organized by the World Veterans Federation. The Hague, November 20-25, 1961*. The Hague: World Veterans Federation, pp. 83-84.

2166 Strøm, Axel (1961). Undersokelse av Norske tidligere konsentrasjonsleirfanger [Examination of Norwegian ex-concentration camp prisoners]. *Tidsskrift for den Norske Laegeforening. Journal of the Norwegian Medical Association*, 81, 803-816.

2167 Strøm, Axel (Ed.) (1968). *Norwegian Concentration Camp Survivors*. Oslo: Universitetsforlaget, and New York: Humanities Press. 186 p.

2168 Strøm, Axel (1968). Method and material. In: Strøm, Axel (Ed.), *Norwegian Concentration Camp Survivors*. Oslo: Universitetsforlaget, and New York: Humanities Press, 11-13.

2169 Strøm, Axel (1968). Time prior to arrest. In: Strøm, Axel (Ed.), *Norwegian Concentration Camp Survivors*. Oslo: Universitetsforlaget, New York: Humanities Press, pp. 14-17.

2170 Strøm, Axel (1968). Work and family life after the war. In: Strøm, Axel (Ed.), *Norwegian Concentration Camp Survivors*. Oslo: Universitetsforlaget, and New York: Humanities Press, pp. 31-35.

2171 Strøm, Axel (1968). Health after war. In: Strøm, Axel (Ed.), *Norwegian Concentration Camp Survivors*. Oslo: Universitetsforlaget, and York: Humanities Press, pp. 36-44.

2172 Strøm, Axel, and Eitinger, Leo (1968). Arrest and imprisonment. In: Strøm, Axel (Ed.), *Norwegian Concentration Camp Survivors*. Oslo: Universitetsforlaget, and New York: Humanities Press, pp. 18-30.

2173 Strøm, Axel; Refsum, S.B.; Eitinger, Leo; Grønvik, Odd; Lønnum, Arve; Engeset, Arne; Osvik, K.; and Rogan, Bjorn (1962). Examination of Norwegian ex-concentration camp prisoners. *Journal of Neuropsychiatry*, 4, 43-62.

2174 Strøm, Axel; Rogan, Bjorn; and Haug, E. (1968). Evaluations and decisions. In: Strøm, Axel (Ed.), *Norwegian Concentration Camp Survivors*. Oslo: Universitetsforlaget, and New York: Humanities Press, pp. 156-169.

2175 Strzelecka, Irena (1984). Pierwszy szpital obozowy w Brzezince [The first concentration camp hospital in Birkenau]. *Przegląd Lekarski*, 41(1), 88-93.

2176 Strzelecka, Irena (1984). Rozwój szpitali obozowych w Oświęcimiu-Brzezince [Development of hospitals in Auschwitz-Birkenau]. *Przegląd Lekarski*, 41(1), 84-88.

2177 Strzelecka, Irena (1985). Oddział Kobieć w Oświęcimiu [Women's division at Auschwitz]. *Przegląd Lekarski*, 42(1), 80-93.

2178 Strzelecka, Irena (1987). Obóz Kwarantanny dla męszczyzn więzionych w Brzezince [Quarantine of male prisoners of Birkenau]. *Przegląd Lekarski*, 44(1), 102-116.

2179 Strzelecka, Irena (1990). Warunki bytowe więźniów w szpitalach obozu oświecimskiego [Living conditions in the hospitals of the Auschwitz concentration camp]. *Przegląd Lekarski*, 47(1), 100-102.

2180 Strzelecka, Irena (1990). Exterminacyjna funkcja szpitali obozowych w KZ Auschwitz [Exterminatory function of the hospitals in the Auschwitz concentration camp]. *Przegląd Lekarski*, 47(1), 103-107.

2181 Strzelecki, A. (1984). Duch więzniów-konspiratórow w obozie w Oswięcimiu [The morale of prisoners-conspirators at Auschwitz]. *Przegląd Lekarski*, 41(1), 93-96.

2182 Suarez, Juan C. (1983). Reflexiones acerca de un sobreviviente de los campos de exterminio [Some reflections of a survivor from a concentration camp]. *Revista de Psicoanalisis*, 40(1), 35-55.

2183 Summerfield, Derek (1993). Psychological survival after concentration camps [Letter]. *British Medical Journal*, 307(6903), 568.

2184 Sun, Majorie (1988). EPA [Environmental Protection Agency] bars use of Nazi data. *Science*, 240(4848), 21.

2185 Susta, A.; Bardfeld, R.; and Kankova, D. (1978). Zur Häuftigkeit und dem Verlauf bestimmter Rheumakrankheiten bei Widerstandskämpfern [The frequency and development of certain rheumatic diseases in resistance fighters]. In: *Medizinische Untersuchungen der Spätfolgen des Krieges und des NS-Regimes bei Jugendlichen und Kindern von ehemaligen KZ-Häftlingen und Verfolgten* [Medical Research of the Late Effects of the War and National Socialism Regime on Youth and Children of Former Concentration Camp Inmates and Persecuted Persons]. Wien: Internationale Föderation der Widerstandskämpfer. [VI Internationaler Medizinischer Kongress der FIR. Prague, 1976].

2186 Susułowska, Maria (1976). Próba interpretacji treści snów byłych więźniów obozów koncentracyjnych [The interpretation of dreams in ex-concentration camp prisoners]. *Przegląd Lekarski*, 33(1), 13-17.

2187 Susułowska, Maria (1985). Interpretation of dreams of former prisoners of concentration camps. *Psychiatria Fennica*, 149-154.

2188 Sway, Marlene (1984). Coping strategies of female Holocaust survivors. *Journal of Sociology and Social Welfare*, 11(4), 939-950.

2189 Swenson, Cynthia-Cupit; and Klingman, Avigdor (1993). Children and war. In: Saylor, Conway F. (Ed.), *Children and Disasters: Issues in Clinical Child Psychology*. New York: Plenum, pp. 137-163.

2190 Syllaba, J. (1978). Flecktyphys in der kleinen Festung Theresienstadt, Bohmen [Typhus exanthematicus in the "little fortress" in Theresienstadt (Terezin), Bohemia]. In: *Medizinische Untersuchungen der Spätfolgen des Krieges und des NS-Regimes bei Jugendlichen und Kindern von ehemaligen KZ-Häftlingen und Verfolgten* [Medical Research of the Late Effects of the War and National Socialism Regime on Youth and Children of Former Concentration Camp Inmates and Persecuted Persons]. Wien: Internationale Föderation der Widerstandskämpfer. [VI Internationaler Medizinischer Kongress der FIR. Prague, 1976].

2191 Sypniewska, Maria (1979). Obrazki z Ravensbrück [Episodes from the Ravensbrück camp]. *Przegląd Lekarski*, 36(1), 175-179.

2192 Szczerbowski, Kazimierz (1970). Wspomnienia pierwszego pisarza "reviru" oświęcimskiego [Reminiscences of the first winter in the sick bay of the Auschwitz concentration camp]. *Przegląd Lekarski*, 26(1), 198-201.

2193 Szczerbowski, Kazimierz (1987). Der erste Schreiber im "Revier" von Auschwitz-Erinnerungen [The first writer of Auschwitz memoirs in the district "Revier"]. In: Hamburger Institut für Sozialforschung (Eds.), *Die Auschwitz-Hefte. Texte der polnischen Zeitschrift "Przegląd Lekarski" über historische, psychische und medizinische Aspekte des Lebens und Sterbens in Auschwitz. Band 1* [The Auschwitz Journal. Text of the Polish Journal "Medical Review" on Historical, Psychic and Medical Aspects of Life and Death in Auschwitz. Volume 1]. Weinheim and Basel: Beltz, pp. 155-158.

2194 Szczerbowski, Kazimierz (1988). W Kancelarii rewiru podczas pierwszych lat Oświęcimia I [In the hospital office during the first few years in the Auschwitz concentration camp]. *Przegląd Lekarski*, 45(1), 125-133.

2195 Szejnman, Michael (1979). Changes in peripheral blood and bone marrow in hunger disease. In: Winick, Myron (Ed.), *Hunger Disease: Studies by the Jewish Physicians in the Warsaw Ghetto*. New York: John Wiley & Sons, pp. 161-199.

2196 Szek, Judit (1991). Estrategias de Sobrevivencia do Ponto de Vista Psicanalitico [Strategies for survival from a psychoanalytic perspective]. *Percurso Revista de Psicanalise*, 3(7), 14-17.

2197 Szemraj-Lochyńska, Alicja, and Kempisty, Czesław (1981). Stan adaptacji do życia na emeryturze nauczycieli akademickich represjonowanych przez hitleryzm [Psychological adaptation of retired university teachers, former victims of Nazi repressive measures]. *Przegląd Lekarski*, 38(1), 33-36.

2198 Szilagyi, Julia; Cserne, Istvan; Peto, Katalin; and Szoke, Gyotgy (1992). A masodik es a harmadik generacio: Holocaust tulelok es gyermekeik [Survivors of the Holocaust: The second and third generation in Hungary]. *Psychiatria Hungarica*, 7(2), 117-129.

2199 Szuszkiewicz, Roman (1971). Dentistry in the Auschwitz concentration camp. In: *Auschwitz Anthology. Vol. 2: In Hell They*

Preserved Human Dignity. Part 1. Warsaw: International Auschwitz Committee, pp. 184-197.

2200 Szwarc, Halina (1965). Chorowośc byłych więźniow Hitlerowskich więzień i obozów koncentracyjnych [The morbidity of ex-prisoners of Hitlerian prisons and concentration camps]. *Przegląd Lekarski*, 21, 38-46.

2201 Szwarc, Halina (1971). The Poznan Center. In: *Auschwitz Anthology. Vol. 3: It Did Not End in Forty-Five. Part 1.* Warsaw: International Auschwitz Committee, pp. 94-104.

2202 Szwarc, Halina (1973). Krankheiten ehemaliger Konzentrationslagerhäftlinge auf der Grundlage der in den Jahren 1964 bis 1966 in der VR Polen durchgeführten Untersuchungen [Diseases among concentration camp prisoners: Investigations carried out in the People's Republic of Poland, 1964-1966]. In: *Ermüdung und vorzeitiges Altern: Folge von Extrembelastungen* [Exhaustion and Premature Aging: Result of Extreme Stress]. Leipzig: Barth, pp. 250-254. [V Internationaler Medizinischer Kongress der FIR. Paris, 21-24 September 1970].

2203 Szwarc, Halina (1978). Vorzeitige Alterung der ehemaligen polnischen KZ Häftlinge und der Kombattanten [Premature aging in Polish ex-concentration camp prisoners and combatants]. In: *Medizinische Untersuchungen der Spätfolgen des Krieges und des NS-Regimes bei Jugendlichen und Kindern von ehemaligen KZ-Häftlingen und Verfolgten* [Medical Research of the Late Effects of the War and National Socialism Regime on Youth and Children of Former Concentration Camp Inmates and Persecuted Persons]. Wien: Internationale Föderation der Widerstandskämpfer. [VI Internationaler Medizinischer Kongress der FIR. Prague, 1976].

2204 Szwarc, Halina (1983). Über die Betreuung und die medizinische Rehabilitation der Naziopfer und Kombattanten [On the treatment and medical rehabilitation of the Nazi victims and resistance fighters]. *Cahiers d'Informations Médicales, Sociales et Juridiques*, 19, 150-154.

2205 Szwarc, Halina (1985). The premature ageing of former KZ-prisoners. *Zeitschrift für Alternsforschung*, 40(4), 209-212.

2206 Szymański, Tadeusz; Szymańska, Danuta; and Śnieżko, Tadeusz (1971). The "hospital" in the family camp for Gypsies in Auschwitz-Birkenau. In: *Auschwitz Anthology. Vol. 2: In Hell They Preserved Human Dignity. Part 2.* Warsaw: International Auschwitz Committee, pp. 1-45.

2207 Szymański, Tadeusz; Szymańska, Danuta; and Śnieszko, Tadeusz (1987). Das "Spital" im Zigeuner-Familienlager in Auschwitz-Birkenau [The "hospital" in the family camp for Gypsies in Auschwitz-Birkenau]. In: Hamburger Institut für Sozialforschung (Eds.), *Die Auschwitz-Hefte. Texte der polnischen Zeitschrift "Przegląd Lekarski" über historische, psychische und medizinische Aspekte des Lebens und Sterbens in Auschwitz. Band 1* [The Auschwitz Journal. Text of the Polish Journal "Medical Review" on Historical, Psychic and Medical Aspects of Life and Death in Auschwitz. Volume 1]. Weinheim and Basel: Beltz, pp. 199-207.

2208 Szymusik, Adam (1962). Poobozowe zaburzenia psychiczne u byłych więźniów obozu koncentracyjnego w Oświęcimiu [Post-camp psychological disturbances among ex-prisoners from the concentration camp Auschwitz]. *Polski Tygodnik Lekarski*, 17, 86-89.

2209 Szymusik, Adam (1972). Post-camp asthenia noticed with former prisoners of the Auschwitz concentration camp. In: *Auschwitz Anthology. Vol. 3: It Did Not End in Forty-Five. Part 2*. Warsaw: International Auschwitz Committee, pp. 207-240.

2210 Szymusik, Adam (1974). Inwalidztwo wojenne byłych więźniów obozów koncentracyjnych [The war disability of ex-concentration camp prisoners]. *Przegląd Lekarski*, 31, 110-112.

2211 Szymusik, Adam (1975). Die Kriegsinvalidität ehemaliger Konzentrationslagerhäftlinge [The war disability of ex-concentration camp prisoners]. *Mitteilungen der FIR*, 9, 10-14.

2212 Szymusik, Adam (1991). Die unauslöslichen Spuren des Terrors: Medizinisch psychiatrische Untersuchungen von ehemaligen KZ-Häftlingen in der Krakauer Psychiatrischen Klinik [The inextinguishable traces of terror: Medical-psychiatric investigation of former concentration camp inmates at the Cracow psychiatric clinic]. In: Stoffels, Hans (Ed.), *Schicksale der Verfolgten: Psychische und somatische Auswirkungen von Terrorherrschaft* [The Fate of Persecuted Persons: Psychic and Somatic Effects of Terror Reign]. Berlin: Springer, pp. 32-41.

2213 Szymusik, Adam (1995). Die Forschungen zum Zustand ehemaliger KZ-Haftlinge in der Psychiatrischen Klinik Krakau: 1959-1990 [Research concerning the condition of former concentration camp inmates in the psychiatric clinic of Cracow: 1959-1990]. In: Hamburger Institut für Sozialforschung (Eds.), *Die Auschwitz-Hefte. Ergänzungsband. Texte der polnischen Zeitschrift "Przegląd Lekarski" über historische, psychische und medizinische Aspekte des Lebens und Sterbens in Auschwitz* [The Auschwitz Journal. Supplementary

Volume. Text of the Polish Journal "Medical Review" on Historical, Psychic and Medical Aspects of Life and Death in Auschwitz]. Weinheim and Basel: Rogner and Bernhard, pp. 14-18.

2214 Szymusik, Adam; Leśniak, Roman; Orwid, Maria; and Teutsch, Aleksander (1978). Untersuchungen an ehemaligen Häftlingen der KZ-lager Auschwitz-Birkenau, durchgeführt an der psychiatrischen Klinik der medizinischen Akademie in Krakow (1959-1976) [Investigations of ex-prisoners of the concentration camps Auschwitz-Birkenau carried out at the psychiatric clinic of the Medical Academy of Cracow (1959-1976)]. In: *Medizinische Untersuchungen der Spätfolgen des Krieges und des NS-Regimes bei Jugendlichen und Kindern von ehemaligen KZ-Häftlingen und Verfolgten [Medical Research of the Late Effects of the War and National Socialism Regime on Youth and Children of Former Concentration Camp Inmates and Persecuted Persons].* Wien: Internationale Föderation der Widerstandskämpfer. [VI Internationaler Medizinischer Kongress der FIR. Prague, 1976].

2215 Tabory, Ephraim, and Weller, Leonard (1987). The impact of cultural context on the mental health of Jewish concentration camp survivors. *Holocaust and Genocide Studies*, 2(2), 299-305.

2216 Tal, Ido (1992). *Tahalichay separatzia-individuatzia v'yecholet **l'intimiut b'kerev banim l'nitzoley hashoah*** **[Separation-individuation** and capacity for intimacy in children of Holocaust survivors]. Unpublished master's thesis, Department of Psychology, Tel Aviv University, Tel Aviv, Israel. 239 pp.

2217 Tal, Kali J. (1991). *Bearing witness: The literature of trauma.* Unpublished doctoral dissertation, Yale University, New Haven, Connecticut, 335 pp. *Dissertation Abstracts International*, 52(7-A), p. 2602. (University Microfilms no. AAC 9136197).

2218 Tanay, Emanuel (1968). Initiation of psychotherapy with survivors of Nazi persecutions. In: Krystal, Henry (Ed.), *Massive Psychic Trauma*. New York: International Universities Press, pp. 219-233.

2219 Tanay, Emanuel (1991). On being a survivor. In: Berger, Alan L. (Ed.), *Bearing Witness to the Holocaust: 1939-1989*. Lewiston, NY: Edwin Mellen, pp. 16-31.

2220 Targowla, René (1950). Sur une forme du syndrome asthénique des déportés et prisoniers de la guerre 1939-1945 [On a form of asthenia syndrome of deportees and prisoners of war]. *Presse Médicale*, 58, 728-730.

2221 Targowla, René (1954). Les sequelles pathologiques de la déportation dans les camps de concentration allemands pendant la deuxième guerre mondiale [The pathological sequelae of deportation to the German concentration camps during World War II]. *Presse Médicale*, 62, 611-613.

2222 Targowla, René (1955). Bericht zur Ausarbeitung einer neuen Rentenabelle für ehemalige Verfolgte, Internierte und Deportierte [Report about the development of a new pension-table for former persecutees, internees and deportees]. In: Michel, Max (Ed.), *Gesundheitsschäden durch Verfolgung und Gefangenschaft und ihre Spätfolgen: Zusammenstellung der Referate und Ergebnisse der Internationalen Sozialmedizinischen Konferenz über die Pathologie der Ehemaligen Deportierten und Internierten, 5-7 Juni 1954 in Kopenhagen* [Health Damages Caused by Persecution and Captivity and the Late Effects: Compilation of the Papers and Results of the International Conference of Social Medicine on the Pathology of Former Deported and Interned Persons, 5-7 June 1954 in Copenhagen]. Frankfurt am Main: Röderberg, pp. 274-280.

2223 Targowla, René (1955). Die neuropsychischen Folgen der Deportation in Deutschen Konzentrationslagern. Syndrom der Asthenie der Deportierten [The neuropsychic results of deportation in German concentration camps. Syndrome of asthenia in deportees]. In: Michel, Max (Ed.), *Gesundheitsschäden durch Verfolgung und Gefangenschaft und ihre Spätfolgen: Zusammenstellung der Referate und Ergebnisse der Internationalen Sozialmedizinischen Konferenz über die Pathologie der Ehemaligen Deportierten und Internierten, 5-7 Juni 1954 in Kopenhagen* [Health Damages Caused by Persecution and Captivity and the Late Effects: Compilation of the Papers and Results of the International Conference of Social Medicine on the Pathology of Former Deported and Interned Persons, 5-7 June 1954 in Copenhagen]. Frankfurt am Main: Röderberg, pp. 30-40.

2224 Tas, J. (1951). Psychical disorders among inmates of concentration camps and repatriates. *Psychiatric Quarterly*, 5, 679-690.

2225 Tauber, Ingrid D. (1980). *Second-generation effects of the Nazi Holocaust: A psychosocial study of a nonclinical sample in North America*. Unpublished doctoral dissertation, California School of Professional Psychology, Berkeley/Alameda, 184 pp. *Dissertation Abstracts International*, 41(12-B), p. 5210. (University Microfilms no. AAC 8110184).

2226 Taufrova, M. (1978). Beziehungen zwischen der psychischen und somatischen Seite der TBC Erkrankung im Konzentrationslager

Ravensbrück und allgemeine Folgerungen, die heute bei der einstellung früherer Lagerhäftlingen zu Krankheiten anwendbar sind [Correlations between the psychic and somatic aspects of TBC in the concentration camp of Ravensbrück: General consequences applicable to the attitude of ex-prisoners to diseases]. In: *Medizinische Untersuchungen der Spätfolgen des Krieges und des NS-Regimes bei Jugendlichen und Kindern von ehemaligen KZ-Häftlingen und Verfolgten* [Medical Research of the Late Effects of the War and National Socialism Regime on Youth and Children of Former Concentration Camp Inmates and Persecuted Persons]. Wien: Internationale Föderation der Widerstandskämpfer. [VI Internationaler Medizinischer Kongress der FIR. Prague, 1976].

2227 Taylor, B. (1975). A doctor against Hitler. *Maryland State Medical Journal*, 24(1), 61-62.

2228 Tec, Nechama (1986). *When Light Pierced the Darkness: Christian Rescue of Jews in Nazi-Occupied Poland*. New York: Oxford University Press. 262 pp.

2229 Tennant, Christopher (1983). Life events and psychological morbidity: The evidence from prospective studies. *Psychological Medicine*, 13(3), 483-486.

2230 Terry, Jack (1984). The damaging effects of the "survivor syndrome." In: Luel, Steven A., and Marcus, Paul (Eds.), *Psychoanalytic Reflections on the Holocaust: Selected Essays*. New York: Ktav, pp. 135-148.

2231 Teutsch, Aleksander (1972). Psychological reactions during psycho-physical stress in the case of 100 former prisoners of Auschwitz-Birkenau. In: *Auschwitz Anthology. Vol. 3: It Did Not End in Forty-Five. Part 2*. Warsaw: International Auschwitz Committee, pp. 143-173.

2232 Teutsch, Aleksander, and Dominik, Malgorzata (1978). Neurosen bei Nachkommen ehemaliger KZ Lagerinsassen [Neuroses in the descendants of ex-concentration camp inmates]. In: *Medizinische Untersuchungen der Spätfolgen des Krieges und des NS-Regimes bei Jugendlichen und Kindern von ehemaligen KZ-Häftlingen und Verfolgten* [Medical Research of the Late Effects of the War and National Socialism Regime on Youth and Children of Former Concentration Camp Inmates and Persecuted Persons]. Wien: Internationale Föderation der Widerstandskämpfer, pp. 74-78. [VI Internationaler Medizinischer Kongress der FIR. Prague, 1976].

2233 Thompson, Lloyd (1947). German concentration camps: Psychological aspects of the camps. *War Medicine*, 1, 466-467.

2234 Thomsen, S.O. (1949). Eftersygdomme hos tidligere koncentrationslejrfanger [Morbid sequelae among ex-concentration camp prisoners]. *Ugeskrift for Laeger*, 111, 665-668.

2235 Thygesen, Paul (Ed.) (1954). *La Déportation dans les Camps de Concentration Allemands et ses Séquelles: Une Analyse médicale et sociale* [Deportation in the German Concentration Camps and its Consequences: A Medical and Social Analysis]. Copenhague: Edité par la Croix Rouge Danoise. 80 pp.

2236 Thygesen, Paul (1955). Allgemeines über die Spätfolgen [General remarks on the late sequelae]. In: Michel, Max (Ed.), *Gesundheitsschäden durch Verfolgung und Gefangenschaft und ihre Spätfolgen: Zusammenstellung der Referate und Ergebnisse der Internationalen Sozialmedizinischen Konferenz über die Pathologie der Ehemaligen Deportierten und Internierten, 5-7 Juni 1954 in Kopenhagen* [Health Damages Caused by Persecution and Captivity and the Late Effects: Compilation of the Papers and Results of the International Conference of Social Medicine on the Pathology of Former Deported and Interned Persons, 5-7 June 1954 in Copenhagen]. Frankfurt am Main: Röderberg, pp. 21-29.

2237 Thygesen, Paul (1973). Late effects of imprisonment in concentration camps during world war II. In: *Physical and Mental Consequences of Imprisonment and Torture: Lectures presented at the Conference at Lysebu, Oslo, October 5-7 1973*. London: Amnesty International, pp. 69-87.

2238 Thygesen, Paul (1979). En lovgivnings intentioner og dens virkninger [The intentions of the law and its consequences]. *Ugeskrift for Laeger*, 141, 1164-1169.

2239 Thygesen, Paul (1980). The concentration camp syndrome. *Danish Medical Bulletin*, 27(4), 224-228.

2240 Thygesen, Paul; Fichez, Louis F.; Laroche, Madeleine; Jaloustre, René; and Sorne, G. (1955). Die psychischen Symptome der Heimkehr [The psychological symptoms of homecoming]. In: Michel, Max (Ed.), *Gesundheitsschäden durch Verfolgung und Gefangenschaft und ihre Spätfolgen: Zusammenstellung der Referate und Ergebnisse der Internationalen Sozialmedizinischen Konferenz über die Pathologie der Ehemaligen Deportierten und Internierten, 5-7 Juni 1954 in Kopenhagen* [Health Damages Caused by Persecution and

Captivity and the Late Effects: Compilation of the Papers and Results of the International Conference of Social Medicine on the Pathology of Former Deported and Interned Persons, 5-7 June 1954 in Copenhagen]. Frankfurt am Main: Röderberg, pp. 52-58.

2241 Thygesen, Paul, and Hermann, Knud (1964). Die Wirkungen des KZ-Syndroms, 19 Jahre danach: Eine medico-soziale Analyse [The influences of the concentration camp syndrome 19 years later: A medical social analysis]. In: *Ätio-Pathogenese und Therapie der Erschöpfung und vorzeitigen Vergreisung* [The Aetiology, Pathogenesis and Therapy of Exhaustion and Premature Aging]. Wien: Verlag der FIR, pp. 311-326. [IV Internationaler Medizinischer Kongress. Bucharest, 22-27 Juni 1964].

2242 Thygesen, Paul; Hermann, Knud; and Willanger, R. (1970). Concentration camp survivors in Denmark: Persecution, disease, disability, compensation. *Danish Medical Bulletin*, 17, 65-108.

2243 Thygesen, Paul; Hermann, Knud; and Willanger, R. (1973). Konzentrationslagerüberlebende in Dänemark [Concentration camp survivors in Denmark]. In: *Ermüdung und vorzeitiges Altern: Folge von Extrembelastungen* [Exhaustion and Premature Aging: Result of Extreme Stress]. Leipzig: Barth, pp. 71-124. [V Internationaler Medizinischer Kongress der FIR. Paris, 21-24 September 1970].

2244 Thygesen, Paul, and Kieler, Jørgen (1952). Introduction. In: Helweg-Larsen, Per; Hoffmeyer, Henrik; Kieler, Jørgen; Hess Thaysen, Eigil; Hess Thaysen, Jørn; Thygesen, Paul; and Hertel Wulff, Munke, *Famine Disease in German Concentration Camps, Complications and Sequelae: With Special Reference to Tuberculosis, Mental Disorders and Social Consequences*. Copenhagen: Ejnar Munksgaard, pp. 13-25. [Also published as *Acta Psychiatrica et Neurologica Scandinavica*, Supplementum 83.]

2245 Thygesen, Paul, and Kieler, Jørgen (1952). Famine disease: Avitaminosis incident to semistarvation. In: Helweg-Larsen, Per; Hoffmeyer, Henrik; Kieler, Jørgen; Hess Thaysen, Eigil; Hess Thaysen, Jørn; Thygesen, Paul; and Hertel Wulff, Munke, *Famine Disease in German Concentration Camps, Complications and Sequelae: With Special Reference to Tuberculosis, Mental Disorders and Social Consequences*. Copenhagen: Ejnar Munksgaard, pp. 207-234. [Also published as *Acta Psychiatrica et Neurologica Scandinavica*, Supplementum 83.]

2246 Thygesen, Paul, and Kieler, Jørgen (1952). Famine disease: Mental deterioration. In: Helweg-Larsen, Per; Hoffmeyer, Henrik; Kieler,

Jørgen; Hess Thaysen, Eigil; Hess Thaysen, Jørn; Thygesen, Paul; and Hertel Wulff, Munke, *Famine Disease in German Concentration Camps, Complications and Sequelae: With Special Reference to Tuberculosis, Mental Disorders and Social Consequences*. Copenhagen: Ejnar Munksgaard, pp. 235-250. [Also published as *Acta Psychiatrica et Neurologica Scandinavica*, Supplementum 83.]

2247 Thygesen, Paul, and Kieler, Jørgen (1952). Famine disease: The Mussulman. In: Helweg-Larsen, Per; Hoffmeyer, Henrik; Kieler, Jørgen; Hess Thaysen, Eigil; Hess Thaysen, Jørn; Thygesen, Paul; and Hertel Wulff, Munke, *Famine Disease in German Concentration Camps, Complications and Sequelae: With Special Reference to Tuberculosis, Mental Disorders and Social Consequences*. Copenhagen: Ejnar Munksgaard, pp. 251-254. [Also published as *Acta Psychiatrica et Neurologica Scandinavica*, Supplementum 83.]

2248 Togel, C. (1990). Bahnstation Treblinka. Zum Schicksal von Sigmund Freud's Schwester Rosa Graf [Treblinka train station: On the fate of Sigmund Freud's sister Rosa Graf]. *Psyche: Zeitschrift für Psychoanalyse und ihre Anwendungen*, 44(11), 1019-1024.

2249 Trachtenberg, Martin, and Davis, Minna (1978). Breaking silence: Serving children of Holocaust survivors. *Journal of Jewish Communal Service*, 54, 294-302.

2250 Trautman, Ernest (1961). Psychiatric and sociological effects of Nazi atrocities on survivors of the extermination camps. *Journal of the American Association of Social Psychiatry*, 118-122.

2251 Trautman, Ernest (1961). Psychiatrische Untersuchungen an Überlebenden der nationalsozialistischen Vernichtungslager 15 Jahre nach der Befreiung [Psychiatric investigations of the Nazi annihilation camp survivors 15 years after their liberation]. *Nervenarzt*, 32, 545-551.

2252 Trautman, Ernest (1964). Fear and panic in Nazi concentration camps: A biosocial evaluation of the chronic anxiety syndrome. *International Journal of Social Psychiatry*, 10(2), 131-141.

2253 Trautman, Ernest (1971). Violence and victims in Nazi concentration camps and the psychopathology of the survivors. *International Psychiatry Clinics*, 9(1), 115-133.

2254 Trebing, G. (1973). Blackfan-Diamond-Syndrom als Folge väterlicher Haftschäden [The Blackfan-Diamond-Syndrome as a result of disturbances caused by persecution of the father]. In: *Ermüdung und* *vorzeitiges Altern: Folge von Extrembelastungen* [Exhaustion and Premature Aging: Result of Extreme Stress]. Leipzig: Barth, pp. 255-258. [V Internationaler Medizinischer Kongress der FIR. Paris, 21-24 September 1970].

2255 Trossman, Bernard (1968). Adolescent children of concentration camp survivors. *Canadian Psychiatric Association Journal*, 13, 121-123.

2256 Tschebotarjow, D. (1961). Wiederherstellungstherapie, Prophylaxe und Behandlung der vorzeitigen Vergreisung bei ehemaligen Kriegsgefangenen und Kriegsinvaliden in der Sowjetunion [Rehabilitation, prevention and therapy of premature aging in ex-prisoners of war and war invalids in the Soviet Union]. In: *Die Behandlung der Asthenie und der vorzeitigen Vergreisung bei ehemaligen Widerstandskämpfern und KZ-Häftlingen* [Treatment of Asthenia and Premature Aging in Former Resistance Fighters and Concentration Camp Inmates]. Wien: Verlag der FIR, pp. 231-238. [III Internationale Medizinische Konferenz. Liege, 17-19 März 1961].

2257 Tuteur, Werner (1966). One hundred concentration camp survivors: Twenty years later. *Israel Annals of Psychiatry and Related Disciplines*, 4(1), 78-90.

2258 Tycho, G. (1969). Discussion of Klaus Hoppe. The emotional reactions of psychiatrists when confronting survivors of persecution. In: Lindon, John A. (Ed.), *Psychoanalytic Forum. Vol. 3.* New York: Science House.

2259 Tyndel, N.M. (1971). Beitrag zur Kasuistik und Psycho-pathologie der während der nationalsozialistischen Verfolgung geborenen Kinder [A contribution to the casuistry and psychopathology of children born during the time of Nazi persecution]. In: Herberg, Hans-Joachim (Ed.), *Spätschäden nach Extrembelastungen* [Late Damage After Extreme Stress]. Herford: Nicolai, pp. 266-269. [II Internationalen Medizinisch-Juristischen Konferenz. Dusseldorf, 1969].

2260 Valent, Paul (1990). Effects of the Holocaust on child survivors. *Australian and New Zealand Journal of Family Therapy*, 1, 12-16.

2261 Valent, Paul (1994). *Child Survivors: Adults Living with Childhood Trauma*. Port Melbourne, Victoria: William Heinemann. 288 pp.

2262 Valkhoff, J. (1982). Psychiatrisering van politieke vluchtelingen en tweede generatie slachtoffers [Making psychiatric patients of political refugees and second generation victims]. *Bulletin de Klientenbond*, 10(4-5), 26-29.

2263 Van-Bork, J.J. (1982). An attempt to clarify a dream-mechanism? Why do people wake up out of an anxiety dream? *International Review of Psycho-Analysis*, 93, 273-277.

2264 Van den Berghe, Gie (1987). *Met de Dood voor de Ogen: Begrip en Onbegrip Tussen Overlevenden van Nazi-Kampen en Buitenstaanders* [Facing Death: Comprehension and Non-Comprehension Between Survivors of the Nazi Camps and Outsiders]. Berchem: EPO. 535 pp.

2265 Van der Hal, Elisheva; Tauber, Yvonne; and Gottesfeld, Johanna (1996). Open groups for children of Holocaust survivors. *International Journal of Group Psychotherapy*, 46(2), 193-208.

2266 Van der Laan, M.C. (1994). Kohut's self-psychologie en de problematiek van tweede generatie-oorlogsgetroffenen [Kohut's self-psychology and the problem of second generation war victims]. *Tijdschrift voor Psychotherapie*, 20, 279-292.

2267 Van der Ploeg, H.M. (1987). Onderzoek naar behandeling van oorlogsslachtoffers met LSD-psychotherapie: Een verslag van vooronderzoek [An investigation of the treatment of war victims with LSD psychotherapy]. *Sectie Medische Psychologie*, 27.

2268 Van Kampen-Bronkhorst, D. (1979). *De Oorlog Duurt Voort, Over de Problematiek van Oorlogsgetroffenen* [The War Goes On, On the Problems of War Victims]. Den Haag: VUGA.

2269 Van Praag, J.P. (1979). Background problems and possibilities of treatment in cases of extreme stress. In: *Israel-Netherlands Symposium on the Impact of Persecution. Jerusalem, 16-24 October 1977*. Rijswijk, The Netherlands: Ministry of Cultural Affairs, Recreation and Social Welfare, pp. 9-17.

2270 Van Ravesteijn, Leopold (1976). De arts geconfronteerd met lijders aan het KZ-syndroom [The physician confronted with patient suffering from the concentration camp syndrome]. *Nederlands Tijdschrift voor Geneeskunde*, 120, 316-318.

2271 Van Ravesteijn, Leopold (1976). Gelaagdheid van herinneringen [The characteristics of memories]. *Tijdschrift voor Psychotherapie*, 5, 195-205.

2272 Van Ravesteijn, Leopold (1976). De traumatische droom [The traumatic dream]. *Tijdschrift voor Psychotherapie*, 2, 1-8.

2273 Van Ravesteijn, Leopold (1978). Gelaagdheid van emoties, het "onzichtbare" schaamtegevoel en het KZ-syndroom [The characteristics of emotions: The "invisible" feelings of shame in the concentration camp syndrome]. *Tijdschrift voor Psychotherapie*, 4(4), 175-185.

2274 Van Tol, D. (1977). KZ-syndroom, rampensyndroom en traumatische neurose [Concentration camp syndrome, disaster syndrome and traumatic neurosis]. *I Medisch Magazine*, 62-71.

2275 Van Veen, A. (1977). *WUV-problemen, doktoraal skriptie over immateriele aspekten van de wet uitkeringen vervolgingsslachtoffers 1940-1945* [WUV problems, Dutch compensation law for the persecuted: Intangible aspects of the WUV 1940-1945]. Unpublished master's thesis, Andragogisch Institut, Rijksuniversiteit Groningen, The Netherlands.

2276 Vegh, Claudine (1979). *Je ne lui ai pas dit au revoir* [I Didn't Say Goodbye]. Paris: Editions Gallimard. 197 pp.

2277 Vegh, Claudine (1981). *Ich Habe Ihnen Nicht Auf Wiedersehn Gesagt. Gesprache Mit Kindern von Deportierten* [I Didn't Say Goodbye: Conversations with Children of the Deportees]. Köln: Kiepenheuer and Witsch.

2278 Vegh, Claudine (1984). *I Didn't Say Goodbye*. New York: E.P. Dutton. 179 pp.

2279 Vella, E.E. (1984). Belsen: Medical aspects of a World War II concentration camp. *Journal of the Royal Army Medical Corps*, 130(1), 34-59.

2280 Venaki, Sophie K.; Nadler, Arie; and Gershoni, Hadas (1985). Sharing the Holocaust experience: Communication behaviors and their consequences in families of ex-partisans and ex-prisoners of concentration camps. *Family Process*, 24(2), 273-280.

2281 Venzlaff, Ulrich (1958). *Die psychoreaktiven Störungen nach entschädigungspflichligen Ereignissen (die sogenannten Unfallneurosen)* [Psychoreactive Disturbances Following Events Liable to Compensation (the So-Called Accident Neurosis)]. Berlin: Springer. 104 pp.

2282 Venzlaff, Ulrich (1959). Grundsätzliche Betrachtungen über die Begutachtung erlebnisbedingter seelischer Störungen nach rassischer und politischer Verfolgung [Prinicipal discussion on the evaluation of psychological disturbances after racial or political persecution]. *Rechtsprechung zum Wiedergutmachungsrecht* 10, 292-298.

2283 Venzlaff, Ulrich (1961). Schizophrenie und Verfolgung [Schizophrenia and persecution]. *Rechtsprechung zum Wiedergutmachungsrecht*, 171-191.

2284 Venzlaff, Ulrich (1962). Untersuchungen an ehemaligen norwegischen Konzentrationslagergefangenen [Investigations on former Norwegian concentration camp prisoners]. *Rechtsprechung zum Wiedergutmachungsrecht,* 7, 295-296.

2285 Venzlaff, Ulrich (1963). Erlebnisintergrund und Dynamik seelischer Verfolgungsschäden [Dynamics and experiences in psychic disturbances caused by persecution]. In: Paul, Helmut, and Herberg, Hans-Joachim (Eds.), *Psychische Spätschäden nach politischer Verfolgung* [Psychological Late Damages Following Political Persecution]. Basel: Karger, pp. 95-109.

2286 Venzlaff, Ulrich (1963). Gutachten zur Frage des Zusammenwirkens erlebnisreaktiver, vegetativer und hormonaler Faktoren bei Verfolgungsschäden [Expert statement on the synergistic action of reactive, vegetative and hormonal factors in disturbances caused by persecution]. In: Paul, Helmut, and Herberg, Hans-Joachim (Eds.), *Psychische Spätschäden nach politischer Verfolgung* [Psychological Late Damages Following Political Persecution]. Basel: Karger, pp. 111-124.

2287 Venzlaff, Ulrich (1964). Mental disorders resulting from racial persecution. *International Journal of Psycho-Analysis*, 45, 617-621.

2288 Venzlaff, Ulrich (1964). Mental disorders resulting from racial persecution outside of concentration camps. *International Journal of Social Psychiatry*, 10(3), 177-183.

2289 Venzlaff, Ulrich (1964). Über die Ursachen seelischer Dauerschäden nach psychomatischen Extrembelastungen [The causes of chronic psychological disturbances after psychosomatic stress]. *Virchow-Pirquet Medical Society*, 24, 23-43.

2290 Venzlaff, Ulrich (1966). Das akute und das chronische Belastungssyndrom [Acute and chronic stress syndromes]. *Medizinische Welt*, 17, 369-376.

2291 Venzlaff, Ulrich (1966). Die Begutachtung psychischer Störungen Verfolgter [The evaluation of psychic disturbances in persecutees]. *Rechtsprechung zum Wiedergutmachungsrecht*, 17, 196-200.

2292 Venzlaff, Ulrich (1967). Akute und chronische psychiatrische syndrome nach Extrembelastungen [Acute and chronic syndromes after extreme stress]. *Medizinische Klinik*, 62, 701-706.

2293 Venzlaff, Ulrich (1967). Psychische Spätschäden nach Gefangenschaft und Verfolgung [Psychic sequelae after imprisonment and persecution]. In: Herberg, Hans-Joachim (Ed.), *Die Beurteilung von Gesundheitsschäden nach Gefangenschaft und Verfolgung* [The Assessment of Health Damages Following Internment and Persecution]. Herford: Nicolai, pp. 93-101. [Internationalen Medizinische-Juristischen Symposiums in Köln].

2294 Venzlaff, Ulrich (1967). Die Sachverständigentätigkeit in der Wiedergutmachung. Bilanz und Ausblick [Specialists' evaluations and the problems of compensation today and in the future]. *Rechtsprechung zum Wiedergutmachungsrecht*, 18, 594-595.

2295 Venzlaff, Ulrich (1968). Erlebnisreaktiver Persönlichkeitswandel: Fiktion oder wirklichkeit? [Personality changes caused by life experiences: fact or fiction?]. *Nervenarzt*, 39, 539-542.

2296 Venzlaff, Ulrich (1968). Forensic psychiatry of schizophrenia in survivors. In: Krystal, Henry (Ed.), *Massive Psychic Trauma*. New York: International Universities Press, pp. 110-125.

2297 Venzlaff, Ulrich (1971). Neurologische-psychiatrische Ursachen von Voralterung und Frühinvalidität nach Konzentrationslagerhäft und Kriegsgefangenschaft [Neurological and psychiatric causes of premature aging and incapacity in prisoners in concentration camps and of war]. In: Herberg, Hans-Joachim (Ed.), *Spätschäden nach Extrembelastungen* [Late Damage After Extreme Stress]. Herford: Nicolai, pp. 82-89. [II Internationalen Medizinische-Juristischen Konferenz. Dusseldorf, 1969].

2298 Venzlaff, Ulrich (1973). Neuropsychiatrische Aspekte der Voralterung Konzentrationslagerüberlebender [Neuropsychiatric aspects of premature aging in concentration camp survivors]. In: *Ermüdung und vorzeitiges Altern: Folge von Extrembelastungen* [Exhaustion and Premature Aging: Result of Extreme Stress]. Leipzig: Barth, pp. 259-265. [V Internationaler Medizinischer Kongress der FIR. Paris, 21-24 September 1970].

2299 Vic-Dupont, Dr.; Fichez, Louis F.; and Weinstein, Dr. (1955). Die Tuberkulose bei den Deportierten [Tuberculosis in deportees]. In: Michel, Max (Ed.), *Gesundheitsschäden durch Verfolgung und Gefangenschaft und ihre Spätfolgen: Zusammenstellung der Referate und Ergebnisse der Internationalen Sozialmedizinischen Konferenz über die Pathologie der Ehemaligen Deportierten und Internierten, 5-7 Juni 1954 in Kopenhagen* [Health Damages Caused by Persecution and Captivity and the Late Effects: Compilation of the Papers and Results of the International Conference of Social Medicine on the Pathology of Former Deported and Interned Persons, 5-7 June 1954 in Copenhagen]. Frankfurt am Main: Röderberg, pp. 91-100.

2300 Villar, H., and Miranda, R. (1964). Efectos alejados, psicopatologicos, medico-legales y sociales de las persecuciones raciales [Late psychopathological, medico-legal and social effects of racial persecution]. *Revista Argentina Neurologica Psiquiatrica*, 1, 289-297.

2301 Villeneuve, A., and Dogan, K. (1971). L'adaptation au milieu contrôlé [Adaptation to a controlled milieu]. *Psychiatry Digest*, 42(1), 8-11.

2302 Virag, Terez (1984). Children of the Holocaust and their children's children: Working through current trauma in the psychotherapeutic process. *Dynamic Psychotherapy*, 2(1), 47-60.

2303 Virag, Terez (1990). A magyarorszagi Holocaust-tulelok leszarmazottainak sajatos lelki strukturaja [The particular psychic structure of the descendants of the survivors of the Holocaust in Hungary]. *Magyar Pszichologiai Szemle*, 46(3-4), 139-154.

2304 Visotsky, Harold M. (1970). Coping behaviors under extreme stress. *Archives of General Psychiatry*, 5, 423-448.

2305 Voeten-Israel, C. (1982). *Kinderen van oorlogsoverlevenden en hun voorgeschiedenis* [Children of war survivors and their history]. Unpublished master's thesis, St. Michielsgestel.

2306 Vogel, Miriam L. (1994). Gender as a factor in the transgenerational transmission of trauma. *Women & Therapy*, 15(2), 35-47.

2307 Volf, Nicka (1993). Jewish children persecuted in the war: 40 years later. In: Kalicanin, Predrag; Bukelic, Jovan; Ispanovic-Radojkovic, Veronika; and Lecic-Tosevski, Dusica L. (Eds.), *The Stresses of War*, Belgrade: Institute for Mental Health, pp. 47-59.

2308 Volkan, Vamik D. (1993). What the Holocaust means to a non-Jewish psychoanalyst. In: Moses, Rafael (Ed.), *Persistent Shadows of the Holocaust: The Meaning to Those Not Directly Affected.* Madison, CT: International Universities Press, pp. 81-105.

2309 Volker, Friedrich (1995). The internalization of Nazism and its effects on German psychoanalysts and their patients. *American Imago*, 52(3), 261-279.

2310 Vuysje, H.G. (1995). A model for integrated psychosocial support of the Jews in the Netherlands. In: Lemberger, John (Ed.), *A Global Perspective on Working with Holocaust Survivors and the Second Generation*. Jerusalem: JDC-Brookdale Institute of Gerontology and Human Development, AMCHA, and JDC-Israel, pp. 93-102.

2311 Wagenaar, Willem A., and Groeneweg, Joop (1990). The memory of concentration camp survivors. *Applied Cognitive Psychology*, 4(2), 77-87.

2312 Waitz, Robert (1961). La pathologie des deportées [The pathology of the deportees]. *La Semaine des Hopitaux de Paris*, 37, 1977-1984.

2313 Waitz, Robert (1972). Pathological changes found with former women prisoners of concentration camps. In: *Auschwitz Anthology. Vol. 3: It Did Not End in Forty-Five. Part 2.* Warsaw, International Auschwitz Committee, pp. 1-41.

2314 Waitz, Robert (1977). *Kind van de Rekening, Jeugdbelevenissen uit de Tweede Wereldoorlog Verteld aan Dick Walda* [Children Who Have to Pay the Piper: Experiences from Children from the Second World War Told to Dick Walda]. Sjaloom: Odijk.

2315 Waitz, Robert, and Ciepielowski, Marian (1965). Doświadczalny dur wysypkowy w obozie koncentracyjnym w Buchenwaldzie [Experimental typhus exanthematicus in the concentration camp of Buchenwald]. *Przegląd Lekarski*, 21(1), 68-69.

2316 Waitz, Robert, and Ciepielowski, Marian (1971). Experimental typhus in the Buchenwald camp. In: *Auschwitz Anthology. Vol. 1: Inhuman Medicine. Part 2.* Warsaw: International Auschwitz Committee, pp. 120-130.

2317 Waldfogel, Shimon (1991). Physical illness in children of Holocaust survivors. *General Hospital Psychiatry*, 13(4), 267-269.

2318 Walisever, Helene B. (1995). *The effect of traumatic loss on attachment and emotional organization: An intergenerational study.*

Unpublished doctoral dissertation, Long Island University, Brookville, New York, 239 pp. *Dissertation Abstracts International*, 56(4-B), p. 2345. (University Microfilms no. AAC 9529748).

2319 Walter, Franciszek K. (1977). W cieniu śmierci. Refleksje z Sachsenhausen [In the shadow of death: Reflections from the Sachsenhausen concentration camp]. *Przegląd Lekarski*, 34(1), 186-190.

2320 Wanderman, Erica (1976). Children and families of Holocaust survivors: A psychological overview. In: Steinitz, Lucy Y., and Szonyi, David M. (Eds.), *Living After the Holocaust: Reflections by the Post-War Generation in America*. New York: Bloch, pp. 115-123.

2321 Wanderman, Erica (1977). *Separation problems, depressive experiences and conception of parents in children of concentration survivors*. Unpublished doctoral dissertation, New York University, 275 pp. *Dissertation Abstracts International*, 41(2-B), p. 704. (University Microfilms no. 80117601).

2322 Wangh, Martin (1962). Psychoanalytische Betrachtungen zur Dynamik und Genese des Vorurteils, des Antisemitismus und des Nazismus [Psychoanalytic views on the dynamics and genesis of prejudice, anti-semitism and Nazism]. *Psyche: Zeitschrift für Psychoanalyse und ihre Anwendungen*, 16, 273-284.

2323 Wangh, Martin (1964). National Socialism and the genocide of the Jews: A psycho-analytic study of a historical event. *International Journal of Psycho-Analysis*, 45(2-3), 386-395.

2324 Wangh, Martin (1968). Discussion of Eddie de Wind, "Begegnung mit dem Tod" [Encounter with Death]. *Psyche: Zeitschrift für Psychoanalyse und ihre Anwendungen*, 22, 447.

2325 Wangh, Martin (1968). A psychogenetic factor in the recurrence of war. *International Journal of Psycho-Analysis*, 49(2-3), 319-323.

2326 Wangh, Martin (1971). Die Beurteilung von Widergutmachungsänspruchen der als Kleinkinder Verfolgten [The evaluation of restitution claims of persecuted children]. In: Herberg, Hans-Joachim (Ed.), *Spätschäden nach Extrembelastungen* [Late Damage After Extreme Stress]. Herford: Nicolai, pp. 270-274. [II Internationalen Medizinisch-Juristischen Konferenz. Dusseldorf, 1969].

2327 Wangh, Martin (1971). Verfolgungsbeschädigte vor deutschen Gutachtern [Persecution casualties facing German restitution experts].

Psyche: Zeitschrift für Psychoanalyse und ihre Anwendungen, 9(25), 716-719.

2328 Wangh, Martin (1983). On obstacles to the working through of the Nazi Holocaust experience and on the consequences of failing to do so. *Israel Journal of Psychiatry and Related Sciences*, 20(1-2), 147-154.

2329 Wangh, Martin (1984). On obstacles to the working-through of the Nazi Holocaust experience and on the consequences of failing to do so. In: Luel, Steven A., and Marcus, Paul (Eds.), *Psychoanalytic Reflections on the Holocaust: Selected Essays*. New York: Ktav, pp. 197-205.

2330 Wardi, Dina (1992). *Memorial Candles: Children of the Holocaust*. London: Tavistock/Routledge. 270 pp.

2331 Wardi, Dina (1994). Bonding and separateness, two major factors in the relations between Holocaust survivors and their children. In: Brink, Terry L. (Ed.), *Holocaust Survivors' Mental Health*. New York: Haworth, pp. 119-131. [Published as a special issue of *Clinical Gerontologist*, 14(3).]

2332 Wardi, Dina (1995). Familial and collective identity in Holocaust survivors and the second generation. In: Lemberger, John (Ed.), *A Global Perspective on Working with Holocaust Survivors and the Second Generation*. Jerusalem: JDC-Brookdale Institute of Gerontology and Human Development, AMCHA, and JDC-Israel, pp. 331-339.

2333 Wardi, Dina, and Litman, Shalom (1981). Les effets uniques de l'holocauste sur la résistance des fils des survivants en psychotherapie de groupe [The unique effects of the Holocaust on the resistance of the children of survivors in group psychotherapy]. *Connexions*, 36, 79-87.

2334 Warnes, Hector (1972). The traumatic syndrome. *Canadian Psychiatric Association Journal*, 17, 391-395.

2335 Weber, D. (1967). Kritisches zur Beurteilungspraxis von Gesundheitsschäden nach Verfolgung [Critical remarks on the evaluation of health damages after persecution]. In: Herberg, Hans-Joachim (Ed.), *Die Beurteilung von Gesundheitsschäden nach Gefangenschaft und Verfolgung* [The Assessment of Health Damages Following Internment and Persecution]. Herford: Nicolai, pp. 52-56. [Internationalen Medizinisch-Juristischen Symposiums in Köln].

2336 Weiler, Liat (1989). *Families of Holocaust survivors adaptation in America and Israel*. Unpublished doctoral dissertation, Hahnemann University of Allied Health Profesions, Philadelphia, Pensylvania, 89 pp. *Dissertation Abstracts International*, 49(12-B), p. 5536. (University Microfilms no. AAC 8904662).

2337 Weinberg, A.A. (1964). On comparative mental health research of Jewish people. *Israel Annals of Psychiatry and Related Disciplines*, 2(1), 27-40.

2338 Weindling, Paul (1991). Medicine in Nazi Germany and its aftermath: Essay review. *Bulletin of the History of Medicine*, 65(3), 416-419.

2339 Weindling, Paul (1992). Psychiatry and the Holocaust. *Psychological Medicine*, 22(1), 1-3.

2340 Weinfeld, Morton, and Sigal, John J. (1986). The effect of the Holocaust on selected socio-political attitudes of adult children of survivors. *Canadian Review of Sociology and Anthropology*, 23(3), 365-382.

2341 Weinfeld, Morton, and Sigal, John J. (1986). Knowledge of the Holocaust among adult children of survivors. *Canadian Journal of Ethnic Studies*, 18, 66-78.

2342 Weinfeld, Morton; Sigal, John J.; and Eaton, William W. (1981). Long-term effects of the Holocaust on selected social attitudes and behaviors of survivors: A cautionary note. *Social Forces*, 60, 1-19.

2343 Weisaeth, Lars, and Eitinger, Leo (1993). Post-traumatic stress phenomena: Common themes across wars, disasters, and traumatic events. In: Wilson, John P., and Raphael, Beverley (Eds.), *International Handbook of Traumatic Stress Syndromes*. New York: Plenum, pp. 69-77.

2344 Weisman, Eric R. (1980). *The rhetoric of Holocaust survivors: A dramatic perspective*. Unpublished doctoral dissertation, Temple University, Philadelphia, Pennsylvania, 399 pp. *Dissertation Abstracts International,* 41(5-A), p. 1840. (University Microfilms no. AAC 8025169).

2345 Weiss, Erwin; O'Connell, Agnes N.; and Siites, Roland (1986). Comparisons of second-generation Holocaust survivors, immigrants, and nonimmigrants on measures of mental health. *Journal of Personality and Social Psychology*, 50(4), 828-831.

2346 Weiss, M. David (1988). Parental uses of authority and discipline by Holocaust survivors. *Family Therapy*, 15(3), 199-209.

2347 Weiss, Micha, and Schindler, Shlomit (1995). Short-term therapy for second generation of Holocaust survivors at AMCHA/Ramat Gan. In: Lemberger, John (Ed.), *A Global Perspective on Working with Holocaust Survivors and the Second Generation*. Jerusalem: JDC-Brookdale Institute of Gerontology and Human Development, AMCHA, and JDC-Israel, pp. 413-422.

2348 Weiss, Sima, and Durst, Natan (1994). Treatment of elderly Holocaust survivors: How do therapists cope? In: Brink, Terry L. (Ed.), *Holocaust Survivors' Mental Health*. New York: Haworth, pp. 81-98. [Published as a special issue of *Clinical Gerontologist*, 14(3).]

2349 Weissmann, Barbara (1986). *Acculturation patterns in survivors of the Holocaust and children of survivors of the Holocaust*. Unpublished doctoral dissertation, California School of Professional Psychology, Los Angeles, 99 pp. *Dissertation Abstracts International*, 47(10-B), p. 4317. (University Microfilms no. AAC 8626133).

2350 Weissmark, Mona S.; Giacomo, Daniel A.; and Kuphal, Ilona (1993). Psychosocial themes in the lives of children of survivors and Nazis. *Journal of Narrative and Life History*, 3(4), 319-335.

2351 Wellers, Georges, and Waitz, Robert (1947). Effet de la misère psychologique prolongée sur l'organisme humain [Effects of prolonged psychological stress on the human organism]. *Journal of Psychology (Paris)*, 39, 59-64.

2352 Wertham, Fredric (1968). Looking at potatoes from below: Administrative mass killings. In: *A Sign for Cain: An Exploration of Human Violence*. London: Robert Hale, pp. 135-152.

2353 Wertham, Fredric (1968). The geranium in the window: The "euthanasia" murders. In: *Sign for Cain: An Exploration of Human Violence*. London: Robert Hale, pp. 153-191.

2354 Wesełucha, Piotr (1969). Obłęd czy metoda? Refleksje poobozowe [Madness or method? Post-concentration camp reflections]. *Przegląd Lekarski*, 25(1), 181-183.

2355 Wesełucha, Piotr (1970). Obóz jako eksperyment psychiatryczny [The concentration camp as an experiment in psychiatry]. *Przegląd Lekarski*, 26(1), 242-246.

2356 Wetterwald, F. (1960). Die urologischen Spätfolgen der Deportation und die damit zusammenhangenden Rückwirkungen des vorzeitigen Alterns [The urological sequelae of deportation and their influence on premature aging]. In: Fichez, Louis F. (Ed.), *Andere Spätfolgen, auf Grund der Beobachtungen bei den ehemaligen Deportierten und Internierten der nazistischen Gefangisse und Vernichtungslager* [Other Belated Consequences, Based on the Observations of Former Deportees and Internees of Nazi Prisons and Death Camps]. Wien: Verlag der FIR, pp. 133-139.

2357 Whiteman, Dorit B. (1993). Holocaust survivors and escapees: Their strengths. *Psychotherapy Patient*, 30(3), 443-451.

2358 Whiteman, Dorit B. (1994). *The Uprooted: A Hitler Legacy - Voices of Those Who Escaped Before the "Final Solution."* New York: Plenum Press Insight Books. 446 pp.

2359 Wibaut, F. (1961). Diseases and disorders resulting from resistance work and imprisonment. In: *International Conference on the Later Effects of Imprisonment and Deportation Organized by the World Veterans Federation. The Hague, November 20-25, 1961*. The Hague: World Veterans Federation, pp. 126-145.

2360 Wickler, D., and Barondess, Jeremiah A. (1993). Bioethics and anti-bioethics in light of Nazi medicine: What must we remember? *Kennedy Institute of Ethics Journal*, 3, 39-55.

2361 Wieder, Jill A. (1985). *Children of Holocaust survivors: Differentiation from family of origin and its relationship to family dynamics*. Unpublished doctoral dissertation, California School of Professional Psychology, Los Angeles, 314 pp. *Dissertation Abstracts International*, 46(11-B), p. 4039. (University Microfilms no. AAC 8522859).

2362 Wieliczański, Henry K. (1964). Spostrzeżenia nad obecnym stanem zdrowia byłych więzniów (obozów) hitlerowskich [Observations on the present health of former Nazi prisoners]. *Przegląd Lekarski*, 21(11).

2363 Wiesel, Elie (1969). *Night*. New York: Avon. 116 pp.

2364 Wiesel, Elie (1986). A singular patient. In: Meier, Levi (Ed.), *Jewish Values in Bioethics*. New York: Human Sciences Press, pp. 103-116.

2365 Wiesel, Elie (1987). *When Memory Brings People Together*. [Speech by Nobel Peace Prize Winner Elie Wiesel of Boston University in Berlin, Germany in the Reichstag on 10 November 1987].

2366 Wiesel, Elie (1990). Out of despair. *American Journal of Psychoanalysis*, 50(2), 97-108.

2367 Wiesel, Elie (1992). *The Forgotten*. New York: Summit. 237 pp.

2368 Wiesner, N.A.F. (1951). *Faith and suffering: A study of the impact of concentration camp experiences on moral and religious attitudes*. Unpublished doctoral dissertation, New School for Social Research, New York. *Dissertation Abstracts International*, vol. W11951, p. 3.

2369 Wijsenbeek, H. (1977). Is there a hiding syndrome? In: *Israel-Netherlands Symposium on the Impact of Persecution, Jerusalem, 16-24 October 1977*. Rijswijk, The Netherlands: Ministry of Cultural Affairs, Recreation and Social Welfare, pp. 68-73.

2370 Wijsenbeek, H. (1981). Forty years later. In: *Israel-Netherlands Symposium on the Impact of Persecution. Dalfsen, Amsterdam, 14-18 April 1980*. Rijswijk, The Netherlands: Ministry of Cultural Affairs, Recreation and Social Welfare, pp. 66-69.

2371 Wilcox, A.J.; Skjaerven, R.; and Irgens, L.M. (1994). Harsh social conditions and perinatal survival: An age-period cohort analysis of the World War II occupation of Norway. *American Journal of Public Health*, 84(9), 1463-1467.

2372 Wilden, H. (1963). Die Entschädigung wegen Schädens an Körper und nach den Vorschriften des Bundesentschädigungsgesetzes (BEG) [Restitution for damages of health according to the German restitution law (BEG)]. *Nervenarzt*, 34, 70-73.

2373 Wilgowicz, Perel (1995). The effects of the Holocaust on the children of former prisoners and survivors. In: Lemberger, John (Ed.), *A Global Perspective on Working with Holocaust Survivors and the Second Generation*. Jerusalem: JDC-Brookdale Institute of Gerontology and Human Development, AMCHA, and JDC-Israel, pp. 423-435.

2374 Willanger, R. (1964). Eine Untersuchung der intellektuellen Reduktion bei ehemaligen Deportierten [An examination of intellectual decline in former deportees]. In: *Ätio-Pathogenese und Therapie der Erschöpfung und vorzeitigen Vergreisung* [The Aetiology, Pathogenesis and Therapy of Exhaustion and Premature Aging]. Wien: Verlag der FIR, pp. 327-333. [IV Internationaler Medizinischer Kongress. Bucharest, 22-27 Juni 1964].

2375 Williams, Robert L.; Medalie, Jack H.; Zyzanski, Stephen J.; Flocke, Susan A.; Yaari, Shlomit; and Goldbourt, Uri (1993). Long-term mortality of Nazi concentration camp survivors. *Journal of Clinical Epidemiology*, 46(6), 573-575.

2376 Wilson, Arnold (1985). On silence and the Holocaust: A contribution to clinical theory. *Psychoanalytic Inquiry*, 5(1), 63-84.

2377 Wilson, Arnold (1990). On silence and the Holocaust: A contribution to clinical theory. In: Fass, Margot L., and Brown, Daniel (Eds.), *Creative Mastery in Hypnosis and Hypnoanalysis: A Festschrift for Erika Fromm*. Hillside, NJ: Lawrence Erlbaum Associates, pp. 263-278.

2378 Wilson, Arnold, and Fromm, Erika (1982). Aftermath of the concentration camp: The second generation. *Journal of the American Academy of Psychoanalysis*, 10(2), 289-313.

2379 Wilson, D.M. (1961). Note presented by the New Zealand Ex-Prisoners of War Association. In: *International Conference on the Later Effects of Imprisonment and Deportation Organized by the World Veterans Federation. The Hague, November 20-25, 1961*. The Hague: World Veterans Federation, pp. 148-149.

2380 Wilson, John P.; Harel, Zev; and Kahana, Boaz (Eds.) (1988). *Human Adaptation to Extreme Stress: From the Holocaust to Vietnam*. New York: Plenum. 397 pp.

2381 Wilson, John P., and Raphael, Beverley (Eds.) (1993). *International Handbook of Traumatic Stress Syndromes*. New York: Plenum. 1011 pp.

2382 Winick, Myron (Ed.) (1979). *Hunger Disease: Studies by the Jewish Physicians in the Warsaw Ghetto*. New York: John Wiley & Sons. 261 p.

2383 Winik, Marta F. (1988). Generation to generation: A discussion with children of Jewish Holocaust Survivors. *Family Therapy*, 15(3), 271-284.

2384 Winkler, G.E. (1959). Neuropsychiatric symptoms in survivors of concentration camps. *Journal of Social Therapy*, 5, 4-11.

2385 Winkler, G.E. (1961). Probleme der psychiatrischen Begutachtung der Opfer der nationalsozialistischen Verfolgung [Problems of psychiatric evaluation of victims of National Socialist persecution]. *Medizinische Welt*, 22, 1226-1232.

2386 Winnik, Heinrich Z. (1966). Concentration camp survivors in Israel. In: David, Henry P. (Ed.), *Migration, Mental Health and Community Services: Proceedings of a Conference Convened by the American Joint Distribution Committee, Co-Sponsored by the World Federation for Mental Health, and Held in Geneva, Switzerland, November 28-30, 1966*. Geneva: American Joint Distribution Committee, pp. 23-33.

2387 Winnik, Heinrich Z. (1966). Holi hanafesh hameuhar (ketotsa'ah mipgi'ot hashoah) [Late mental disorder (due to persecution in the Holocaust)]. *Harefuah*, 70(5), 175-178.

2388 Winnik, Heinrich Z. (1967). Further comments concerning problems of late psychopathological effects of Nazi persecution and their therapy. *Israel Annals of Psychiatry and Related Disciplines*, 5(1), 1-16.

2389 Winnik, Heinrich Z. (1967). Psychiatric disturbances of Holocaust "Shoah" survivors. A symposium of the Israel psychoanalytic society. *Israel Annals of Psychiatry and Related Disciplines*, 5(1), 91-100.

2390 Winnik, Heinrich Z. (1968). Contribution to symposium on psychic traumatization through social catastrophe. *International Journal of Psycho-Analysis*, 49(2-3), 298-301.

2391 Winnik, Heinrich Z. (1968). Psychological problems after severe mental stress. In: Lopez Ibor, Juan J. (Ed.), *Proceedings. Fourth World Congress of Psychiatry, Madrid, 5-11 September 1966. Vol. 2*. New York: Excerpta Medica Foundation.

2392 Winnik, Heinrich Z. (1969). Second thoughts about "psychic trauma." *Israel Annals of Psychiatry and Related Disciplines*, 7(1), 82-95.

2393 Winnik, Heinrich Z. (1979). The impact of persecution (general background of the problem in Israel). In: *Israel-Netherlands Symposium on the Impact of Persecution. Jerusalem, 16-24 October 1977*. Rijswijk, The Netherlands: Ministry of Cultural Affairs, Recreation and Social Welfare, pp. 18-24.

2394 Winnik, Heinrich Z. (1981). On the impact of persecution: Introductory remarks to the 2nd Netherland-Israel Symposium. In: *Israel-Netherlands Symposium on the Impact of Persecution. Dalfsen, Amsterdam, 14-18 April 1980*. Rijswijk, The Netherlands: Ministry of Cultural Affairs, Recreation and Social Welfare, pp. 9-14.

2395 Winters Behr, S. (1993). *Hidden child survivors of the Holocaust: Lifting the veil*. Unpublished master's thesis, Antioch University, Yellow Springs, Ohio.

2396 Wishny, Stephen L. (1980). Children of the Holocaust and their relevancy to probation: Pre-sentence investigation and planning. *Federal Probation*, 44(4), 12-15.

2397 Withuis, Jolande (1990). De gevoelige erfenis van de jaren, '40-'45 [The sensitive legacy of 1940-1945]. *Amsterdams Sociologisch Tijdschrift*, 17(3), 128-144.

2398 Witkowski, Józef (1972). Dzierzana - Sytuacja sanitarna w hitlerowskim obozie dla dzieci w Lodzi [Dzierzana - Sanitary conditions in the Lodz concentration camp for children]. *Przegląd Lekarski*, 29(1), 151-157.

2399 Witkowski, Józef (1972). Moringen - hitlerowski obózdla maloletnich [Moringen - The Nazi concentration camp for juveniles]. *Przegląd Lekarski*, 29(1), 137-139.

2400 Witkowski, Józef (1975). Sytuacja sanitarna w obozie w Myslowicach [Sanitary conditions prevailing at the Myslowice camp]. *Przegląd Lekarski*, 32(1), 96-107.

2401 Witkowski, Józef (1979). Warunki sanitarne robotników w przymusowych w "Festung Breslau" [Sanitary conditions prevailing among compulsory laborers in "Festung Breslau"]. *Przegląd Lekarski*, 36(1), 61-73.

2402 Witkowski, Józef (1980). Małoletni więźnie w Gross-Rosen [Juvenile prisoners in Gross-Rosen]. *Przegląd Lekarski*, 37(1), 118-128.

2403 Witusik, Władysław (1973). Somatisch-pathologische Veränderungen des Sehorgans bei ehemaligen Konzentrationslagerhäftlingen [Somato-pathological changes of the visual system in former prisoners of concentration camps]. In: *Ermüdung und vorzeitiges Altern: Folge von Extrembelastungen* [Exhaustion and Premature Aging: Result of Extreme Stress]. Leipzig: Barth, pp. 125-136. [V Internationaler Medizinischer der FIR. Paris, 21-24 September 1970].

2404 Witusik, Władysław (1976). Augenkrankheiten bei ehemaligen Konzentrationslagerhäftlingen [Diseases of the eye in former prisoners of concentration camps]. In: *Medizinische Untersuchungen der Spätfolgen des Krieges und des NS-Regimes bei Jugendlichen und Kindern von ehemaligen KZ-Häftlingen und Verfolgten* [Medical Research of the Late Effects of the War and National Socialism

Regime on Youth and Children of Former Concentration Camp Inmates and Persecuted Persons]. Wien: Internationale Föderation der Widerstandskämpfer. [VI Internationaler Medizinischer Kongress der FIR. Prague, 1976].

2405 Witusik, Władysław, and Witusik, Romuald A. (1968). Ślady następstw chorobowych związanych z pobytem w więźieniach i obozach koncentracyjnch [Pathological sequelae caused by incarceration in prisons and concentration camps]. *Przegląd Lekarski*, 25, 56-64.

2406 Witusik, Władysław, and Witusik, Romuald A. (1971). The Auschwitz environment. In: *Auschwitz Anthology. Vol. 3: It Did Not End in Forty-Five. Part 1.* Warsaw: International Auschwitz Committee, pp. 105-151.

2407 Wlazłowski, Zbigniew (1967). Szpital w obozie koncentracyjnym Gusen [Hospital in the concentration camp Gusen]. *Przegląd Lekarski*, 23(1), 112-121.

2408 Wlazłowski, Zbigniew (1968). Gruźlica pluc i postepowanie z chorymi na grużicę [Pulmonary tuberculosis and treatment of tuberculosis in the concentration camp of Gusen]. *Przegląd Lekarski*, 24(1), 98-101.

2409 Włodarska, Helena (1970). Ze szpitala kobiecego obozu w Brzezince [The women's hospital at the Brzezinka concentration camp]. *Przegląd Lekarski*, 26(1), 213-216.

2410 Wohlfahrt, S. (1964). KZ-offrens nuvarande situation [The present situation of concentration camp victims]. *Lakartidningen*, 61, 4107-4124.

2411 Wohlfahrt, S. (1966). Aer det humant att tvinga KZ offer resa till Vaesttyskyland foer laekarundersoekning? [Is it humane to force concentration camp victims to travel to West Germany for medical examinations?]. *Lakartidningen*, 63, 631-637.

2412 Wojtasik, Władysław (1969). Zmiany chorobowe u byłych więźniów obozow koncentracyjnych ze środowiska kieleckiego [Pathological findings in the former concentration camp inmates from the County of Kielc (Poland)]. *Przegląd Lekarski*, 25, 18-24.

2413 Wojtasik, Władysław (1971). Zmiany elektrokardiograficzne u 105 byłych więźniów obozów koncentracyjnych (ze srodowiska Kieleckiego) [Electrocardiographic findings in 105 ex-concentration camp prisoners (from the County of Kielc)]. *Przegląd Lekarski*, 28, 10-12.

2414 Wojtasik, Władysław (1973). Zmiany chorobowe u byłych więźniów obozów koncentracyjnych (z powiatow Wloszczowskiego I Staszowskiego w Kieleckiem) [Pathological findings of ex-concentration camp prisoners (from Wloszczow and Staszow in the County of Kielc]. *Przegląd Lekarski*, 30, 21-29.

2415 Wojtasik, Władysław (1974). Najczęstsze zmiany chorobowe w układzie krążenia u mieszkajacych na Kieleczyźnie byłych więźniów obozow Hitlerowskich [The most frequent pathological changes in the circulatory system of former Hitler-camp prisoners living in the Kielc area]. *Przegląd Lekarski*, 31(1), 75-82.

2416 Wojtasik, Władysław (1976). Nadciśnienie tętnicze a miażdzyca-uwagi na podstawie badań byłych więźniów obozów hitlerowskich [Hypertonia and arteriosclerosis. Some remarks on the investigation of ex-prisoners in the Hitlerian concentration camps]. *Przegląd Lekarski*, 33(1), 80-84.

2417 Wokski, Józef (1978). Z życia w obocie Koncentracynym w Dachau [Life at the Dachau concentration camp]. *Przegląd Lekarski*, 35(1), 172-174.

2418 Wolf, B. (1971). *Tismonet hahistaglut shel nitzoley hashoah: Trumah l'patalogiah ham'oocheret shel hashoah* [The Adaptation Syndrome of the Holocaust Survivors: A Contribution to the Delayed Pathology of the Holocaust]. Ramat Gan, Israel: No publisher. 78 pp.

2419 Wolffheim, Nelly (1958). Kinder aus Konzentrationslagern; Mitteilungen über die Nachwirkungen des KZ Aufenthaltes auf Kinder und Jugendliche [Children from concentration camps: Reports on the aftereffects of the stay in concentration camps in children and juveniles]. *Praxis der Kinderpsychologie und Kinderpsychiatrie*, 7, 302-312.

2420 Wolffheim, Nelly (1959). Kinder aus Konzentrationslagern: Mitteilungen uber die Nachwirkungen des KZ-Aufenthaltes auf Kinder und Jugendliche [Children from concentration camps: Reports on the aftereffects of the stay in concentration camps in children and juveniles]. *Praxis der Kinderpsychologie und Kinderpsychiatrie*, 8, 20-27.

2421 Wolken, Otto (1971). Liberation of the Auschwitz-Birkenau concentration camp. In: *Auschwitz Anthology. Vol. 2: In Hell They*

Preserved Human Dignity. Part 2. Warsaw: International Auschwitz Committee, pp. 97-122.

2422 Wolken, Otto (1971). What I think of children. In: *Auschwitz Anthology. Vol. 2: In Hell They Preserved Human Dignity. Part 2.* Warsaw: International Auschwitz Committee, pp. 13-20.

2423 Wolken, Otto (1987). Die Befreiung von Auschwitz-Birkenau [The liberation of Auschwitz-Birkenau]. In: Hamburger Institut für Sozialforschung (Eds.), *Die Auschwitz-Hefte. Texte der polnischen Zeitschrift "Przegląd Lekarski" über historische, psychische und medizinische Aspekte des Lebens und Sterbens in Auschwitz. Band 2* [The Auschwitz Journal. Text of the Polish Journal "Medical Review" on Historical, Psychic and Medical Aspects of Life and Death in Auschwitz. Volume 2]. Weinheim and Basel: Beltz, pp. 261-265.

2424 Worms, Robert (1955). Rückfälle des Typhus exanthematicus (Brillsche Krankheit) bei ehemaligen Deportierten [Recurrence of typhus (Brill's disease) in former deportees]. In: Michel, Max (Ed.), *Gesundheitsschäden durch Verfolgung und Gefangenschaft und ihre Spätfolgen: Zusammenstellung der Referate und Ergebnisse der Internationalen Sozialmedizinischen Konferenz über die Pathologie der Ehemaligen Deportierten und Internierten, 5-7 Juni 1954 in Kopenhagen* [Health Damages Caused by Persecution and Captivity and the Late Effects: Compilation of the Papers and Results of the International Conference of Social Medicine on the Pathology of Former Deported and Interned Persons, 5-7 June 1954 in Copenhagen]. Frankfurt am Main: Röderberg, pp. 209-215.

2425 Wreschner Rustow, Margrit M. (1989). *Identity and trauma: Jewish children saved by Christians during the Holocaust.* Unpublished doctoral dissertation, Union for Experimenting Colleges and Universities, Cincinnati, Ohio, 202 pp. *Dissertation Abstracts International*, 49(8-B), p. 3099. (University Microfilms no. AAC 8821938).

2426 Wulff, E. (1978). Zur Frage der wesentlichen Mitverursachung schizophrener Psychosen durch Verfolgungsbedingte Extrembelastungen [On the problem of essential contribution to schizophrenia psychoses through extreme stress due to persecution]. In: *Medizinische Untersuchungen der Spätfolgen des Krieges und des NS-Regimes bei Jugendlichen und Kindern von ehemaligen KZ-Häftlingen und Verfolgten* [Medical Research of the Late Effects of the War and National Socialism Regime on Youth and Children of Former Concentration Camp Inmates and Persecuted Persons]. Wien: Internationale Föderation der Widerstandskämpfer. [VI Internationaler Medizinischer Kongress der FIR. Prague, 1976].

2427 Wyschogrod, Edith (1988). Man-made mass death and changing concept of self. *American Journal of Psycho-Analysis*, 48(1), 25-34.

2428 Yaari, A.; Adler, R.; and Eisenberg, E. (1996). Holocaust survivors and their pain. *International Journal of Psychology*, 31(3-4), 4818.

2429 Yeheskel, Ayala (1995). The intimate environment and the sense of coherence among Holocaust survivors. *Social Work in Health Care*, 20(3), 25-35.

2430 Yehuda, Rachel; Elkin, Abbie; Binder-Brynes, Karen; Kahana, Boaz; Southwick, Steven M.; Schmeidler, James; and Giller, Earl L. (1996). Dissociation in aging Holocaust survivors. *American Journal of Psychiatry*, 153(7), 935-940.

2431 Yehuda, Rachel; Giller, Earl L.; Southwick, Steven M.; Kahana, Boaz; Boisoneau, David; Ma, Xiaowan; and Mason, John W. (1994). Relationship between catecholamine excretion and PTSD symptoms in Vietnam combat veterans and Holocaust survivors. In: Murburg, M. Michele (Ed.), *Progress in Psychiatry. No. 42: Catecholamine Function in Post-Traumatic Stress Disorder: Emerging Concepts*. Washington, D.C.: American Psychiatric Press, pp. 203-219.

2432 Yehuda, Rachel; Kahana, Boaz; Binder-Brynes, Karen; Southwick, Steven M.; Mason, John W.; and Giller, Earl L. (1995). Low urinary cortisol excretion in Holocaust survivors with post-traumatic stress disorder. *American Journal of Psychiatry*, 152(7), 982-986.

2433 Yehuda, Rachel; Kahana, Boaz; Schmeidler, James; Southwick, Steven M.; Wilson, Skye; and Giller, Earl L. (1995). Impact of cumulative lifetime trauma and recent stress on current post-traumatic stress disorder symptoms in Holocaust survivors. *American Journal of Psychiatry*, 152(12), 1815-1818.

2434 Yehuda, Rachel; Kahana, Boaz; Southwick, Steven M.; and Giller, Earl L. (1994). Depressive features in Holocaust survivors with post-traumatic stress disorder. *Journal of Traumatic Stress*, 7(4), 699-704.

2435 Yehuda, Rachel; Resnick, Heidi; Kahana, Boaz; and Giller, Earl L. (1993). Long-lasting hormonal alterations to extreme stress in humans: Normative or maladaptive? *Psychosomatic Medicine*, 55(3), 287-297.

2436 Yuchtman-Yaar, Ephraim, and Menahem, Gila (1992). Socioeconomic achievements of Holocaust survivors in Israel: The first and second generation. *Contemporary Jewry*, 13, 95-122.

2437 Zabłocki, Jan (1977). W rewirze obozu w Sachsenhausen [The sick bay at the Sachsenhausen concentration camp]. *Przegląd Lekarski*, 34(1), 193-194.

2438 Zagórska, Ewa (1981). Nad zeszytami Oświęcimia [Medical review issues dealing with Auschwitz]. *Przegląd Lekarski*, 38, 224-229.

2439 Zasacki, Stanisław (1978). Laboratorium szpitala obozu w Brzezince [The laboratory at the sick-bay in Birkenau]. *Przegląd Lekarski*, 35(1), 158-160.

2440 Zawodzińska, Celina (1974). Kilka refleksji z lat uwięzienia [Reminiscences from concentration camps]. *Przegląd Lekarski*, 31, 213-217.

2441 Zbowid, Warschau (1955). Stellungnahme der polnischen Organisation der Widerstandskämpfer und Opfer des Naziterrors zu den Konferenzthemen von Kopenhagen [The attitude of the Polish organizations of resistance fighters and persecution victims to the themes of the conference in Copenhagen]. In: Michel, Max (Ed.), *Gesundheitsschäden durch Verfolgung und Gefangenschaft und ihre Spätfolgen: Zusammenstellung der Referate und Ergebnisse der Internationalen Sozialmedizinischen Konferenz über die Pathologie der Ehemaligen Deportierten und Internierten, 5-7 Juni 1954 in Kopenhagen* [Health Damages Caused by Persecution and Captivity and the Late Effects: Compilation of the Papers and Results of the International Conference of Social Medicine on the Pathology of Former Deported and Interned Persons, 5-7 June 1954 in Copenhagen]. Frankfurt am Main: Röderberg, pp. 84-90.

2442 Zdawski, Tadeusz (1971). The Szczecin center. In: *Auschwitz Anthology. Vol. 3: It Did Not End in Forty-Five. Part 1*. Warsaw: International Auschwitz Committee, pp. 163-170.

2443 Zdawski, Tadeusz (1986). Wstępne sprawozdanie o psychiatrycznych studiach nad byłych więźniami hitlerowskich obozów obszar Szczecina) [Preliminary reports of psychiatric studies of former prisoners of Nazi concentration camps (Szczecin area)]. *Przegląd Lekarski*, 24, 64-65.

2444 Zechovoy, Amnon (1986). *Orientatziat zman v'yachasim beyn ishim etzel nitzoley shoah dor rishon v'sheyni* [Time orientation and interpersonal relations among Holocaust survivors: First and second generation]. Unpublished master's thesis, Department of Psychology, Tel Aviv University, Tel Aviv, Israel. 100 pp.

2445 Zelechowski, Janet (1979). Z rewiru w Dachau [The Dachau concentration camp and its hospital]. *Przegląd Lekarski*, 36, 163-164.

2446 Zeleznikow, Janet, and Lang, Moshe (1989). Separation crises and the Holocaust. *Australian and New Zealand Journal of Family Therapy*, 10(1), 31-32.

2447 Zellermayer, Julius (1968). The psychosocial effect of the Eichmann trial on Israeli society. *Psychiatry Digest*, 13-23.

2448 Zielina, Jan (1966). Wynik badań lekarskich byłych więźniów hitlerowskich więzień i obozów koncentracyknych [The results of medical investigations of ex-concentration camp prisoners]. *Przegląd Lekarski*, 23(1), 49-51.

2449 Zielina, Jan (1971). Block No. 9 of the Auschwitz I camp hospital. In: *Auschwitz Anthology. Vol. 2: In Hell They Preserved Human Dignity. Part 1*. Warsaw: International Auschwitz Committee, pp. 198-208.

2450 Zielina, Jan (1971). The Cieszyn center. In: *Auschwitz Anthology. Vol. 3: It Did Not End in Forty-Five. Part 1*. Warsaw: International Auschwitz Committee, pp. 191-199.

2451 Zilberfein, Felice S. (1994). *Children of Holocaust survivors: Separation obstacles, attachments and anxiety*. Unpublished doctoral dissertation, New York University, 177 pp. *Dissertation Abstracts International*, 56(10-B), p. 541. (University Microfilms no. AAC 9514309).

2452 Zilberfein, Felice S. (1995). Children of Holocaust survivors: Separation obstacles, attachments, and anxiety. In: Lemberger, John (Ed.), *A Global Perspective on Working with Holocaust Survivors and the Second Generation*. Jerusalem: JDC-Brookdale Institute of Gerontology and Human Development, AMCHA, and JDC-Israel, pp. 341-376.

2453 Zilberfein, Felice S. (1996). Children of Holocaust survivors: Separation obstacles, attachments, and anxiety. *Social Work in Health Care*, 23(3), 35-55.

2454 Zilberfein, Felice S., and Eskin, Vivian (1992). Helping Holocaust survivors with the impact of illness and hospitalization. *Social Work in Health Care*, 18(1), 59-70.

2455 Zlotogorski, Zoli (1981). *Offspring of concentration camp survivors: The relationship of perceptions of family cohesion and adaptability* *to levels of ego functioning*. Unpublished doctoral dissertation, Michigan State University, East Lansing, 135 pp. *Dissertation Abstracts International*, 42(8-B), p. 3452. (University Microfilms no. AAC 8202541).

2456 Zlotogorski, Zoli (1983). Offspring of concentration camp survivors: The relationship of perceptions of family cohesion and adaptability to levels of ego functioning. *Comprehensive Psychiatry*, 24(4), 345-354.

2457 Zlotogorski, Zoli (1985). Offspring of concentration camp survivors: A study of levels of ego functioning. *Israel Journal of Psychiatry and Related Sciences*, 22(3), 201-209.

2458 Zobel, Jakob (1955). Zahnschäden als Häftfolge [Tooth damages as results of imprisonment]. In: Michel, Max (Ed.), *Gesundheitsschäden durch Verfolgung und Gefangenschaft und ihre Spätfolgen: Zusammenstellung der Referate und Ergebnisse der Internationalen Sozialmedizinischen Konferenz über die Pathologie der Ehemaligen Deportierten und Internierten, 5-7 Juni 1954 in Kopenhagen* [Health Damages Caused by Persecution and Captivity and the Late Effects: Compilation of the Papers and Results of the International Conference of Social Medicine on the Pathology of Former Deported and Interned Persons, 5-7 June 1954 in Copenhagen]. Frankfurt am Main: Röderberg, pp. 226-227.

2459 Zuckerman, Alan S. (1984). The limits of political behavior: Individual calculations and survival. *Political Psychology*, 5(1), 37-52.

2460 Żukowski, Wojciech; Turska-Karbowska, Grażyna; Gizler, Maria; and Orleska, Irena (1987). Der Zustand der "Konzentrationslager-Kinder" auf Grund der Untersuchungen des Niederschlesischen Zentrums für Medizinische Diagnostik [The condition of concentration camp children based on investigations of the Center for Medical Diagnostics of Lower Silesia]. In: Hamburger Institut für Sozialforschung (Eds.), *Die Auschwitz-Hefte. Texte der polnischen Zeitschrift "Przegląd Lekarski" über historische, psychische und medizinische Aspekte des Lebens und Sterbens in Auschwitz. Band 2* [The Auschwitz Journal. Text of the Polish Journal "Medical Review" on Historical, Psychic and Medical Aspects of Life and Death in Auschwitz. Volume 2]. Weinheim and Basel: Beltz, pp. 81-88.

2461 Zwerling, Israel (1983). Psychiatric studies of the Holocaust. *Contemporary Psychiatry*, 2(2), 134-138.

Selected Annotated Bibliography

Selected Annotated Bibliography

Aziz, Philippe (1976). *Doctors of Death*. Geneva: Ferni Publishers. 1014 pp.

Each volume in this four-volume series, has a distinct title. Volume 1: *Karl Brandt, the Third Reich's Man in White*; Volume 2: *Joseph Mengele, the Evil Doctor*; Volume 3: *When Man Became a Guinea Pig for Death*; and Volume 4: *In the Beginning Was the Master Race*. While the titles appear specific, actually Aziz's work explores the entire range of medical involvement in genocidal death.

The details of what transpired within the Nazi medical machinery confirm the horrors experienced and witnessed by the very few survivors of "medical" experiments and other atrocities. This series contains valuable information and insights.

Bastiaans, Jan (1957). *Psychosomatische Gevolgen van Onderdrukking en Verzet* [Psychosomatic Sequelae of Persecution and Resistance]. Amsterdam: Noord-Hollandsche Uitgevers Maatschappij. 485 pp.

A pioneer in the treatment of victims of war, Bastiaans studied primarily ex-members of the Dutch resistance, many of whom spent time in various concentration camps. In the English summary of the book (pp. 467-472), Bastiaans states that "in previously well balanced and healthy people, neuropsychiatric and psychosomatic syndromes only manifest themselves after more severe stress than in less stabilized and adapted people. When it can be shown that certain sequelae of war stress are genetically related to disturbances of childhood one must still attach *great value to the stresses of the war period...*" (p. 470) [emphasis by Robert Krell].

Bastiaans very early attributed to massive trauma the power to cause illness in otherwise well people. In fact, in his introduction (which may not have been generally available since it was published in Dutch), Bastiaans finds it understandable that those who were spared the atrocities (including doctors) would prefer to avoid the reality presented by these particular patients. Bastiaans also intimates that the extraordinary stress experienced by concentration camp inmates will not be found in the medical-psychiatric literature to that time, yet cites the works of doctor-inmates, Elie A. Cohen (1952) and Eddy de Wind (1946).

Bergmann, Martin S., and Jucovy, Milton E. (Eds.) (1982). *Generations of the Holocaust*. New York: Basic. 338 pp. [1990 edition, New York: Columbia University Press. 356 pp.]

This book is the product of a working group devoted to the psychoanalytic study of the effect of the Holocaust on the second generation. The study group's case material was utilized to derive the various insights noted.

The prelude is comparatively strong in addressing the incredible oversight and failure to provide psychologic assistance after liberation, the viability of theoretical psychoanalysis to deal with such overwhelming trauma, and the complexity of the psychopathology encountered.

Survivors as parents faced an immediate and conscious dilemma, whether to protect their children from the stories of horror, or not. At an unconscious level, a variety of emotions were unleashed upon children; unresolved loss, chronic bereavement, smothering overprotectiveness or affective distance, the sharing of a world filled with danger and aggression. There are four sections, one which sets the background, the survivors' children, the persecutors' children and theoretical and clinical aspects. The patient accounts are compelling, some of the therapeutic approaches mystifying but basically well intentioned. There is much to be learned.

Boder, David P. (1949). *I Did Not Interview the Dead*. Urbana, IL: University of Illinois Press. 220 pp.

Boder collected some of the earliest known interviews of survivors. He wire recorded 120 hours of testimony from 70 people in the summer of 1946. On the basis of the transcribed narratives, he devised the Traumatic Index, 12 experiences assumed to have traumatizing effects. Eight interviews comprise this remarkable volume of eyewitness accounts.

At times the questions reveal the interviewer's inability to believe what he is being told. In at least one case (the narrative of Abe Mohnblum), the survivor's challenge to trained psychologists is dramatic for he claims that his experiences defy psychologic understanding which is challenged by the interviewer.

In the field of massive psychic trauma, this is a pioneering contribution.

Braham, Randolph L. (Ed.) (1988). *The Psychological Perspectives of the Holocaust and its Aftermath*. Boulder, CO: Social Science Monographs; New York: Csengeri Institute for Holocaust Studies of the Graduate School and University Center of the City University of New York. 225 pp.

This volume is based on a conference held at The City University of New York on May 4-5, 1987. This well-edited work includes an impressive series of papers/chapters focusing on mental health issues for survivors and their children.

Cocks, Geoffrey (1985). *Psychotherapy in the Third Reich: The Göring Institute*. New York and Oxford: Oxford University Press. 326 pp.

This intriguing work describes the disintegration of psychiatry and psychoanalysis in Nazi Germany. The Berlin Psychoanalytic Institute, the world's first, founded in 1920, disappeared in 1936. While Jews and others fled, prominent psychiatrists who remained became involved in "racializing" medicine and psychiatry.

Cocks describes not only the functioning (or dysfunctioning) of psychotherapy during the Nazi period, but its resurrection in post-war Germany.

This book is of interest in the historical machinations which ultimately delivered to other shores the best and brightest minds and which in Germany itself wreaked havoc in fulfilling its racial mission.

Davidson, Shamai (1992). *Holding on to Humanity - The Message of Holocaust Survivors: The Shamai Davidson Papers*. (Ed. Charny, Israel W.) New York: New York University Press. 243 pp. (Paperback edition: 1995).

Charny's introduction to this seminal work is itself a most enlightening and insightful commentary on survivors. In recounting Davidson's struggle with the general notion that the vast majority of survivors were indeed damaged while ensuring that this neither necessarily implied psychopathology nor diminished in any way the individual survivor's creative accomplishments, Charny provides invaluable insights into the nature of massive trauma.

These insights should be required reading for mental health professionals. With such an auspicious beginning, this book then reveals the treasure of Shamai Davidson's lifetime of observations. Davidson states that survivors who insisted on telling of their trauma had their experiences converted into psychiatric symptoms to be dealt with by the "expert." Since the experts themselves exercised denial in facing the Holocaust experience, they avoided the topic even in long-term psychotherapy and psychoanalysis.

Davidson's depth of understanding is evident in his analysis of feelings held towards the survivor in Israeli society. In the process of his discussion, Davidson points the way to dealing with victims of massive trauma. For example, he set up counselling services for non-clinical survivors. Free from stigmatization, Holocaust survivors began to offer their unexpressed feelings in order to heal. Trauma survivors should not have to experience breakdowns in order to receive assistance.

Throughout his writings, Davidson provides thoughtful and relevant contributions to the treatment of victims generally, and to Holocaust survivors specifically.

Dicks, Henry V. (1972). *Licensed Mass Murder: A Socio-Psychological Study of Some SS Killers*. New York: Basic. 283 pp.

This ambitious work attempts to understand and analyze, through case studies, the Nazi mind of the Nazi murderers.

The author draws interesting conclusions from his in-depth interviews, mainly how easily the paranoid dynamic descends in a climate which encourages the unlimited exercise of power over the powerless. There are examples of men able to murder in unimaginably cruel ways who then relish their contacts with their own wives and children. Dicks concludes that the eight SS interviewed were not simply primitive, compulsive psychopaths nor were they insane. He comments on their ability to "split off" part of their personalities.

Dimsdale, Joel E. (Ed.) (1980). *Survivors, Victims, and Perpetrators: Essays on the Nazi Holocaust*. Washington, D.C.: Hemisphere. 474 pp.

The most thorough overview of the psychiatric implications of the Holocaust in its time, this book is an extraordinary collection of important information. The range of contents provides the reader with knowledge about "The Setting" (Hillberg), "The Victim" (Lifton, Eitinger, Chodoff, etc.) and "The Perpetrator."

The chapters dealing with the victim are especially compelling in attempting to provide information about the survivor's post-war world and the struggle to cope as well as offering therapeutic approaches to the survivor and his or her family. Particularly relevant are the articles on coping behavior of survivors and the social behavior of concentration camp inmates. Much of what is written reflects commonly held myths about issues of adaptation both in the concentration camp universe and outside it.

Dwork, Deborah (1991). *Children with a Star: Jewish Youth in Nazi Europe*. New Haven, CT: Yale University Press. 354 pp.

The author of this major study examines the experiences of Jewish children in the face of persecution, terror and death. For this information she draws on the accounts of child survivors. Only eleven percent of European Jewish children alive in 1939, survived the war.

The few child survivors represented here, through their eyewitness accounts recalled forty years later, provide a statement about the lasting impact of their traumatic memories and their clarity of recall. While describing the horrendous fate of others, children and adults, their recollections also provide insights into their functioning today.

The examination of Jewish childhood in Nazi-occupied Europe clarifies, once and for all, the nature of true genocide. Children, just beginning their lives, and who could not affect in any way political or religious affairs, were hunted and murdered.

Eitinger, Leo (1972). *Concentration Camp Survivors in Norway and Israel.* The Hague: Martinus Nijhoff. 199 pp. (First published in 1964 by Universitetsforlaget, Oslo).

Eitinger's book is a landmark work but seriously flawed. He investigated the concentration camp syndrome (C.C.S.) in 2 groups of former camp inmates. His stated purpose was to examine whether the severe psychic and physical stress situations to which human beings were exposed in the concentration camps have had lasting psychological results. While Dr. Eitinger's descriptions of patients and their ordeals are straightforward and relevant, his conclusions are not.

Amongst Israeli survivors who are "schizophrenic," he carefully avoids blaming the illness on captivity. This leaves the reader wondering how a schizophrenic person could have survived a concentration camp.

He fails to connect the "neuroses" of 20 patients from the "Israel Neurotic Group" to their war experiences. Yet he describes one patient who lost both parents and five siblings by age 19, another who lost his wife and two sons, and a third who lost her husband but whose two children were saved in hiding.

Eitinger is on firmer ground when relating organic cerebral changes to psychiatric illness in the Norwegian group.

While swinging back and forth inconclusively, Eitinger continues to make valuable observations. Of one survivor he notes (p. 160), "It is obvious that experiences of the traumatic magnitude we are dealing with here, must act almost independently of the premorbid personality." After discussing possible connections with organicity he adds once again, "It would be within the bounds of reason to assume that psychic trauma of a serious and chronic nature could also be responsible for changes which resemble the concentration camp syndrome."

Eitinger denoted certain factors as "cumulative tainting" including head injuries, encephalitis and spotted fever and concluded that "a sum of injurious somatic factors may be regarded as the reason for the changes which have taken place." He nevertheless points out that Jews with such injuries/illnesses had no chance to survive.

Epstein, Helen (1988). *Children of the Holocaust: Conversations with Sons and Daughters of Survivors*. New York: Penguin. 356 pp.

First published in 1979, Helen Epstein's book signalled the beginning of the psychological self-scrutiny by children of survivors of the impact of Holocaust trauma in survivor families. Her accounts reveal themes common to the "Second Generation," and much of her book is devoted to impressions and clinical studies done by psychologists and psychiatrists.

While the revelations were often healing to the children of survivors in terms of feeling less alone with their parentally derived Holocaust preoccupations, the survivor-parents were distressed to know that they had unwittingly transmitted pieces of their trauma.

The title of the book turned out to be misleading in that there *are* children of the Holocaust, namely those who directly experienced the Holocaust during childhood and survived.

Felman, Shoshana, and Laub, Dori (1992). *Testimony: Crises of Witnessing in Literature, Psychoanalysis, and History*. New York: Routledge. 294 pp.

The authors each contribute book chapters, some previously published as separate articles. One is an interpreter of texts and a literary critic, the other an interpreter of people and a therapist to survivors of trauma.

This interesting collaboration provides insights into students' reactions to survivor testimony and the risks of listening to traumatic narratives of the extremes of human suffering. The book explores literary and visual sources to examine perspectives on the meaning of testimony.

Frankl, Viktor E. (1986). *The Doctor and the Soul: From Psychotherapy to Logotherapy*. New York: Vintage. 318 pp.

This book was originally published in 1946 in Vienna where Frankl was born in 1905. Dr. Frankl was already a Doctor of Medicine and Doctor of Philosophy prior to his imprisonment in Auschwitz and Dachau.

His thinking integrates a blend of the traditional psychiatric knowledge of his time with the experience of the camps to formulate an existential therapy, which he named *logotherapy*.

Frankl divided the reactions of the camp inmate into three phases: reception into the camp, actual camp life and post-liberation. His exploration of the psychology of the concentration camp is a valuable contribution but obviously limited to his particular experience (Frankl writes about his fellow inmates, male prisoners). Yet from these experiences, he is uniquely qualified to comment on the meaning of life, death, suffering, work and love - the topics which he discusses. Frankl's writings about the search for meaning in life have proven very influential in contemporary theology and philosophy.

Gallagher, Hugh G. (1990). *By Trust Betrayed: Patients, Physicians and the License to Kill in the Third Reich*. New York: Henry Holt. 342 pp.

The author provides a detailed look at the "Aktion T-4" program, the program for murder of children deemed "life unworthy of life." He examines T-4 in relation to doctors, lawyers and the Church and their complicity or silence on these matters.

Particularly compelling is the chapter "Aktion T-4 Sequelae 1945-88," which demonstrates the degree to which information about German/Nazi medicine was suppressed in Germany after the war. Alexander Mitscherlich was denounced as a traitor to his country for publishing an accurate account of the Nuremberg trial of doctors (See *Doctors of Infamy* by Mitscherlich).

Gershon, Karen (Ed.) (1966). *We Came as Children: A Collective Autobiography*. London: Gollancz. 176 pp.
The writer interviewed thirty persons who had been brought to safety in England from Europe. These children's transports (kinder transports) succeeded in delivering nearly 10,000 children before the outbreak of war. Most were deeply affected by subsequent events as they became witness across the Channel to the murder of their families, confirmed only after the war. Some came with a parent or parents but each story of the child refugees attests to the impact of the catastrophic events which unfolded.

Gill, Anton (1988). *The Journey Back From Hell: Conversations With Concentration Camp Survivors*. New York: William Morrow. 494 pp.
This book is a fount of psychologic and psychiatric information because Gill has interviewed some of the most knowledgable people in the field. There are interviews with Dr. Jan Bastiaans, the Dutch psychiatrist-founder of a hospital devoted to the treatment of war victims, Dr. Elie Cohen, a Dutch psychiatrist-survivor who wrote *Human Behavior in the Concentration Camp*, and Dr. Leo Eitinger, survivor of Auschwitz and the first psychiatrist to conduct comparative studies on Jewish and non-Jewish survivors of concentration camps.
The insights explored are invaluable. Gill also devotes several chapters to issues which bear directly on medical and psychological findings including, "Some Effects of the KZ on the Mind," "In Denmark, Healers and Fighters" and "Healers."
This book contains a discussion of the classic work of Thygesen and Hermann (1951-52) who examined Danish resistance fighters and who found that 63% were symptomatic with a constellation of symptoms labelled the KZ syndrome - the definitive forerunner of PTSD. Although the Danes emphasized the effects of famine, it was the combination of famine and severe emotional stress that caused the syndrome. It should also be noted that these survivors of camps were not primarily in the most severe camps nor specifically targeted for death.

Goldstein, Jacob; Lukoff, Irving F.; and Strauss, Herbert A. (1991). *Individuelles und kollektives Verhalten in Nazi Konzentrationslagern: Soziologische und psychologische Studien zu Berichten ungarisch-jüdischer Überlebender* [Individual and Collective Behavior in Nazi Concentration Camps: Sociological and Psychological Studies and Research on Hungarian-Jewish Survivors]. Frankfurt am Main and New York: Campus. 198 pp.
This book written in German, does not indicate the primary source but

must have originated in New York (the place of work of all three authors) and is based on 507 interviews of concentration camp survivors who returned to Budapest after the war. The interviews were deposited in the Archives of YIVO (Yidishn Visnshaftlikhn Instituts) and formed the foundation for the observations offered.

Hass, Aaron (1995). *The Aftermath: Living with the Holocaust*. New York: Cambridge University Press. 213 pp.

The author, in examining the clinical literature on survivors, found a discrepancy between their descriptions as depressed and dysfunctional, when in fact he experienced their resilience. He finds Holocaust survivors to be like other people except for their special knowledge of evil and vulnerability.

Hass interviewed 58 Jewish survivors and utilizes eyewitness accounts to illustrate the manner in which some survivors adapted and have coped to this day. He decries the focus on psychopathology and because of that view discusses such issues as "survivor guilt" in a more measured manner than most. There is a wealth of material, some of it contradictory. While warning against assumptions about the transmission of trauma to the children, there are many examples offered of precisely that transmission.

Basically this book is an ambitious work which provides insights into important aspects of the survivor's existence, survival after survival.

Keilson, Hans, and Sarphatie, Herman R. (1992). *Sequential Traumatization in Children: A Clinical and Statistical Follow-Up Study on the Fate of the Jewish War Orphans in the Netherlands*. Jerusalem: Magnes. 463 pp.

This book, first published in German (1979) by Ferdinand Enke Verlag, examines the disruption of life in critical developmental stages of children. Of approximately 140,000 Dutch Jews, about 15% survived, including 3,500 children of which 1417 were re-united with a surviving parent. It is the 2,000 orphans which Keilson examines. The study was started in 1967 and completed ten years later.

Keilson divides the persecution into three phases, the events leading up to the persecution, the time spent in a concentration camp or in hiding and the post-war period with its attendant difficulties.

The author's observations on trauma are very valuable and predate, by many years, similar contemporary observations. The details of the many case studies are not only heart-rending but quite accurately reflect the inner psychic realities of severely traumatized children.

Kestenberg, Judith S., and Fogelman, Eva (Eds.) (1994). *Children during the Nazi Reign: Psychological Perspective on the Interview Process*. Westport, CT: Praeger. 221 pp.

The editors have compiled a series of articles of varying quality on interviews conducted with child survivors of the Holocaust. The impact of the interviews is examined in terms of the interviewee's psychologic well-being. Interestingly, there is considerable self-scrutiny by interviewers of their own reactions.

On the whole, child survivors report satisfaction with attempts to relate their accounts and to recapture whatever memories remain to them of their earliest traumatic experiences. Some memorable accounts are offered.

The shortest chapter, "On Being Interviewed About the Holocaust" - 3 pages, is actually most important for it addresses the issue of the comparative value of audio taping versus audiovisual taping. If there were time for only one possible medium, which would it be?

Kren, George, and Rappoport, Leon (1994). *The Holocaust and the Crisis of Human Behavior.* New York: Holmes & Meier. 176 pp.

Kren and Rappoport's book is a powerful reminder of the Holocaust as a breach in human existence. They dispel a number of myths, for example, that traditional German anti-Semitism was a major cause of the Holocaust. Anti-Semitism was everywhere in Russia and Poland but only Germany made it state policy. The psychological dimensions of this unique genocide are discussed as is genocide as social policy. The authors raise the powerful challenges to culture and civilization that are exposed in light of the Holocaust.

Kren and Rappoport save some ammunition for the failure of science which is usually thought of as objective, amoral and devoted to the common good. In the Holocaust, science served mass murder and was invoked as the justification for the elimination of the "bacteria" while providing the technological means, "Zyklon B."

Krystal, Henry (Ed.) (1968). *Massive Psychic Trauma.* New York: International Universities Press. 369 pp.

The contents of this book came from the Wayne State University Workshops on The Late Sequelae of Massive Psychic Trauma.

Because of its nature, it is an uneven work with both many valuable insights and considerable chaff. Historically, this book did serve to galvanize further work in the field. A major issue that is raised there is the Krystal and Niederland hypothesis "that the major pathogenic force is survivor guilt." They closely related features of depression to survivor guilt and then noted that "92 percent (of 151 patients) expressed self-reproach for failing to save their relatives."

At various times the authors demonstrate a great depth of understanding such as in their observations that survivors of persecution are suspected of unfair play or collaboration and that therefore "we tend to blame the survivor for the guilt of the perpetrator." However, there are flaws in their work such as in the discussion of the "two pathogenic forces in survivors of Nazi persecution," namely survivor guilt and problems of aggression. The theoretic connection of these "pathogenic forces" to the experience of the survivor does not really fit the reality of the Holocaust. For example, the authors offer that "survivor guilt is a form of pathological mourning in which the survivor is stuck in a magnification of the guilt which is present in every bereaved person. "What is pathologic mourning? How does the loss of an 87 year old mother due to illness (normal mourning of up to one year) compare with the murder of parents, wife and children, brothers and sisters at one time, some of the murders witnessed by the survivor? It cannot be a magnification of *normal* bereavement. There is *nothing* normal to be found and comparisons of language, particularly the theoretic, fail. The authors redeem themselves partially when acknowledging that the dreams in survivors' nightmares, cannot be completely explained theoretically.

Krystal, Henry (1990). *Integration and Self-Healing: Affect, Trauma, Alexithymia*. Ann Arbor, MI: Analytic Press.

This is an erudite book, written many years after Krystal's initial contributions to "Massive Psychic Trauma," but nonetheless it ultimately disappoints where survivors are concerned. The chapter on trauma and affect provides a valuable discourse on the nature of trauma and its understanding. While explaining the psychologic phenomenon of helplessness in face of overwhelming and inevitable danger, Krystal falls into the trap of describing this as the reason why European Jews "obeyed orders in an automaton-like fashion, took off their clothes, and together with their children descended into a pit..." The reason for obeying orders in the face of machineguns lay in the fact that there was no escape, and resistance resulted in the murder of children in front of parents, the rape of daughters in front of fathers, the mutilation and torture of grandparents before one's eyes. To cooperate with one's inevitable murder is not tantamount to suicide as Krystal intimates. Here Krystal follows Bettelheim into an arena of thought which defies both reality and the imagination.

Where Krystal, who himself is a survivor, shines as a psychoanalyst is in the posing of incisive questions, e.g., "What happens to people who surrender to what they experience as overwhelming danger, but do not die?" And in examining childhood trauma, "How can we imagine the child's *timeless* horror?" His discussion of early trauma is masterful, particularly the notion that "among the *direct* effects of severe childhood trauma in adults is lifelong *dread* of the traumatic state and the *expectation* of it."

Lagnado, Lucette Matalon, and Dekel, Sheila Cohn (1991). *Children of the Flames: Dr. Josef Mengele and the Untold Story of the Twins at Auschwitz*. New York and London: Penguin. 320 pp.

Human medical experimentation reached its horrendous zenith at the hands of Mengele. This book focuses on Mengele's obsession with twins upon whom he conducted medical atrocities. Of an estimated 3,000 twins who passed through his "laboratories," only 100 are known to have survived. They live with the medical and psychologic consequences of the experiments.

The authors interviewed survivor twins and found that the younger they were, with less conscious memory, the greater their burdens as adults. Their terror was mixed with child-like adulation, for Mengele "saved" them from the gas chambers and played with them sometimes.

Mengele's medical career is chronicled: M.D. (University of Frankfurt) and Ph.D. in Anthropology (University of Munich), with post-graduate work at the Verschuer's Institute at the University of Frankfurt. As a physician in power at Auschwitz, the testimonies to his cruelty defy belief. This book must be read by physicians-in-training as a warning to what is now known to be possible.

Langer, Lawrence (1991). *Holocaust Testimonies: The Ruins of Memory.* New Haven: Yale University Press. 216 pp.

Langer explores the vagaries of memory, and therewith language, through an examination of audiovisual testimonies of Holocaust survivors. He shows that memory shared with an interviewer is different from that committed in writing. His thoughtful and careful work surpasses in psychological depth much of what is written by those with psychologic and psychiatric training. Langer certainly reaffirms the commitment to listen, and to listen very well to the narrative of survivors. Langer proves himself a great teacher because he is such a good student.

Lemberger, John (Ed.) (1995). *A Global Perspective on Working with Holocaust Survivors and the Second Generation.* Jerusalem: JDC-Brookdale Institute of Gerontology and Human Development, AMCHA, and JDC-Israel. 459 pp.

This volume comprises a collection of the proceedings of a conference held July 3-4, 1994 in Jerusalem. It is an uneven work in that there are articles of high quality and some that might have been omitted. A useful appendix of article abstracts serves as a guide to the papers of particular interest to the reader. There is much of value, including contributions by Dasberg, Durst, Hassan, Hass and Wardi among others. It is heartening to see in one collection the efforts of many sensitive and thoughtful professionals who work with survivors and their families.

Lifton, Robert Jay (1986). *The Nazi Doctors: Medical Killing and the Psychology of Genocide.* New York: Basic. 576 pp.

Lifton, a psychiatrist, examines the role of the Nazi doctors in the killing process. He interviewed twenty-nine men (twenty-eight physicians and one pharmacist) involved at high levels of Nazi medicine, twelve former prominent Nazi non-medical professionals and eighty former Auschwitz prisoners (over one-half doctors) who had worked in medical blocks. Lifton describes how the murder of Jews became a therapeutic imperative, that it was the elimination of a deadly disease afflicting the Aryan race.

Nazi doctors presided over the murder of most of the million victims at Auschwitz, a process initiated by doctors who participated in direct medical killing of those deemed "life unworthy of life."

This book traces the development of racial and Nazi-medical ideology, offers insights as to what made it psychologically possible for physicians to participate in and justify mass murder, and raises disturbing questions for the medical profession.

Lifton, Robert Jay, and Markusen, Eric (1990). *The Genocidal Mentality: Nazi Holocaust and Nuclear Threat*. New York: Basic. 346 pp.

The link between Auschwitz and Hiroshima is made explicit through the authors' contention that the attempt to annihilate the Jewish people through genocidal murder made genocide possible on an even larger scale with the advent of nuclear weapons. The mind set which led to genocide of the Jews could become the mind set to justify nuclear war, with its enormous potential for mass death.

Lifton's studies on Nazi doctors and their capacity for "psychic numbing" and "doubling," methods for distancing themselves from murder and rationalizing killing as medical healing (of Aryan societies), forms the framework for examining similar mechanisms in those who come to share a genocidal mentality.

It is a powerful work in that the psychologic consequences derived from observations of perpetrators and victims of the Holocaust are applied to the political and social dimensions of the contemporary world.

Luel, Steven A., and Marcus, Paul (Eds.) (1984). *Psychoanalytic Reflections on the Holocaust: Selected Essays*. New York: Ktav. 238 pp.

This book comprises a series of thought-provoking essays, primarily by psychoanalysts, concerning psychoanalysis and the Holocaust. With the exception of reprinted articles by Krystal, "Integration and Self-Healing in Post-traumatic States" and Lifton's "Medicalized Killing in Auschwitz," the articles are original contributions.

Particularly compelling is the introduction by the co-editors which hints at the silence which predominated within the psychoanalytic profession. Psychoanalysis and psychoanalytic theory are profoundly challenged by the events of the Holocaust.

The concluding chapter is a round-table discussion which provides insights that the Holocaust has not influenced psychoanalytic technique, and that psychoanalysis has not re-examined critically concepts such as that of survivor guilt.

With respect to treatment, the entire question of the original psychoanalytic model of trauma is opened to question. The issues raised are genuinely worth consideration. This book is a valuable contribution to an area of thought which was in fact strengthened through the escape of refugees from Nazism.

Macardle, Dorothy (1949). *Children of Europe: A Study of the Children of Liberated Countries: Their Wartime Experiences, Their Reactions, and Their Needs, With a Note on Germany*. London: Gollancz. 349 pp.

This virtually unknown book is one of the most informative works on the psychologic consequences for child victims of the Holocaust. The author's words are most meaningful. In her foreword she states, "Official definitions are scrupulously colorless, and one may well fail to guess the misery masked by such terms as 'displaced person,' or 'unidentified' or 'war-handicapped' or - supreme understatement to cover total bereavement and desolation - 'unaccompanied child'" (p. 11).

A little further she writes, "I talked with child-psychologists in many countries. They are appalled by the dimensions of the problem which is gradually being revealed. A hundred experts are needed for each one who exists. They are working intensively, and are exploring what is in many respects a new field, for never has childhood been so assailed and tormented since the beginning of man" (p. 13).

She describes as the first victims the children of Germany who were taught to be Nazis within a framework of twisted ideology. She then chronicles the violations of country upon country, beginning with Czechoslovakia, Poland, Greece and Yugoslavia, then Norway and the West.

Macardle estimates the numbers of murdered Jewish children at about 2 million. While uncertain and stating that accuracy is impossible, she is certain that one million were deliberately killed by German governmental ordinance, the others having died of starvation and hardship.

Her observations on trauma in childhood are described in chapters entitled "Casualties," "Lost Children" and "Out of the Nazi Camps." She includes commentary on famine in children of Nazi-occupied Europe, including German children as well as those children kidnapped for the "Lebensbern" centers to be raised as the most desirable Aryans.

The last few chapters are devoted to an examination of the prospects of psychological health and a summation of the prevailing conditions for children at that time. In describing a children's village organized to treat the child victims of war, Macardle writes, "A few hundred are receiving the healing and atonement that millions need" (p. 312).

Marcus, Paul, and Rosenberg, Alan (1989). *Healing Their Wounds: Psychotherapy With Holocaust Survivors and Their Families*. New York: Praeger. 304 pp.

This finely edited book reflects the best of contemporary thinking with respect to Holocaust survivors. Much can be learned from it for the treatment of victims generally. For example, Janet Hadda's chapter, "Mourning the Yiddish Language and Some Implications for Treatment," should alert mental health professionals to the disruption of self-identity caused by the loss of a meaningful language and its unique usage.

Rabbi Martin Cohen's, "The Rabbi and the Holocaust Survivor," proposes the healing encounter of survivor and Rabbi studying together in an attempt to unravel the mysteries of how we can accept the concept of a loving God in light of the Holocaust experience. Here too are therapeutic implications for traumatized victims from other cultures and religions. The reimmersion in once meaningful traditions may assist in one's confrontation with despair.

The editors included a sufficient number of viewpoints to provide a satisfying perspective on the complex clinical challenge posed by Holocaust survivors.

Marks, Jane (1993). *The Hidden Children: The Secret Survivors of the Holocaust*. New York: Fawcett Columbine. 308pp.

The child survivor accounts offered are powerful testimonies to the memory of children, and to their resilience. In addition to the eyewitness revelations, the author has added two interesting chapters on the Hidden Child experience, one by Nechama Tec, the other by Eva Fogelman.

Matussek, Paul (1975). *Internment in Concentration Camps and its Consequences*. New York: Springer. 269 pp.

This translation by Derek and Inge Jordan of the 1971 German edition, "Die Konzentrationslagerhaft und ihre Folgen," offers the details of an extraordinary study. From the names of 210,811 victims of persecution compiled at the Regional Indemnification Office in Munich, every 40th name was selected (5,270 names) and further reduced to 737 persons still living in Munich.

The difficulties with collecting data are enumerated. As in many psychiatric books and articles, this one also relies on a number of descriptive eyewitness accounts, brief and evocative. The research observations are valuable. For example, early writers assumed that the "hasty" marriages of persecutees in response to post-war bereavement and loneliness would be conflict-ridden. The researchers found no definite correlation with later marital harmony, although they did confirm the phenomenon of early marriage.

In his Foreword, Hans Strupp describes the analysis of the clinical data as "sophisticated and sensitive" and states "it is rare that a research report becomes a deeply moving document." This book does.

Miklos, Nyiszli (1960). *Auschwitz: A Doctor's Eyewitness Account*. New York: Fawcett Crest. 160 pp.

This book's importance lies in the offering of an eyewitness account by a doctor who participated in Mengele's dark experiments in order to survive. In that alone, there are lessons. The horrors of Auschwitz are laid bare whether or not Dr. Nyiszli participated.

For survivors of the Holocaust and their psychological well-being, the more important part of this book may be Bruno Bettelheim's Foreword. In it he expounds his philosophy about the victim's role in their victimization to such a degree one would think Jews devised the means to their "final solution." Bettelheim helped set the tone for much of what transpired with respect to the psychologic understanding of the survivor. Read him at his worst, in 1960!

Nyiszli describes despair; disbelief and denial in a world designed by the perpetrators, not its victims. He describes what was done and thereby leaves a record also of what was done to the few who managed to survive.

Mitscherlich, Alexander, and Mielke, Fred (1949). *Doctors of Infamy: The Story of the Nazi Medical Crimes*. New York: Henry Schuman. 172 pp.

This classic book contains an opening statement by Andrew C. Ivy who was Medical Scientific Consultant to the Prosecution, Military Tribunal No. 1, Nuremberg. His indictment of the medical profession is strong and perhaps correct. "Had the profession taken a strong stand against the mass killing of sick Germans before the war, it is conceivable that the entire idea and techniques of death factories for genocide would not have materialized" (p. xi).

The authors describe the various experiments conducted by physicians and their helpers including the gruesome deliberate murders for the collection of skulls of Jews to be sent to the Professor of Anatomy at Strasbourg University. Of 23 defendants on trial at Nuremberg, seven were hanged, four of whom were physicians.

Moskovitz, Sarah (1983). *Love Despite Hate: Child Survivors of the Holocaust and Their Adult Lives*. New York: Shocken. 245 pp.

This book is the product of a series of minor miracles, and no small measure of knowledge and dedication. Over one million Jewish children were murdered by the Nazis. Of fifteen thousand children who passed through Theresienstadt, one hundred survived. In Auschwitz, of tens of thousands of children, five hundred remained at the time of liberation, some just barely alive.

The miracle is that any survived. Of three hundred children assembled from the camps, hiding places, and orphanages in preparation for their flight to England, only seventeen were under the age of eight. Moskovitz writes, "It was difficult to find child survivors. They were rare, these little ones who had been strong enough to survive disease, separation from parents, the traumatic conditions of ghettoisation, and the death camps themselves" (p. 5). Of these children, twelve from Terezin, five from Auschwitz, and several from hiding and orphanages arrived in Lingfield, England in 1945. Their ages: three to eleven.

A second miracle took place. They were received and cared for by Alice Goldberger, a loving, intelligent, attentive woman who made it her life's work to provide for the children whose shattered lives required reconstruction. There was no guide for her; there were no precedents to match the horrors experienced by these children. She lived day in and day out with children subjected to shattering losses and constant terror.

Which brings us to the third miracle; the chance meeting of Alice Goldberger and Sarah Moskovitz. Moskovitz, a developmental psychologist, wondered how Alice had created binding ties with children who had every reason not to trust. And a thought even more challenging, "What were they like today?" Dr. Moskovitz set out to interview twenty-four of these "survivor children," most of them citizens of the United States and Israel, nearly thirty-five years after their arrival in England.

What has happened to them forms the core of this powerful document, a recounting of their stories with remarkable compassion and insight.

Samuel Schwartz was not yet two when he arrived at Terezin, without a parent. As a liberated four year old, he asked every adult he encountered, "Bist due mein?" [Are you mine?]. In 1978, at age thirty-seven, Samuel has a wife and three children. His mother survived the war, but could not care for him and no mother-son relationship developed. During Dr. Moskovitz's interview, Samuel's four year old son, Robbie, left the room and returned to show a book by Dr. Seuss, "Are You My Mother?"

Magda Lieberman was eleven when she came to England. In 1977, she is living in Israel with her husband. A son is seventeen, a daughter newly married. During the war Magda had protected and saved her eight year old niece, Hedi, and five year old nephew, Fritz. Hedi wrote a special letter to Magda for her daughter's wedding. It said, "You have taught us right from wrong. You have taught us to know honesty from dishonesty. You have taught us to distinguish the important from the superficial." A tribute to an "eleven year old mother."

Julius Hamburger was nine. He had protected and fed four little girls who arrived with him from Auschwitz. Two spoke only Yiddish, the other two Italian. Of Julius' family of twelve children, his parents and seven sisters and brothers perished. Now named Uri, he lives in Israel with his wife and two children. He had never again seen the four girls for whom he cared. The two Italian girls live in Padua and Brussels, each married with two children. The two Yiddish-speaking girls live in London with husbands and children in orthodox Jewish homes.

Twenty-four lives, twenty-four stories, each movingly related with extraordinary sensitivity and insight. Dr. Moskovitz reveals herself by including her questions, her comments, and interventions. For the reader who is also a therapist, the author's style and skill in conducting these difficult interviews also makes her book worth reading.

But underlying the accounts of the lives of these troubled children, now grown up, are themes which not only defy the imagination but also defy contemporary thinking and research in child psychology, child psychiatry and infant development. A thorough reading casts some doubts on long-held theories in respect to early childhood, loss of parents, and multiple foster experiences. As adults, they now live productive lives despite having been deprived in childhood of parenting, food, and safety, as well as being subjected to severe abuse and unimaginable stress. There were no suicides. Only one of twenty-four is receiving care in a psychiatric hospital.

The author writes, "Despite the severest deprivation in early childhood, these people are neither living a greedy, me-first style of life, nor are they seeking gain at the expense of others. None express the idea that the world owes them a living for all they have suffered. On the contrary, most of their lives are marked by an active compassion for others..." (p. 23).

The book is a unique contribution to contemporary literature and should be widely read.

Müller-Hill, Benno (1988). *Murderous Science: Elimination by Scientific Selection of Jews, Gypsies, and Others, Germany 1933-1945*. New York: Oxford University Press. 208 pp.

This remarkable book, translated from the German by George R. Fraser, opens with a calendar chronicling important events. For example: "Spring 1937. A decision is made that all German colored children are to be illegally sterilized. After the prerequisite expert reports are provided by Dr. Abel, Dr. Schade, and Professor Fischer, the sterilizations are carried out" (p. 11).

The author notes a bond between anthropologists and psychiatrists, the former identifying inferior non-Germans, the latter identifying inferior Germans. Inferior beings were to be eliminated.

There is a compelling description of physicians involved in murder, their selection of human "material" for anthropological and psychiatric research and reports on conversations with some of the perpetrators, their assistants, or offspring.

Perl, Gisella (1984). *I Was a Doctor in Auschwitz*. Salem, NH: Ayer. 189 pp.

Perl's book was first published in 1948 by International Universities Press of New York. Through a series of concise chapters, the author conveys the extremes of horror in Auschwitz as its camp gynecologist.

She saw everything, she heard everything. As a physician she was forced to operate under conditions so primitive as to defy imagination. Witnessing the torture of pregnant women, Dr. Perl began to abort them in order to save their lives. She "worked" with Josef Mengele and witnessed first-hand his sadism.

Through her descriptions of inmates and their names, Dr. Perl honors the victims, avoiding nameless numbers.

Incredibly she worked again as an obstetrician at Jerusalem's Shaare Zedeck Hospital, delivering babies.

Proctor, Robert (1988). *Racial Hygiene: Medicine Under the Nazis*. Cambridge, MA: Harvard University Press. 414 pp.

This work is a well researched and documented account of the origins of "racialist medicine." Some of the statistics cited are compelling. Roughly half of all German physicians joined the Nazi party (p. 66). From January 1933 to the end of 1939, 319,900 of Germany's Jews fled the Reich. By May 1935, 20% of Jewish physicians had left the Reich (pp. 152-153).

The Epilogue on Post-war Legacies again emphasizes the struggle over knowledge, memory and responsibility.

Schwarberg, Günter (1984). *The Murders at Bullenhuser Damm: The SS Doctor and the Children*. Bloomington, IN: Indiana University Press. 178 pp.

This book first published in German in 1980, now translated by Erma Baber Rosenfeld with Alvin H. Rosenfeld, describes the murder of 20 Jewish children under age 12 with injections of tubercle bacilli. Dr. Kurt Heissmeyer needed to submit a scientific paper for promotion to professor of Medicine.

The Jewish children from Holland, Poland, France and Italy became Heissmeyer's "guinea pigs," and indeed the children and an equal number of guinea pigs were injected with the same substances. After being subjected to various experiments, the children were hanged April 20, 1945 and cremated on April 21, 1945.

Incredibly, there are medical pictures of the children at the Neuengamme concentration camp.

Segev, Tom (1994). *The Seventh Million: The Israelis and the Holocaust*. New York: Hill and Wang. 593 pp.

This extraordinary book describes the impact of the catastrophe perpetrated upon Jews who, after Germany's defeat, made their way to Palestine (prior to 1947) and to the newly re-established Israel post-1948. The *Seventh Million* tells the story of the Zionist response to the Nazis, the Yishuv's response to the arrival of the first refugees, to the destruction of European Jewry, and to the arriving survivors of that destruction.

There are some distinct peculiarities, not least of which is the author's thesis that the Holocaust shaped the collective identity of the new Israel. Yet, if anything, the established Zionist identity did not allow survivors sufficient political input to "shape" Israel, which the author confirms when documenting the non-compassionate response to new post-war arrivals.

While there is much to praise, there is much to critique. This massive work does not chronicle the psychologic consequences of survivorhood in the land where such consequences were assumed to be healed by living in Israel. The achievement of Statehood proved not enough to heal the traumas of Nazi persecution, but for some it was a partial-answer.

Segev begins his book with the story of the writer Yehiel De-Nur (Ka-Tzetnik), whose books are extremely disturbing for they describe what really happened inside the camps. De-Nur received psychiatric treatment from Dr. Jan Bastiaans in Holland (therapy which enabled him to escape his total seclusion and actually agree to a television interview).

In a sense, the book follows the path of a patient (country) in denial to a gradual and painful accommodation to the past, some of it brought home by powerful events such as the Eichman trial and the threats of the 1967 and 1973 wars on Israel.

Sigal, John, and Weinfeld, Morton (1989). *Trauma and Rebirth: Intergenerational Effects of the Holocaust*. New York: Praeger. 204 pp.

Sigal and Weinfeld selected a random sample of Jewish Holocaust survivors who reside in Montreal, and compared them with Montreal Jews who were pre-war immigrants and to Montreal Jews who were native born. Long-term harmful effects were noted in the Holocaust survivors. It was also possible to distinguish personality types as related to the consequences of persecution.

Such findings are tempered by the thoughtful and measured discussions of the various conclusions drawn by these authors/researchers. The authors conclude that despite the profound psychological and physical handicaps there was little impairment in the work place or evidence for non-participation in communal activities. A similar absence of impaired functioning was noted in the Second Generation, the offspring of survivors.

These observations of apparent normality in the general population stand in stark contrast to the voluminous clinical literature describing the psychopathology of survivors and their children. Of special interest is the fact that children of survivors rated their parents in one third of the sample as providing positive attributes such as a strengthening of their Jewish identification and their positive feelings towards family. The authors believe that the focus on psychopathology derives from a subgroup where the interaction of parental personality profile, the nature of the wartime experience and the family interaction, provided the ingredients to definable psychopathology. It is from this group that clinicians seem to have generalized to the entire population.

The introductory chapters, particularly chapter II which provides an overview of research on survivors and their families, are especially worthwhile. Unfortunately there are many typos which are distracting to the careful reader. The discussions are reasoned and informative, with an occasional weak speculative comment. For example, the authors surmise that among survivors of Nazi persecution, Canadian Jewish community organizations are held in low repute for what they did not do to combat increasing anti-Semitism in Nazi Germany or for insufficient action to save threatened Jews during wartime. In examining this point, the authors have missed the more likely explanation freely offered to anyone who asks. The majority who shy away from the organized community (beyond that of their own Synagogue congregation) do so because of the absence (perceived or real) of communal assistance upon arrival. Few felt genuinely welcome.

One note of caution. Although the results are in some sense a tribute to the courage and resilience of the Holocaust survivor families, nevertheless the unbearable trauma and a lifetime of bereavement have taken a serious toll. The clinician must remain alert to those who are seriously affected and whose problems surface in the latter stages of life: depression, recaptured grief or retriggered mourning require assistance with a view to the ever-present dimension of their Holocaust experience.

Stein, André (1993). *Hidden Children: Forgotten Survivors of the Holocaust.* New York: Penguin. 273 pp.

There are ten child survivor stories as told to André Stein. Each stands alone. Together they are a powerful testament to survival. Each "child" reveals much of his or her psychological make-up.

Strøm, Axel (Ed.) (1968). *Norwegian Concentration Camp Survivors.* Oslo: Universitetsforlaget, and New York: Humanities Press. 186 pp.

This book reflects an investigation of Norwegian former political prisoners during 1940-1945, conducted from 1957-1963. Of 100 prisoners described in reports published in 1961 and 1962, 85 had KZ Syndrome (read PTSD-Chronic). All had organic brain disease and encephalopathy. Most were tortured so severely, that mere survival was miraculous. And these men were non-Jews.

On the basis of this study alone, Jewish survivors should never have had to prove "damage" in order to receive restitution payments.

Valent, Paul (1993). *Child Survivors: Adults Living with Childhood Trauma.* Port Melbourne, Victoria: William Heinemann. 288 pp.

Paul Valent, himself a child survivor and psychiatrist, sensitively captures the essence of ten child survivor stories. Each is followed by a comment from the author which places in perspective some of the adaptive mechanisms in place during the war and after. It is an enriched and enriching offering.

Wardi, Dina (1992). *Memorial Candles - Children of the Holocaust.* New York: Tavistock/Routledge. 270 pp.

The title of this book implies the transmission of the traumas of Holocaust survivor parents to their offspring who, in effect, become the repository of memory and hope - memorial candles.

The author illustrates themes which burden the sons and daughters of Holocaust survivors and for which they may seek treatment. Her vast experience includes individual and group psychotherapy with dozens of second generation individuals. Vignettes and the personal perspectives and words offered by eyewitnesses and participants in therapy are enlightening. In families where there are several children, one may be selected to serve as the "memorial candle" protecting the other siblings from similar pressures. Issues of separation and abandonment are exceedingly complex and individuation generally delayed. Wardi discusses in detail several controversial concepts concerning identification, aggression, self-esteem and concludes with the therapeutic implications of "parting from the role of memorial candle."

Whiteman, Dorit Bader (1993). *The Uprooted: A Hitler Legacy. Voices of Those Who Escaped Before the "Final Solution."* New York: Plenum Press Insight Books. 446 pp.

This book has important psychologic implications, for it demonstrates the psychiatric consequences for those who seemed to have escaped. However, those who barely left Nazi Europe in time also lost entire families and were the victims of dispossession and displacement. These victims were silenced in that their personal experiences could not compare with those caught in Nazi-occupied Europe.

The escapees find voice in this remarkable work through the 190 accounts on which it is based: The author wisely allows the escapees to tell their stories and the profound lasting effects of their traumatic memories are captured from the past and in later life.

Whiteman, a psychologist, provides a valuable overview on "the emotional aftermath," in Part Four of her book.

Wiesel, Elie (1992). *The Forgotten.* New York: Summit Books. 237 pp.

This is Elie Wiesel's thirty-sixth book and it seems a work of contradiction. After all, the title reflects the antithesis of Wiesel's major theme of remembering and remembrance.

The forgotten. Why should he, so devoted to memory, write about forgetting? It was Wiesel who stated "Remember, for in remembering there is hope."

There is no contradiction. In tackling the issue of loss of memory, Wiesel emphasizes precisely the commitment to memory.

Elhanan Rosenbaum is losing his prodigious and searing memory. Orphaned during the war, he became a partisan fighter who witnessed an act of vengeance which haunts him to the end. The disease which robs Elhanan's mind compels his son Malkiel to record his father's memories and visit the Roumanian village, the home of his father and the scene of the crime.

It is there that Malkiel finds the truths which salvage not only his father's failing memory but his own. For what might be forgotten could no longer be when the son becomes the repository of his father's recollections.

As in so many of Wiesel's novels, wisdom comes not from the expected sources - the teachers, the doctors, the professors - wisdom often belongs to the beggars or those deemed to be mad. And here it is the gravedigger, the Roumanian Jew in the village of Feherfaler, who carries

Index of Names

The Index of Names contains all authors and editors cited in this book. There are three types of entries in the Index of Names. Entries to references that appear at the end of the two opening chapters are cited, for example, as **1:22**, with 1 refering to the chapter number and 22, the reference number. All entries in the main Bibliography of Medical and Psychological Effects of the Holocaust appear by citation number. Finally, all references in the Selected Annotated Bibliography appear as **SAB-317** with 317, the page number of the annotated citation.

FSC
www.fsc.org
MIX
Papier | Fördert
gute Waldnutzung
FSC® C083411

Kolibri 360 GmbH
Ferdinand-Jühlke-Straße 7
99095 Erfurt, Deutschland
produktsicherheit@kolibri360.de